NVQs for Dental Nurses

SECOND EDITION

Carole Hollins BDS

General Dental Practitioner
Member of the Panel of Examiners, National Examining Board for Dental Nurses

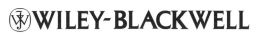
WILEY-BLACKWELL

A John Wiley & Sons, Ltd., Publication

This edition first published 2009
© 2009 Carole Hollins
© 2003 Blackwell Munksgaard

Blackwell Publishing was acquired by John Wiley & Sons in February 2007. Blackwell's publishing programme
has been merged with Wiley's global Scientific, Technical, and Medical business to form Wiley-Blackwell.

First published 2003
Second edition published 2009

Registered office
John Wiley & Sons Ltd, The Atrium, Southern Gate, Chichester, West Sussex, PO19 8SQ, United Kingdom

Editorial offices
9600 Garsington Road, Oxford, OX4 2DQ, United Kingdom
2121 State Avenue, Ames, Iowa 50014-8300, USA

For details of our global editorial offices, for customer services and for information about how to apply
for permission to reuse the copyright material in this book please see our website at www.wiley.com/
wiley-blackwell.

Library of Congress Cataloging-in-Publication Data
Hollins, Carole.
    NVQs for dental nurses / Carole Hollins. — 2nd ed.
        p. ; cm.
    National vocational qualifications for dental nurses
    Includes bibliographical references and index.
    ISBN 978-1-4051-9256-9 (pbk. : alk. paper)   1. Dental assistants—Outlines, syllabi, etc.
I. Title.   II. Title: National vocational qualifications for dental nurses.
    [DNLM: 1. Dental Assistants—Examination Questions.   Wu 18.2 H741n 2009]
    RK60.5.H65 2009
    617.6′0233—dc22
                                                                            2009012271

A catalogue record for this book is available from the British Library.

Set in 9.5/12pt Palatino by Graphicraft Limited, Hong Kong
Printed in Singapore

1   2009

Contents

Introduction to the Second Edition

This textbook has been written for those Dental Nurses studying to qualify as Dental Care Professionals (DCPs) via the National Vocational Qualification (NVQ) route. It is the second edition, and its writing has been prompted by the recent changes to the structure of the Level 3 NVQ qualification in dental nursing, as well as the introduction of compulsory registration of all DCPs with the General Dental Council.

The updated NVQ qualification consists of 11 units, all of which are mandatory, and which have incorporated the changes to dentistry and relevant legislation since the first edition. Nine of them cover the general areas of dental practice in which the majority of dental nurses will work, while the other two units cover the concept of 'life-long learning' and basic life support. This book provides the underpinning theoretical knowledge required to study and understand all of the areas of dental nursing covered by the NVQ qualification, while the workplace competencies are achieved at the chairside as witnessed assessments.

In addition, the final chapter introduces information on the new Vocationally Related Qualification (VRQ), which has replaced the Independant Assessment as the written examination of the NVQ qualification. Examples of question styles are included, but not the answers – it is hoped that the readership will enjoy discovering these as they read the text book and learn the subject of dental nursing!

Carole Hollins

Acknowledgements

Grateful thanks are extended once again to the staff and patients of Kidsgrove dental practice for their eager participation in posing for various photographs – who said attending for dental treatment couldn't be fun!

I especially wish to thank Tracey Evans for her unstinting help, support and 'modelling skills' during the writing and compilation of the book; she is a dental nurse and tutor *par excellence*, and an inspiration to student dental nurses throughout Stoke-on-Trent.

I also thank the General Dental Council for their very kind permission to reproduce their Standards Guidance document in part, and express huge appreciation again to various other illustrators for their ongoing support.

Finally, to all of the staff at Wiley-Blackwell, a huge 'thank you' for their continued and very friendly help and support throughout the writing of this book.

1 The N/SVQ

The concept of qualification by N/SVQ has been developed around the recognition of the competence of candidates to perform a range of tasks to the standards required for their successful employment. For this qualification, the candidates will be dental nurses who are employed by any of the following employers:

- General dental practices, either National Health Service (NHS), private or 'mixed'
- Community dental clinics
- Dental departments within general hospitals
- Dental teaching hospitals
- Dental corporate bodies
- The armed forces

Formal qualifications are not required by candidates wishing to undertake this N/SVQ in Dental Nursing, but they must be employed in a suitable dental workplace where the necessary opportunities to gain evidence for the completion of the qualification are provided. As the dental workplace can be a hazardous environment for numerous reasons, the qualification is not approved for any candidates under the age of 16 years.

This dental nursing qualification is specifically involved with direct chairside tasks and the support provided to dentists and dental care professionals (DCPs; such as hygienists and therapists) during a range of dental treatments. However, considerable underpinning knowledge of topics such as anatomy, dental instruments and materials, and dental equipment is also required. The theoretical knowledge needed in these areas should be provided by formal classroom teaching.

The decision on whether a candidate is deemed to be 'competent' or 'not yet competent' in a given task is determined by the assessment of evidence produced by the candidate to show that they can perform each of the tasks covered by the qualification, in a competent manner in the workplace. The assessments are carried out by trained and qualified assessors, and for this qualification an assessor is a dentist, qualified DCPs or another professional who is competent and qualified in certain areas of healthcare, such as a radiographer.

The evidence considered acceptable can be produced either directly or indirectly. Examples of each are given below.

Direct evidence:

- Observation in the workplace by an assessor
- Observation and testimony by a named expert witness (dentist, registered DCP)
- Observation of a simulated task by an assessor (such as basic life support)
- Observation and testimony by a witness (such as a patient)

Indirect evidence:

- Performance reports from a workplace mentor (dentist, senior DCP)
- Professional discussions and questioning by an assessor
- Written assignments, homework, presentations and case studies

The N/SVQ in Dental Nursing qualification consists of 11 mandatory units:

- Unit 1 – Ensure your own actions reduce the risk to health and safety (ENTOA)
- Unit 2 – Reflect on and develop your practice (HSC33)
- Unit 3 – Provide Basic Life Support (CHS36)
- Unit 4 – Prepare and maintain environments, instruments and equipment for clinical dental procedures (OH1)
- Unit 5 – Offer information and support to individuals on the protection of their oral health (OH2)
- Unit 6 – Provide chair side support during the assessment of patients' oral health (OH3)
- Unit 7 – Contribute to the production of dental radiographs (OH4)
- Unit 8 – Provide chairside support during the prevention and control of periodontal disease and caries, and the restoration of cavities (OH5)
- Unit 9 – Provide chairside support during the provision of fixed and removable appliances (OH6)
- Unit 10 – Provide chair side support during non-surgical endodontic treatment (OH7)
- Unit 11 – Provide chair side support during the extraction of teeth and minor oral surgery (OH8)

The first unit and the last eight form the basis of general dental practice, while the second and third units have been added to cover areas of competence that are necessary in accordance with the National Occupational Standards for dental nursing. Each unit is made up of a number of 'elements of competence', which describe all of the tasks that the dental nurse must be able to carry out competently. Every element of all 11 units must be carried out competently to achieve the N/SVQ qualification. In addition, the factual knowledge evidence from various areas of the 11 units is tested in the form of a written Vocationally Related Qualification (VRQ), and this will also have to be successfully completed before the dental nurse can register as a qualified DCP with the General Dental Council.

The four broad sections of the N/SVQ syllabus to be covered by the VRQ are discussed in detail in Chapter 13, and are summarised below:

- Principles of infection control in the dental environment
- Assessment of oral health and treatment planning
- Dental radiography
- Scientific principles in the management of plaque-related diseases

It can be seen then, success in the N/SVQ requires evidence of competency in all of the chairside tasks, as well as proof of knowledge and understanding of the underpinning information required to carry out the tasks to a consistent standard.

To assist the dental nurse in completing the N/SVQ successfully, City & Guilds provide the necessary paperwork for candidates to build a portfolio of performance evidence, which provides a record of their competence in the workplace. To be able to cover the whole range of tasks in which the dental nurse must be assessed, each element of competence is accompanied by the following information:

- **Scope** – suggestions and guidance on possible areas that may be covered in each workforce competence, often linked to key words from the City & Guilds glossary provided at the beginning of each unit
- **Performance criteria** – these provide descriptions of all the specific areas of the overall task that must be addressed, and the standard of performance that is acceptable for each
- **Knowledge specification** – the theoretical information that must be known and understood by the dental nurse, so that they can apply it to their workplace tasks and perform them to a consistently high standard.

This textbook is designed to provide the required theoretical information to cover the knowledge specifications of all 11 units, so that the dental nurse has a thorough understanding of their role in the dental team, and can perform the necessary tasks to an acceptable standard at all times.

Knowledge specifications

Each of the 11 units is covered chapter by chapter in the book, and the table of contents lists those areas of the dental nursing syllabus that are discussed in each chapter. Where the same information is required in several units, it is discussed fully in the chapter to which it is initially referred, and then summarised in any relevant later chapters.

Several knowledge specifications of one unit may be repeated in others because they are relevant to both. An example of this occurs in Units 6 and 8, which both refer to the dental nurse requiring 'a factual knowledge of the primary and secondary dentition and the average dates of eruption'. The knowledge specification is covered in detail in Unit 6, where it is referred to initially, and is then summarised in Unit 8 where it is referred to again. It is hoped that this will help to minimise the amount of cross-referencing required by the reader.

Each of the knowledge specifications fall into one of the following descriptions, which indicates the depth of understanding that the candidate needs to acquire:

- Factual knowledge
- Working knowledge
- Factual awareness
- Working understanding

These can be interpreted and explained as follows:

- **Factual knowledge**:
    - Give a description of the subject, based on stated facts
    - The stated facts are written and reported elsewhere (such as in other textbooks) and are irrefutable, that is, they are correct and are not able to be disproved
    - An example is 'a factual knowledge of the development of dental plaque and methods for controlling it' (Unit 5, K2)

- **Working knowledge**:
    - Show understanding of the subject by being able to explain it in the context of the dental workplace
    - This will involve giving details around the subject, and may be based on one's personal interpretation of the information involved
    - There will also be an element of personal experience within the explanation
    - An example is 'a working knowledge of the different types of disclosing agents available' (Unit 5, K14)
    - The extent of the working knowledge shown will be dependent on the range of personal experience of the subject

- **Factual awareness**:
    - Show knowledge of the subject by identification of the key points
    - This indicates the ability to discover the knowledge by observation or by analysis, rather than by personal experience
    - This will involve the ability to identify the factual points clearly, to prove the understanding of the subject
    - An example is 'a factual awareness of the priorities in life support' (Unit 3, K2)

- **Working understanding**:
    - Show an understanding of the subject by the ability to reason
    - This shows the ability to discover and interpret the knowledge by demonstration

– An example is 'a working understanding of what to do in the event of foreign body obstruction of an individual's airway' (Unit 3, K6)

These explanations indicate the depth of understanding that is required by the
candidate for each of the knowledge specifications throughout this N/SVQ
qualification. A full list of the knowledge specifications covered by each unit is
given at the start of each chapter. Chapter 13 is devoted to an explanation of the
VRQ, the subjects it covers, and examples of the style of questions that may appear
in the written paper. The answers can all be found within the text of the book.

The book also contains numerous diagrams and photographs to help illustrate
key points referred to in the text. In addition to the glossary provided by City &
Guilds in their portfolio documentation, a 'Glossary of Terms' has been included
in the end of this book to give descriptive definitions of key words and phrases
used within the text and that have specific meaning here.

2 Unit 1: Ensure Your Own Actions Reduce the Risk to Health and Safety (ENTOA)

Knowledge specifications

K1 – A working knowledge of your legal duties for health and safety in the workplace as required by current Health and Safety legislation

K2 – A working knowledge of your duties for health and safety as defined by any specific legislation covering your job role

K3 – A working knowledge of the hazards that may exist in your workplace

K4 – A working knowledge of the particular health and safety risks which may be present in your own job role and the precautions you must take

K5 – A working knowledge of the importance of remaining alert to the presence of hazards in the whole workplace

K6 – A working knowledge of the importance of dealing with or promptly reporting risks

K7 – A working knowledge of the requirements and guidance on the precautions

K8 – A working knowledge of agreed workplace policies relating to controlling risks to health and safety

K9 – A working knowledge of responsibilities for health and safety in your job description

K10 – A working knowledge of the responsible persons to whom to report health and safety matters

K11 – A working knowledge of the specific workplace policies covering your job role

K12 – A working knowledge of suppliers' and manufacturers' instructions for the safe use of equipment, materials and products

K13 – A working knowledge of safe working practices for your own job role

K14 – A working knowledge of the importance of personal presentation in maintaining health and safety in the workplace

K15 – A working knowledge of the importance of personal conduct in maintaining the health and safety of yourself and others

K16 – A working knowledge of your scope and responsibility for rectifying risks

K17 – A working knowledge of workplace procedures for dealing with risks which you are not able to handle yourself

All employers, including dental practitioners, have responsibilities towards their staff and any other persons on their premises in relation to safe working practices and safety at work. These are governed by the **Health and Safety at Work Act 1974**.

In the dental workplace, 'any other persons' include: patients and their escorts, visiting utility workers, such as postal deliverers and meter readers, and visitors such as repair and maintenance personnel.

The aim of the Act with specific reference to the dental workplace is to protect all persons at work, and in particular:

■ Provide and maintain safe equipment, appliances and systems of work
■ Ensure dangerous or potentially harmful substances are handled and stored safely (see COSHH regulations, later)
■ Maintain the place of work (including its entrance and exit) in a safe condition
■ Provide a safe working environment for employees, with no risks to health and adequate facilities for their welfare
■ Provide necessary teaching, training and supervision to ensure Health and Safety is complied with

All work places must also have a current Health and Safety Law poster on display within the premises, for all staff to see (Figure 2.1).

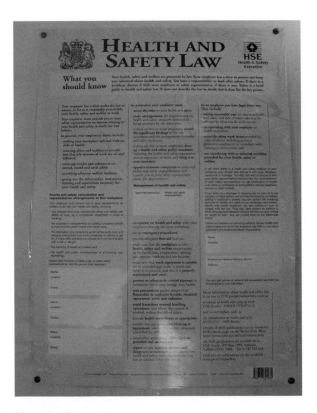

Figure 2.1 Health and safety poster.

Employers' responsibilities

Under the Act, all employers must ensure, as far as is reasonably practicable, that the health and safety of all persons on the premises is protected – and this must be achieved by carrying out a **risk assessment** of the workplace activities that occur on the premises. This is a specific requirement under the **Management of Health and Safety at Work Regulations 1999.**

A risk assessment is merely a detailed examination of the normal day-to-day activities that occur in the workplace in an effort to identify those that have the potential to cause harm to anyone on the premises – these are called the **hazards**. Once the hazards have been identified, a set of **precautions** can be determined that will prevent or minimise the risk associated with each hazard, thereby ensuring the safety of all those on the premises.

Recording the findings of the risk assessment is considered 'best practice', but is a legal requirement for all employers with five or more employees. As any relevant laws and regulations are updated, areas of the risk assessment may need to be reconsidered and updated too.

A typical process of risk assessment in the workplace can be summarised as follows:

- **Find the hazards**
- **Determine who is at risk of harm, and why**
- **Evaluate the risk of harm, and if additional precautions need to be taken to prevent harm**
- **Record the findings of the risk assessment**
- **Review the assessment regularly, and update it as necessary**

Employees' responsibilities

All employees are legally required to take reasonable care for their own and others' health and safety, and to co-operate with their employer to this effect while carrying out their normal workplace activities. Indeed, it is an offence for an employee to intentionally break the workplace rules and policies in relation to health and safety, whether this causes harm to themselves or others, or not.

As the majority of dental nurses training in practices tend to be young persons, the following two sets of regulations are also pertinent to dental practices:

- Health and Safety (Young Persons) Regulations 1997
- Management of Health and Safety at Work Regulations 1992

These regulations stipulate that the risk assessment of the dental workplace carried out must take into account the following points:

- The inexperience and immaturity of young persons
- Their lack of awareness of risks to their health and safety

- The fitting and layout of the practice and surgery
- The nature, degree and duration of any exposure to biological, chemical or physical agents
- The form, range, use and handling of work equipment
- The way in which processes and activities are organised
- Any health and safety training given, or intended to be given

Compliance with Health and Safety Law in the dental workplace involves all of the following, and all except those relating to ionising radiation will be covered in this Unit.

(1) Fire regulations
(2) COSHH – Control Of Substances Hazardous to Health
(3) RIDDOR – Reporting of Injuries, Diseases and Dangerous Occurrences Regulations
(4) Safe disposal of hazardous and special waste
(5) Manual handling
(6) Ionising radiation legislation
(7) Maintaining security in the workplace

(1) Fire regulations

Fire is a daily hazard that can occur in any workplace environment, but a risk assessment of the dental workplace will identify several specific fire hazards, as follows:

- **Flammable vapours and gases** – emergency oxygen cylinders, cleaning solvents, portable gas canisters
- **Naked flames** – used at the chairside for various dental procedures
- **Pressure vessels** – autoclaves and compressors, both of which can explode
- **Waste storage** – hazardous biological waste stored on the premises, often in the form of paper products and other flammable materials

In addition, all dental equipment is electrically operated and may short circuit, malfunction or spark and cause a fire at any time, especially if not serviced and maintained correctly.

Larger electrical items of dental equipment, such as the dental chair and inspection light, or autoclaves, have to be serviced and maintained by trained personnel on a regular basis. However, smaller portable items such as curing lights can be inspected for electrical safety by a general electrician, in a process known as portable appliance testing (PAT). This should be carried out annually, with each appliance having the plug, fuse size and wiring inspected for wear and tear. If all is well, a sticky label is applied to indicate that the appliance is PAT compliant, and the due date of the next PAT inspection (Figure 2.2).

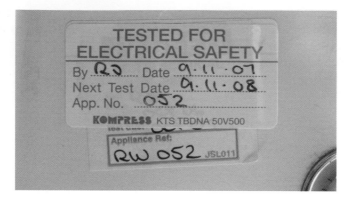

Figure 2.2 PAT label on electrical item.

In general, the commonest causes of fire in the workplace are:

- Faulty electrical supply or equipment
- Faulty heating equipment, or heating equipment used in a dangerous manner (such as heating equipment placed close to combustible materials)
- Flammable vapours and gases

Recent legislation (July 2007) to ban cigarette smoking in enclosed public places and the workplace has reduced the risk of fire from this source considerably.

Fire precautions in the workplace are governed by the **Fire Precautions Regulations 1997**, and require the employer to assess what fire precautions are needed by carrying out a risk assessment of the premises (as described previously) and by complying with the following.

Emergency routes and exits:

- Must be kept free of obstruction to allow immediate evacuation from the premises (thus, they should *not* be locked during work time)
- Should lead directly to a place of safety
- Should be clearly indicated by green 'Fire Exit' signs and pictogram of running man (Figure 2.3)

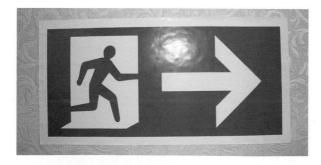

Figure 2.3 Fire exit pictogram.

■ Emergency instructions for evacuation of the premises in the event of a fire should be posted in easy to see areas, such as at reception and in waiting rooms (Figure 2.4)

■ Emergency lighting should be provided if necessary

■ Emergency doors should open in the direction of escape, and must not be electrically operated so that they can open immediately

■ No sliding or revolving doors should be used as fire exits

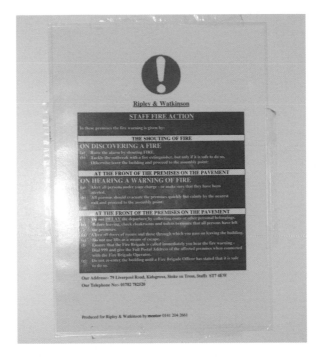

Figure 2.4 Fire instructions.

Fire safety inspectors also advise:

■ Fitting smoke detectors and alarms

■ Training staff in the use of fire extinguishers and fire blankets

■ Having at least two types of extinguisher in the dental workplace

Fire extinguishers vary depending on the type of fire that they are designed to fight; fires are classified as follows:

■ **Class A fire** – caused by the ignition of carbon-containing items, such as paper, wood and textiles

■ **Class B fire** – caused by flammable liquids, such as oils, solvents and petrol

- **Class C fire** – caused by flammable gases, such as domestic gas, butane, liquid petroleum gas (LPG)
- **Class D fire** – caused by reactive metals that oxidise in air, such as sodium and magnesium
- **Class E fire** – caused by electrical components and equipment
- **Class F fire** – caused by liquid fats, such as used in kitchens, restaurants

In the dental workplace, the likeliest causes of fire shown above suggest that extinguishers to fight fire classes A, B, C and E should be available. The content of each fire extinguisher varies, depending on its recommended use, and is identifiable by a coloured label on the extinguisher. The extinguishers themselves are now all red in colour so that they can be easily located. (Figure 2.5)

The labels themselves are coded as follows:

- Red (water) extinguisher – for use on all except electrical fires
- Black (carbon dioxide) extinguisher – for use on all fires
- Blue (dry powder) extinguisher – for use on all fires

Fire extinguishers must be inspected yearly and replaced as necessary, and dental practices should have a written fire safety policy with which all staff are familiar, so that a set procedure is known and followed by all.

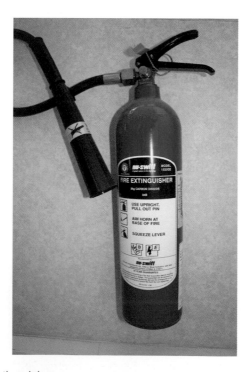

Figure 2.5 A fire extinguisher.

(2) COSHH (Control Of Substances Hazardous to Health)

COSHH is a legal requirement for employers, whereby all chemicals and potentially hazardous substances used in the workplace are assessed for risk of injury to staff, so that reports can be written for each and kept updated for quick reference in the case of accident or injury. Problems are only likely to occur if the substances and materials are not handled and used correctly, so it is very important that all members of staff are made aware of the hazards involved, and the correct handling of the substances.

Hazardous substances include any that have been labelled as **dangerous** by the manufacturer, and these are easily recognised by the use of a universal system of symbols which indicate the specific hazard of the substance. So, they may be classed as 'toxic', 'harmful', 'corrosive' or 'irritant' (Figure 2.6).

Know your hazardous chemical products. Below are the four health categories:

TOXIC
– can cause damage to health at low levels
for example, mercury is toxic by inhalation

HARMFUL
– can cause damage to health
for example, some disinfectants /tray adhesives are harmful by inhalation

CORROSIVE
– may destroy living tissue on contact
for example, phosphoric acid (etchant) causes burns in contact with skin

IRRITANT
– may cause inflammation to skin and/or eyes, nose and throat
for example, some disinfectants and x-ray developer can irritate the eyes and skin

Note:
For packaged hazardous chemical products, the label (depending on the size) should contain a symbol (as above) and simple information about the hazard and the precautions required. The Safety Data Sheet will provide more detailed information and the supplier is obliged to provide this if the substance is hazardous to health and is used at work.

Figure 2.6 COSHH hazard signs. Source: *Levison's Textbook for Dental Nurses*, 10th edn, C. Hollins, 2008, Wiley-Blackwell.

These symbols will appear on the substance packaging, along with information on the actions to take in the event of an accident; all of this information will be included in the COSHH report of each substance.

Other hazardous substances found specifically in the dental workplace are:

- **Ionising radiation** – as it has a maximum exposure limit
- **Micro-organisms** – present on all items and equipment contaminated by the body fluids of patients

The COSHH assessment will follow the stages set out below for each of the substances:

(1) **Identify** those substances which are hazardous, by reading the manufacturers' leaflets, which should accompany the product
(2) Identify **who** may be harmed – usually all persons using the substance
Identify **how** they may be harmed – breathing in, irritant to eyes or skin, etc.
(3) **Evaluate** the risk of the substance
(4) Determine whether **health monitoring** is required (mercury exposure, for example)
(5) **Control the risks**, or reduce them as far as possible
(6) **Inform** all staff of the risks (show sheets and sign to say they have read and understood them)
(7) **Record** the assessment and review and **update** it regularly

Each substance will have the relevant details entered onto an evaluation sheet, set out in the same way for ease of reference (Figure 2.7). The evaluation sheets for all substances used in the workplace should be kept in several folders throughout the premises, for ease of access by all staff. The evaluation sheets of those substances posing serious harm if misused or involved in spillages should also be kept in an 'emergency file', with medical emergency details included.

The COSHH regulations were amended most recently in 2004, to outline the principles of 'best practice' that every workplace is expected to adhere to in an effort to control the exposure of staff to substances hazardous to health. Their particular relevance to the dental workplace is as follows:

- Activities must be designed and operated to minimise the emission, release and spread of substances hazardous to health
- All relevant routes of exposure must always be taken into account when developing control measures
- The most effective and reliable method of minimising the escape and spread of any hazardous substance must be adopted by the dental workplace, in line with current legislation
- Suitable personal protective equipment (PPE) must be provided by the employer for use by all those handling hazardous substances, where adequate control of exposure cannot be achieved by other means alone

Name of Substance				
Hazardous Ingredients				
Used for				
By whom				
Frequency				
Amount				
Nature of Risks	Chemical	Flammable	Poisonous	Biological
Exposure Limits	OES (MEL if applicable)		ppm	mg m^{-3}
	Long term (8 hr TWA)		–	
			–	
Other				
Health Effects				
Eye contact				
Skin contact				
Inhalation				
Ingestion				
Precautions for Safe Handling and Use				
Spillage				
Waste disposal				
Storage				
Control Measures				
Ventilation				
Eye protection				
Respiratory protection				
Gloves				
Health monitoring				
Staff training				
Other				
First Aid Measures				
Eye contact				
Skin contact				
Inhalation				
Ingestion				

Dentists and staff members to sign to confirm these Control Measures are carried out:

1	4	7
2	5	8
3	6	9

Figure 2.7 Example of COSHH assessment sheet. Source: *Levison's Textbook for Dental Nurses*, 10th edn, C. Hollins, 2008, Wiley-Blackwell.

- Methods of control must be regularly reviewed, amended and updated as necessary, in line with current legislation
- All staff must be informed and trained in the correct handling and use of all hazardous substances that they are likely to come across while performing their daily duties

To comply with these principles of 'best practice', the dental workplace has to consider the following control measures in an effort to reduce the risks to staff when handling any substances hazardous to health.

- If possible, the hazardous substance must be substituted for one that is considered to be less hazardous
- If possible, isolation methods should be adopted so that the hazard is controlled
- Ensure that adequate ventilation is provided in areas where hazardous substances that give off toxic fumes are used
- Ensure all the necessary PPE is available for all staff
- Adopt good housekeeping techniques throughout the dental workplace, and ensure all staff abide by them
- Ensure that all staff are suitably trained in the handling of hazardous substances that they come across in the dental workplace
- Have the correct procedures in place in the event of an accident involving a hazardous substance, to be followed by all staff
- Regularly record all reviews of the existing procedures, and update them as necessary in line with current legislation

Three hazardous substances used in the dental workplace on a daily basis by most staff require special mention in relation to COSHH. These are:

- Mercury
- Acid etchant
- Bleach (and other disinfectants)

Mercury

Mercury is a liquid metal that is mixed with various metal powders to form dental amalgam – this is a material used to fill teeth (see Unit 8). It is classed as a hazardous substance because it is toxic, and it can enter the body in the following ways:

- **Inhalation** – toxic vapours are released from uncovered sources at room temperature and above, and are particularly hazardous because they are colourless and odourless and therefore difficult to detect
- **Absorption** – particles can be absorbed through the skin, nail beds, and the eye membranes, and eventually become lodged in the kidneys
- **Ingestion** – particles can contaminate foodstuffs and drinks, and be taken into the digestive system and eventually lodge in the kidneys

Dental amalgam is still the commonest material used to fill teeth, so mercury is present in significant amounts in the majority of dental workplaces. Exposure to the hazards mercury poses cannot easily be avoided, but the risks can be minimised by following simple rules designed to limit the chances of staff contact.

Inhalation

- Ensure that the workplace is adequately ventilated and kept at a reasonable working temperature, so that fumes do not build up
- Avoid placing mercury and waste amalgam near heat sources (including sunny windowsills), as more fumes are given off at higher temperatures
- Use capsulated amalgam so that bottles of mercury do not have to be stored on the premises
- Store all waste amalgam in special sealed tubs containing a mercury-absorbing chemical (Figure 2.8)
- Similarly, used amalgam capsules must be stored in special sealed tubs, as it is likely that tiny amounts of mercury will remain in them after use (Figure 2.9)

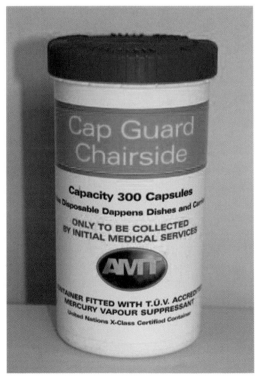

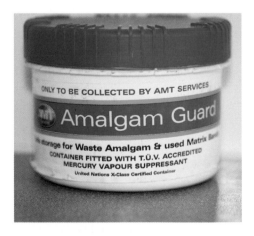

Figure 2.8 Waste amalgam tub.

Figure 2.9 Waste amalgam capsule tub.

- Ensure every trace of amalgam is removed from instruments before they are sterilised in the autoclave, otherwise fumes will be released as the autoclave heats up
- If a mercury spillage occurs, wear appropriate PPE including a face mask, to avoid inhalation

Absorption

- Always wear the correct PPE when handling amalgam capsules and waste amalgam, to avoid skin, nail and eye contact
- Open-toed shoes must not be worn in the surgery area, to avoid absorption through the feet if any amalgam or mercury is spilled
- Always wear safety goggles or a face visor when old amalgam fillings are being removed, so that stray specks do not enter the eyes
- If a mercury spillage occurs, wear gloves and safety goggles to avoid skin or eye contact

Ingestion

- Food and drink must never be consumed in the surgery environment
- Stocks of mercury and amalgam capsules must not be stored within the staff rest room
- Waste amalgam containers must not be stored within the staff rest room

Handling of mercury spillages

The use of capsulated amalgam products will limit the likelihood of a large mercury spillage, but the capsules themselves can rupture during use, releasing liquid mercury into the environment although on a much smaller scale. All spillages of mercury, no matter how small, must be reported to the senior dentist and recorded in the workplace 'Accident Book'. This will provide a written record of any accident or incident that has occurred on the premises, and that could have potentially harmed someone. It must include the following details:

- The date and location of where the accident/incident occurred
- Who was affected
- The names of any witnesses
- Details of the accident/incident
- Actions taken to assist those affected

In the unfortunate event of any long-term health effects, this report will provide valuable evidence about whether correct procedures were followed, and whether the accident/incident was avoidable or not.

If mercury is spilled, it tends to form into liquid globules or small balls. In this shape, the liquid can easily roll around and be difficult to pick up, indeed larger globules often break into smaller ones when attempts are made to handle them. The correct actions to take after a mercury spillage are therefore very important, to prevent further contamination and spread into the workplace environment.

If a small spillage occurs:

(1) Wear suitable PPE
(2) Suck up small globules into a disposable plastic syringe or a dedicated bulb aspirator
(3) Put the particles into the waste amalgam special waste container

Never use the dental suction unit, or the vacuum cleaner, to suck up spilt mercury – their use will release toxic mercury vapours into the workplace. Alternatively, the lead foils present in intra-oral x-ray film packets can be used to gather the globules together and scoop them up. However, since they too are now classed as toxic special waste, their handling and use in this manner should be avoided if possible.

To avoid the release of small globules into the workplace, the amalgamator machine (Figure 2.10) should have a lid on and be stood on a foil tray to collect any spillages without them contaminating the workplace. Any globules collected by these methods can be simply tipped into the waste amalgam store.

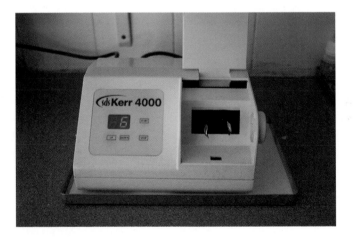

Figure 2.10 An amalgamator.

If a larger spillage occurs:

(1) Wear suitable PPE
(2) Open windows to ventilate the area
(3) Inform senior staff
(4) Use the contents of the mercury spillage kit to control the spread of the spillage (Figure 2.11)

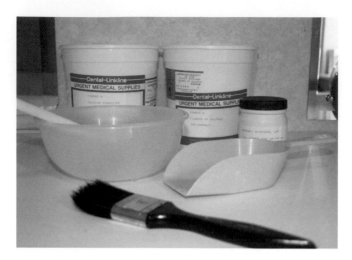

Figure 2.11 Mercury spillage kit.

(5)   Mix the powders of **flowers of sulphur** and **calcium hydroxide** with water to make a paste, and paint this around the spillage to contain it
(6)   The remaining paste can be painted over the spillage
(7)   Once dry, the contaminated paste and spillage are wiped up thoroughly with damp paper towels, and disposed of in the waste amalgam store

If the size of the spillage is significant, such as a full bottle of mercury, or if globules rolled into inaccessible areas, the work area must be sealed off and closed down. The Health and Safety Executive must be informed of the spillage, and Environmental Health will attend to clear away the contamination professionally and safely.

Acid etchant

Acid etchant is used during the placement of composite (tooth-coloured) fillings (see Unit 8). As the name suggests, it is acidic and can therefore chemically burn soft tissues, such as within the patient's mouth or the skin of those handling the substance. The material itself is 33% phosphoric acid, in either a liquid or gel form.

All staff handling the etchant must be wearing the correct PPE, and when placed within the patient's mouth it must be confined to the tooth undergoing restoration. Very careful aspiration must be used while the material is washed off the tooth, so that it does not fall elsewhere and burn the patient's oral mucosa. To aid this, the acid etchant is usually brightly coloured so that it is easily visible – for instance some manufacturers produce a bright pink liquid and others a bright blue gel.

The manufacturer's instructions for use, contained within the packaging of the material, will show the necessary symbol indicating a hazardous substance, and will provide details of the first-aid actions to take if an accident occurs, in accordance with COSHH regulations.

Bleach (and other disinfectants)

All disinfectants have a huge role to play in the decontamination of work areas and fixed equipment in the dental practice. Bleach, which is **sodium hypochlorite**, is used in many situations:

- 10% fresh solution is used to disinfect all non-metallic, non-fabric surfaces within the surgery
- 10% fresh solution is used to disinfect impressions and removable prostheses before transferring between the patient and the laboratory
- 50% fresh solution is used to clean away blood spillages within the surgery

Other disinfectants include a variety of aldehydes and isopropyl alcohol products, often sold as spray solutions or pre-soaked wipes.

Bleach has an unpleasant taste and smell, and is chemically irritant to soft tissues. It can cause tissue damage to the mouth and digestive tract, the eyes, and the lungs if strong vapours are inhaled. Appropriate PPE must be worn whenever it is handled, and fresh solutions made daily for the uses indicated above should be held in lidded containers so that the noxious chlorine vapours do not become overpowering.

Disinfectant bottles of any solutions used will show the necessary hazardous substance symbol, and give the necessary first-aid actions in the event of an accident, in line with COSHH regulations (Figure 2.12).

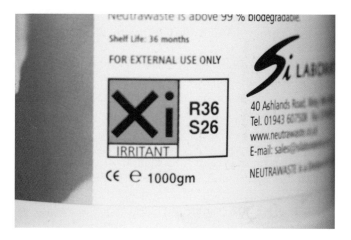

Figure 2.12 Hazardous substance label.

(3) RIDDOR (Reporting of Injuries, Diseases and Dangerous Occurrences Regulations)

In addition to any minor accidents or incidents that may occur in the workplace, a separate set of regulations exist that cover those accidents and incidents classi- fied as 'significant events'. All workplaces have a duty to report these signific- ant events to the Health and Safety Executive, which will investigate the matter and determine if correct procedures were followed, if the event was avoidable or not, and ultimately if an employer is legally to blame and therefore liable to prosecution.

Major injuries that must be reported are:

■ Fractures of the skull, the spine or the pelvis
■ Fractures of the long bones of an arm or leg
■ Amputation of a hand or foot, or the loss of sight in one eye
■ Hypoxia (oxygen starvation) severe enough to produce unconsciousness
■ Any other injury requiring 24 hours hospital admission, unless for observation only

The notifiable dangerous occurrences which require reporting to the Health and Safety Executive are:

■ Explosion, collapse or burst of an autoclave or compressor
■ Electrical short circuit or overload causing more than 24 hours of stoppage
■ Explosion or a fire due to gases or flammable products causing more than 24 hours of stoppage
■ Uncontrolled release or escape of mercury vapour (a major mercury spillage)
■ Any accident involving inhalation/ingestion/absorption of a substance caus- ing hypoxia requiring medical treatment
■ Any case of acute ill health due to exposure to pathogens or infectious materials

All other accidents occurring on the premises, no matter how minor and whether involving staff or patients, should be recorded in the 'Accident Book'. This also includes any violent assaults or attacks occurring on the premises, and these should also be reported to the police.

Compliance by all staff with Health and Safety laws should avoid the occurrence of a significant event on the premises, although sometimes purely unavoidable incidents can occur, even at a fully compliant workplace. Investigation of these incidents by the Health and Safety Executive often results in a change to recom- mended working practice, thereby reducing the chances of a similar event occur- ring again. This is called 'significant event analysis' and illustrates successful risk assessment in action.

Besides the obvious hazards associated with the dental workplace, more general hazards and risks that require consideration are:

- **Surgery** – no trailing wires from electrical equipment, good ventilation at all times, all chemicals stored away safely and securely when not in use
- **Reception and waiting room** – no trailing wires from electrical equipment, heaters surrounded with a guard to prevent burns, floor uncluttered to avoid trips, display cabinets not overloaded
- **Kitchen and staff rest room** – kept hygienically clean and tidy, no storage of stock or waste materials in food fridge, cupboards not overloaded, all equipment PAT tested
- **Store rooms** – no access to anyone except staff members, floors uncluttered
- **Stairs** – double handrails for ease of use, uncluttered steps, stair covering kept in good repair

(4) Safe disposal of hazardous and special waste

There are three types of waste produced by all dental workplaces:

- Non-hazardous waste – normal household waste, paper, etc.
- Hazardous waste – all waste, including sharps, that is contaminated by body fluids (especially saliva and blood)
- Special waste – specific hazardous waste produced by dental workplaces:
    - Amalgam and amalgam capsules, containing **mercury** which is toxic
    - **Radiograph fixer** and **developer** solutions, which are toxic
    - **Lead foil** from radiograph film packets, which is toxic
    - Partially discharged **local anaesthetic cartridges**, which contain some local anaesthetic solution and is a medicine
    - Out-of-date **emergency drugs**, which are medicines

Non-hazardous waste

Non-hazardous waste is produced at reception and in staff rest room areas, rather than in the clinical areas. It is normal household waste, consisting of paper, writing or computer products, waste food and its containers, packaging of stock deliveries, etc. It is no more of a hazard in the workplace than it is in the home, and therefore requires no special disposal.

Hazardous waste

The definition of hazardous waste is 'any items that are potentially contaminated with body fluids', and this encompasses all of the following dental waste:

- Extracted teeth that do not contain amalgam fillings
- All disposable items contaminated with saliva or blood
- All disposable items which have come into contact with a patient

■   All paper products used to clean the surgery after treating each patient
■   All covers used during the treatment of each patient

Those items that are not sharp must be disposed off in yellow/orange hazardous waste sacks, which are sealed with identifying tags and must be collected only by a hazardous waste handling company. They must be stored safely at the dental workplace before collection, away from possible contact with the public, and must be incinerated once they have been removed from the premises.

Some hazardous waste products are sharp and may cause penetrating injuries and infection. They are particularly dangerous in the transfer of pathogenic microorganisms. They include all of the following:

■   Scalpel blades
■   Suture needles
■   Local anaesthetic needles
■   Empty glass local anaesthetic cartridges
■   Empty glass ampoules of drugs
■   Endodontic hand instruments (used in root canal treatments)
■   Metal matrix bands
■   Orthodontic archwires (used for dental braces)

These items must be disposed of in rigid 'sharps bins', coloured yellow and with a puncture-proof base and a sealable lid that cannot be reopened once closed. They must be sealed once they are three-quarters full (Figure 2.13).

Ideally, the sharps items should be placed in these bins directly by the dentist rather than the dental nurse, to avoid having to pass sharp items between each other and thereby reducing the risk of a sharps injury.

If a 'dirty' sharps injury does occur, the immediate hazard to the casualty is the transfer of a blood-borne infection from the patient. The most serious of these are hepatitis B or C, and acquired immune deficiency syndrome (AIDS). Staff vaccinated against hepatitis B will be protected from the disease, but the other two diseases are both fatal and it is vital that the correct procedure is followed when a 'dirty' sharps injury occurs, as follows:

(1)   Stop work immediately and squeeze the wound to encourage bleeding
(2)   Wash the wound under warm running water to encourage more bleeding
(3)   Dry and dress the wound with a waterproof dressing
(4)   Check the patient's medical history to determine if there is a serious risk of infection
(5)   If so, Occupational Health must be contacted immediately for advice regarding the need for blood tests and anti-viral treatment
(6)   The incident must be recorded in the workplace 'Accident Book', and a risk assessment carried out to determine if procedures need to be changed
(7)   If the casualty does contract a serious infection, the Health and Safety Executive must be notified in accordance with RIDDOR

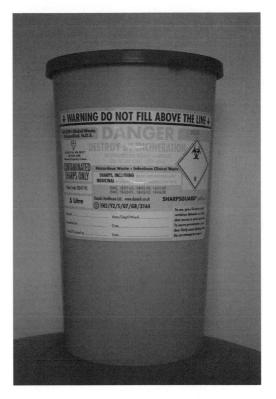

Figure 2.13 A sharps box. Source: *Levison's Textbook for Dental Nurses*, 10th edn, C. Hollins, 2008, Wiley-Blackwell.

The Environmental Regulations that are in force with regard to hazardous waste are summarised below:

- Environmental Protection Act 1990 – the duty of care is on the dentist to store hazardous waste safely and securely, and to arrange for its correct disposal, by incineration
- Environmental Protection Regulations 1991 – the collector of the waste must have a certificate of registration, and supply transfer notes which must be signed by both parties. Repeat collections can be covered by one note per year, and the transfer notes must be kept for two years
- Carriage of Dangerous Goods Regulations 1996 – updated from 1 January 2002 so that yellow/orange sacks must be stored and transported in United Nations (UN)-approved rigid containers, and sharps boxes must comply with BS 7320 standards

Special waste

All waste classed as special is potentially harmful but cannot be disposed off by incineration as other hazardous waste can. Further regulations governing their safe disposal are as follows:

- Consignment notes must be used and signed at each stage of the disposal process
- These notes must be kept for three years
- An additional levy is payable by the producer of the waste, the dentist
- Radiographic developer and fixer may still be disposed of via the sewers with the written permission of the relevant water company
- Waste amalgam and capsules can no longer be posted to recycling companies, but they can still be collected from the dental premises if transfer and consignment notes are produced and signed accordingly, and the collector has the relevant certificate of registration

Otherwise, separate containers provided by the waste collector must be used to store each type of special waste on the premises for up to six months, before collection (Figure 2.14).

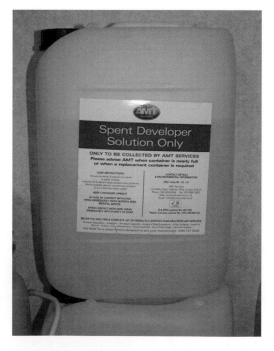

Figure 2.14 Developer waste container.

In particular, the containers used to store waste amalgam and amalgam capsules must contain a mercury-absorbing chemical, to avoid vapour release. All other special waste containers must be of a rigid plastic design, shaped so as not to fall over and spill their contents easily, and clearly labelled with their contents. They must be stored in an area of the workplace that has no public access, to avoid accidents.

(5) Manual handling

In the majority of dental workplaces, the usual manual handling that occurs is the transport of boxes containing stock items, or the movement of waste containers in and out of storage. Hospital departments and dental clinics may also require staff to be involved with the movement of disabled, sedated or unconscious patients too, and separate and specific training must be given in these areas by the employer.

Lifting heavy or awkward items incorrectly can result in all kinds of injuries to staff, and employers must ensure that, as far as reasonably practicable, they adhere to the regulations laid down in the Manual Handling Operations Regulations 1992. These were further revised in 2002, and state:

- All hazardous manual handling should be avoided, as far as is reasonably practicable
- Any hazardous manual handling that cannot be avoided must be correctly assessed
- All efforts must then be made to reduce the risk of injury as far as possible

While carrying out an assessment of any manual handling and lifting that has to be carried out in the dental workplace, the following points must be considered when deciding whether the task is hazardous or not:

- The weight and dimensions of the object being moved or lifted
- The likelihood of staff having to reach, bend, twist or stoop while moving or handling the object
- The frequency of the task
- The likelihood of excessive movements being required, such as pushing or pulling
- The distance that the object has to be moved
- The need for the object to be carried up or down the stairs
- The physical ability of the staff involved in moving and handling
- The existence of any medical conditions that contraindicate staff moving or handling objects (this includes pregnancy)
- The need for any training to be given in the correct techniques of moving and handling

If each point is taken separately, it can be seen that much can be done to avoid injury to staff during moving and handling activities.

Weight and dimensions

The heavier the load and the greater its dimensions, the more difficult will be its handling and the more likely injury will occur, so consider the following:

- Split the load to make it lighter
- Ask other staff to help while lifting and moving it
- Use a trolley or other handling aids, if available

Awkward movements and frequency

Examples include twisting etc. while lifting or moving a load. The more times the move is carried out, the more likely it is to cause injury, so consider the following:

- Clear the path of travel before lifting, to avoid having to twist etc.
- Move the feet to change direction, rather than twisting etc.
- When precise positioning is required, put the load down then adjust its position
- When loads have to be moved frequently, use a trolley or other handling aid to avoid straining the back

Excessive movements

Pushing and pulling lighter loads is not usually a problem, but when heavier loads are involved they must either be split into smaller units first or a trolley or other handling aid must be used. In most instances, large boxes of stock can be opened and put into their place of storage individually, to avoid having to push or pull them into position.

Distance and stairs

It makes sense to move objects the minimum distance whenever possible, and to avoid having to carry them up and down stairs manually. The place of storage for stock should be carefully considered, to avoid repetitive strain injuries to staff, and a lift must always be used if available. Otherwise, a trolley or other handling aid needs to be provided.

Physical ability and medical conditions

Elderly or unfit staff are more likely to injure themselves while moving and handling, by over-estimating their own capabilities. The following must be considered:

- Elderly staff tend not to be as strong as younger staff, and may have less stamina to hold a load for any length of time
- Overweight staff will find it difficult to hold loads as close to their centre of gravity as they need to for stability, and this will put unnecessary strain on their arms and back

- Short staff will lift and carry loads less easily than taller staff
- Male staff tend to be stronger than female staff, although this cannot be assumed
- Various medical conditions will prevent some staff from being capable of moving and handling objects without risking injury to themselves, such as back problems, heart and respiratory conditions, hernias, etc.
- Pregnant staff should not be involved in moving and handling heavy objects

Training

A correct handling technique should be taught to all staff involved in moving and lifting objects in the dental workplace, and this may involve the following:

- Sending the staff (and the employer) on a well-run training course to learn the best posture to adopt while lifting and moving loads
- Acquiring trolleys and other handling aids for the premises
- Changing the location of storage rooms, to make them closer to the delivery point and ideally at ground level
- Acquiring more storage cupboards or shelves at waist height for heavier items
- Acquiring step ladders for the placement of light loads in storage spaces above shoulder level

(6) Ionising radiation legislation

The type of ionising radiation used in dentistry is 'x-rays', an invaluable tool for accurate diagnosis of some dental problems, but their misuse or overuse can be dangerous to staff and patients alike. The legislation concerning the safe use of x-rays in the dental workplace is fully covered in Unit 7 – Contribute to the Production of Dental Images.

(7) Security in the workplace

Although it is unlikely that dental practices will have just one or two members on the premises during normal working hours, this situation can occur during holiday times or when several staff are attending courses so no patient appointments are set. In the interests of staff safety, it would be advisable for the premises to be locked during these times so that staff are not left vulnerable and open to attack.

All employers have a responsibility to maintain the security of both the workplace premises and the safety and security of their staff. In addition, all staff have a responsibility to uphold the security procedures that have been put into place by their employer, to ensure that the safety of the workforce and the security of the premises is never compromised.

Maintaining security during the day

Security of the premises and the safety of the staff during the day are achieved by ensuring that the premises are only accessed by those who have a right of entry. This is more difficult to achieve in large hospital departments and dental clinics than it is in general practice, where the majority of people attending are regular patients who are known by the staff.

However, procedures must be in place to ensure that all visitors to the premises have to pass through a reception point, so that they can be seen and identified by staff. Several methods can be used to achieve this:

- Locked entry point with a speaker phone
- Fire exits that can only be opened from inside the premises
- Entry way that has to pass directly through reception, so that all visitors have to report there
- CCTV system
- Trained staff manning reception at all times, with an appointments system in place to identify any unexpected visitors to the premises
- Security screening in place so that the reception area cannot be breached
- Panic button in case any threatening behaviour occurs

When expected visitors attend, such as booked patients, maintenance or repair workers, or stock sales representatives, they will be checked off against the appointment book and then usually held in the reception waiting area.

Patients will have appointment details to be confirmed, while others will have usually phoned to book their attendance with a staff member. In any instance, the following should be the norm to eliminate the risk of any violence towards staff.

- Ensure all staff are trained to be caring and sympathetic towards patients
- All visitors to the workplace should be treated with respect, and spoken to courteously. This is especially important when a patient attends unexpectedly, or without an appointment, and highlights the need for a robust dental emergency policy to be in place
- Ensure all staff are aware of the practice protocols in relation to assault and violence towards themselves
- Ensure all patients are aware of these too – this should be nothing less than a statement of 'zero tolerance' in cases of violence towards staff

While working at reception, it is important that all cashboxes or tills are out of the reach of other persons and are locked unless in actual use. This reduces the risk of opportunistic thieves attempting to steal from the premises. Similarly, all patient records, whether written or computerised, must be held securely and out of view of anyone attending the premises – the confidentiality of patient details is a legal requirement in the dental workplace. Filing cabinets or the record storage room should be locked at the end of each day, and computer records should be password protected. In larger dental workplaces, passwords are often only given to senior staff members.

Staff rooms should not be accessible to anyone except staff, and can be made so by the use of security code entry systems. Ideally, lockers should be provided for all staff too, so that valuables and personal belongings are never at risk of being stolen.

Maintaining security out of hours

It is of great importance that the dental workplace is always securely locked when not in use. Not only are there expensive but portable items of equipment on the premises, but also drugs, syringes and needles, which may attract break-ins by drug users for instance.

Several methods of maintaining the security of the premises are available, as follows:

- Adequate alarm system in place, which is ideally manned by a security company, so that unusual entry times or alarm activation can be acted upon immediately
- Only senior staff should be given the alarm code, to reduce the number of persons who may open the premises
- Similarly, key holder numbers must be kept to a minimum
- The loss of a key by any member of staff must be reported to the employer immediately
- All keys must be handed in when staff leave their employment
- Ensure that alarms are set correctly at the end of each day, so that break-ins are detected immediately
- Change the alarm code on a regular basis, and ensure that only senior staff are notified of the new code
- Ensure that all monies are banked daily, to remove the incentive for opportunist burglary
- Ensure that all doors are locked and bolted at the end of each day, especially the fire exits
- All windows should have locks on them, and be closed and locked at the end of each day
- Ground floor windows are usually required to have metal screens placed over them by insurance companies
- Most dental employers will have a policy in place to limit access to the premises by staff to their normal working hours only, and this must be upheld by all

3 Unit 2: Reflect on and Develop Your Practice (HSC33)

Knowledge specifications

Values

K1 – A working knowledge of legal and organisational requirements on equality, diversity, discrimination and rights when working with individuals and others to improve your knowledge and practice

K2 – A working knowledge of dilemmas and conflicts that you may face in your practice

Legislation and organisational policy and procedures

K3 – A working knowledge of codes of practice and conduct, and standards and guidance relevant to your own role and the roles, responsibilities, accountability and duties of others about personal and professional development

K4 – A working knowledge of current local, UK and European legislation, and organisational requirements, procedures and practices for accessing training and undertaking personal and professional development activities

K5 – A working knowledge of the purpose of, and arrangements for your supervision and appraisal

Theory and practice

K6 – A working knowledge of how and where to access information and support on knowledge and best practice relevant to your area of work, the individuals and key people with whom you work and the skills and knowledge you need to practice effectively

K7 – A working knowledge of principles underpinning personal and professional development and reflective practice

K8 – A working knowledge of how to work in partnership with individuals, key people and others to enable you to develop and enhance your knowledge and practice

> **K9** – A working knowledge of development opportunities that can enhance your practice
> **K10** – A working knowledge of lessons learned from inquiries into serious failure of health and social care practice, and from successful interventions
> **K11** – A working knowledge of approaches to learning that will allow you to transfer your knowledge and skills to new and unfamiliar contexts

The dental profession is undergoing reform with the start of the legal regulation of all members of the dental team, including dental nurses. All members other than dentists are now known as 'dental care professionals', or DCPs, and compulsory registration with the General Dental Council (GDC) is now the norm, once qualification has been achieved.

However, as with dentists, all DCPs will be expected to develop a system of lifelong learning and continuing professional development, so that as dentistry and dental nursing evolves and develops, new skills and information will need to be understood and practised by all. Qualification and compulsory registration are now the basic requirement for becoming a dental nurse, rather than their end goal of achievement.

History of dental nursing

Basic dental treatment was available even in ancient times, but the concept of the dentist being assisted by another person – now referred to as the dental nurse – is a more modern one. All dentists will agree that a second pair of hands in the surgery is invaluable in providing a high standard of oral health care to patients, but it was the introduction of a formal qualification in 'Dental Surgery Assisting' (as it was initially called) in 1943 that began the necessary development of training pathways for these individuals.

The inception of the National Examining Board for Dental Nurses some 65 years ago sowed the seeds for the creation and development of the huge organisation it is today, with over 3000 candidates taking the National Certificate qualification each year. In addition, the Level 3 National Vocational Qualification in Oral Health Care was introduced more recently, to accommodate the learning requirements of those choosing a more work-based training programme in dental nursing. Together, the two qualifications produce trained and competent dental nurses in the UK of a calibre envied elsewhere.

Following the introduction of compulsory qualification and registration of DCPs with the GDC in August 2008, dental nurses are now recognised as a profession in their own right, with training opportunities to increase their knowledge and skills in a variety of areas:

- Oral health education
- Dental sedation nursing

- Special care dental nursing
- Orthodontic nursing
- Dental radiography

As dentistry and dental nursing continue to develop and evolve, it is likely that more post-registration qualifications for dental nurses will be introduced with time. As always, dental nurses may also choose to take more formal career decisions, and train to become dental hygienists and dental therapists – two more invaluable members of the modern dental team.

General Dental Council

The GDC is the governing body of the whole dental profession, and it has a legal duty to protect patients and to regulate the dental team. It issues guidance on the standards to be maintained by all dental professionals (including dental nurses), and sets outs the principles that each team member is expected to follow, whether routinely treating patients or not.

Statutory registration of dental nurses – standards guidance

The series of booklets issued by the GDC that lay down the standards expected of all those now able to register with them are summarised below. On qualification and acceptance onto the DCP register, all dental nurses will receive their own copy of these booklets (Figure 3.1).

As a dental professional, you are responsible for making sure you do the following.

- **Be familiar with and understand**:
  - Current standards which affect your work
  - Relevant guidelines issued by organisations other than the GDC
  - Available sources of evidence that support current standards
- **Apply your up-to-date knowledge and skills ethically**

You are also personally responsible for following the **principles of practice in dentistry**, as stated by the GDC. This means always doing the following:

- Putting patients' interests first and acting to protect them
- Respecting patients' dignity and choices
- Protecting the confidentiality of patients' information
- Co-operating with other team members and other healthcare colleagues in the interests of the patients
- Maintaining your professional knowledge and competence
- Being trustworthy

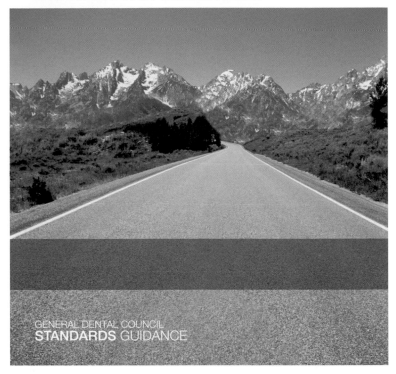

Figure 3.1 GDC Standards Guidance document. Reproduced with kind permission from the General Dental Council (www.gdc-uk.org).

Each of the above points is covered in more detail within the GDC booklets, and all dental nurses will be expected to familiarise themselves with their content upon registration. For unqualified dental nurses, each point is briefly explained below for the sake of completeness.

Put patients' interests first and act to protect them

- Put patients' interests first before your own or those of any colleague, organisation or business
- Follow these principles when handling questions and complaints from patients, and in all other aspects of non-clinical service
- Work within your knowledge, professional competence and physical abilities
- Respect the patient's right to complain
- Take action if you believe patients might be at risk because of your health (or a colleague's)
- Do not make any claims that could mislead patients

Respect patients' dignity and choices

- Treat patients politely and with respect
- Recognise and promote patients' responsibility for making decisions about their dental care
- Promote equal opportunities for all patients, and do not discriminate
- Communicate effectively with patients
- Maintain appropriate boundaries in the relationships you have with patients

Protect the confidentiality of patients' information

- Treat information about patients as confidential and only use it for the purposes for which it is given
- Prevent information from being accidentally revealed by keeping information secure at all times
- Take appropriate advice on revealing information in an exceptional circumstance without consent before doing so

Co-operate with others in the interests of patients

- Respect the role of others in caring for patients
- Do not discriminate against other team members
- Communicate effectively with other team members in the interests of patients

Maintain your professional knowledge and competence

- Develop and update your knowledge and skills throughout your working life
- Reflect on your knowledge and skills, and identify both your strengths and weaknesses
- Provide a good standard of care based on up-to-date evidence and guidance
- Follow all the laws and regulations which affect your work

Be trustworthy

- Always act honestly and fairly
- Apply these principles to all professional relationships and activities
- Maintain appropriate standards of personal behaviour in all walks of life

The GDC states that every dental professional is responsible for ensuring they are familiar with and understand:

- Current standards which affect their work
- Relevant guidelines issued by organisations other than the GDC
- Available sources of evidence that support current standards

The GDC also stipulates that every dental professional must apply their up-to-date knowledge and skills ethically.

The points stated above indicate that the standards and guidelines are open to improvement and change with time; so what was considered a reasonable standard at the time of a dental nurse's initial training and inception into the profession may not be considered to be so now. The only way of determining if change has occurred is for the dental nurse to regularly update their knowledge and skills, in part by reflecting on and evaluating their day-to-day actions and outcomes (see later). This then allows the dental nurse to develop their training and skills, and progress accordingly.

Factors that may influence development and progression

The factors that may influence the development of a dental nurse include the following:

- Their own personal values and beliefs
- The rights of patients
- Employment legislation

Values and beliefs

The dental nurse's values and beliefs will have been influenced and developed largely by their immediate social circle, this will include family, friends and work colleagues. When others (especially patients) are prejudged about their own values and beliefs by the dental nurse before forming a working relationship with them, then the dental nurse has shown **prejudice**. Unfortunately, this is usually a negative expression or opinion with regard to the patient's age, race, sex, appearance, religion, disability, etc.

If the prejudice extends to the dental nurse treating others unfairly or less favourably than they should, then that person has been **discriminated against** by the dental nurse. This is in direct contradiction to one of the GDC's stated principles of practice: to 'respect the patients' dignity and choices'. This means that patients have the right to:

- Be treated with dignity and respect
- Be responsible for making decisions about their care
- Be treated fairly and in line with the law, so that equal opportunities are promoted for all
- Not be discriminated against for any reason
- Communicated with in a manner suitable for them to make informed decisions about their care
- Expect that appropriate boundaries will be maintained by all DCPs

There are various laws now in place to ensure that discrimination does not occur and that **equal opportunities** are promoted at all times, and for all persons.

Rights of patients

The first principle of all DCPs is to be responsible for 'putting patients' interests first and acting to protect them', in accordance with the GDC guidance on the professional standards expected of the profession. This means that all DCPs have a duty of care to always act in a professional manner, whether dealing with patients directly or not. In other words, this embraces the other principles laid down by the GDC with respect to the standards expected of the profession, and gives the patients the right to expect all of the following:

- All dental professionals will act only within the remit of their training, and patients will be referred elsewhere for further treatment when necessary
- Accurate and full records will be kept of all patients attending for treatment, and these will be easily accessible to the patient as necessary
- The right to make a complaint about the care received, if necessary, which will be correctly handled by the profession
- Not to be misled in any way to accept treatment that is not in their best interests
- All information held in their records will be treated as confidential, and only used for the purposes for which it was given
- That the dental team will cooperate with each other at all times to put the interests of the patient first
- That the dental team will maintain their professional knowledge and competence, and keep them updated as necessary
- That all pertinent laws and regulations that affect the provision of dental care will be upheld by all, at all times
- That all members of the dental team are trustworthy, and appropriate standards of personal behaviour are always maintained

Employment legislation

There are many laws and regulations that govern the safe delivery of dental care, but the two main acts that relate to DCPs are:

- **The Dentists Act**
- **Health and Safety at Work Act**

The requirements laid down in the Dentists Act have been broadly covered previously, and the Health and Safety Act dictates that all DCPs are responsible for the safety of patients and work colleagues, as well as themselves, while at the work premises (see Unit 1). This means that all 'in-house' policies and protocols determined by the employer are important documents in their own rights that must be adhered to by all employees, as they are based on current legislation.

A **policy** in these terms then is a course of action that has been adopted by the workplace – so an infection control policy is the individualised manner that the workplace has developed to ensure that infection is controlled adequately on the premises. This may vary from workplace to workplace; a policy suitable for a hospital department for example, will not be suitable for a general practice, and vice versa.

When the policy has been agreed upon and put into writing as the course of action to be followed, it will be signed by all employees to show that they have given their agreement to follow its terms, and it then becomes a **protocol** – a draft of terms agreed and signed by all parties as a code of conduct, or procedure. Both protocols and policies would usually be introduced and dealt with during the induction training of all new employees, and updated as necessary. Failure to agree to the terms laid down, or to follow them correctly is likely to jeopardise their employment.

Other legislation that is pertinent to dental practice is covered in Unit 1, Unit 4 and Unit 7, and includes the following;

■ The Fire Precautions (Workplace) Regulations
■ The Health and Safety (First Aid) Regulations
■ Control of Substances Hazardous to Health (COSHH)
■ Reporting of Injuries, Diseases and Dangerous Occurrences Regulations (RIDDOR)
■ Environmental Protection Act (Controlled Waste Regulations)
■ Ionising Radiation Regulations (IRR99)
■ Ionising Radiation (Medical Exposure) Regulations (IRR(ME)2000)

Reflective practice

Career and future development decisions can only be made after a period of **reflection** has been undergone by the dental nurse, to determine the following:

■ Their own limitations and effectiveness in their current role
■ How to act upon any shortcomings or areas of development that are then identified

Dental practice, like any other workplace environment, changes with time. The obvious areas of change will be those that are covered by legislation, as some laws are updated and others become obsolete. The initial qualification of a dental nurse, and then the induction training received at the start of employment, is not static but is subject to constant change. This may happen when any of the following occur:

■ New legislation is passed
■ New treatment techniques are developed
■ New materials are developed

- A change in the patient base of the workplace occurs
- A change in employer occurs
- A change in work colleagues occurs, as some staff leave and new members are employed
- A change in working conditions occurs

Any of these events may open up new opportunities for learning new skills and information.

Formal learning

Now that compulsory registration of dental nurses has begun, registrants will have to carry out some form of update training on a regular basis, as a condition of their continued registration. This is referred to as **continuing professional development** (CPD), and has been compulsory for other GDC registrants for some time.

Any new learning is easier if it is made interesting and relevant to the learner, but without some guidance in place it would be human nature for DCPs to confine their CPD just to areas of particular interest to themselves. The GDC states that certain areas of update must be covered by all, and the CPD must be **verifiable** (that is, easily proved that it has been carried out) by the issuing of certificates at the end of the learning session.

The areas of update that are compulsory for dental nurses are called core subjects. These are:

- **Medical emergencies**
- **Disinfection and decontamination**
- **Radiography and radiological protection**

For those dental nurses dealing with patients on a regular basis, the following will also have to be covered:

- **Legal and ethical issues**
- **Complaints handling**

Learning in the workplace

On a less formal basis, learning can occur on a regular basis within the work environment by the dental nurse reflecting on their work performance – by constantly analysing, constructively criticising and evaluating themselves. The aim is to recognise their own shortcomings and act upon them to improve their overall work performance.

However, it is human nature to be subjective and tend towards being either overly critical or overly lenient when reflecting on your own performance, as your ideas are based on the perception you have of yourself. More constructive analysis is that carried out by others, especially more experienced colleagues who have gone through the process themselves previously. This is the basis for an **appraisal**

system within the workplace, where a senior colleague acts as a **mentor** for a more junior colleague, and gives verbal and written feedback on their performance (see later).

Mentoring can be carried out on a daily basis initially, with new employees being 'shadowed' by senior colleagues so that problems and shortfalls can be identified and addressed early in the learning process.

The two main types of reflection that occur are:

- **Reflection in action** – occurs as a situation happens
- **Reflection on action** – occurs after the event

Reflection on action is also referred to as hindsight.

Reflection enables the dental nurse to think about how learning occurs, especially from experience, so that their work performance becomes more effective. It should produce a thinking professional who can react effectively and appropriately to changing circumstances to produce a successful outcome for the patient and the dental team. It is the duty of the employer to ensure that changes in legislation are followed and referred to in updated policies, but it is the duty of the dental nurse to ensure that the updates are known of, understood, and adhered to. An example of reflection on action in the dental nurse context is given below.

Compare the competence of a dental nurse when nursing for a certain procedure for the first time compared to their competence when nursing for the same procedure for the fourth or fifth time. Obviously they will feel more comfortable as experience is gained, because subconsciously their own techniques are bettered after each event. In other words, 'practice makes perfect'.

So for instance, when aspirating for an oral surgery procedure, the first time the following may occur:

- Unsure of all the instrument identifications, as some may be being handled for the first time
- Aspiration is not fully effective, as there is uncertainty about when to intervene without blocking the operator's vision
- Hesitant when handling some instruments
- Concentrating so much on the procedure that the patient is forgotten

Whereas when aspirating for the fourth or fifth time:

- Instruments are now known because they are more familiar
- Aspiration is more effective, perhaps by learning from the first patient choking and the dentist being unable to see clearly
- Confident when handling instruments because they are more familiar
- Able to monitor and reassure the patient at the same time

Reflection on action occurs by being able to think back over the procedure at a later date. This allows realisation and identification of any problems encountered to occur, with the natural continuation of thought being to recognise how to improve next time. Most of us carry out this second type of reflection on a regular basis, for example when driving home from work and 'going over' the day's events in our minds, or by discussing our day with a family member, friend or colleague.

However, we often forget the full impact of our thoughts unless we write them down at the time, and review them at a later date. Therefore, it would be prudent for the dental nurse to keep a diary, or portfolio, on a daily or at least weekly basis. This helps to organise and clarify the thoughts, so that the reason why problems occurred can be discovered, and **action plans** can be developed to prevent their recurrence.

A suggested layout of a diary or portfolio could be:

- **Describe** the event
- **Record** your emotions and thoughts
- **Evaluate** the event – giving both good and bad points
- **Critically analyse** the event – why did it happen?
- Reach a **conclusion** – what could have been done differently?
- **Develop an action plan** – what will be done differently next time?

After going through this process, it is relatively easy to determine whether a gap in your knowledge has been identified.

It can be seen that the points suggested above follow those used when carrying out a **risk assessment** following an event, such as an injury occurring in the workplace or a chemical spillage. When a serious event happens, such as any covered by RIDDOR for example, the evaluation process is often referred to as a **significant event analysis**. The key aim of any analysis is to identify what went wrong, and how to prevent it reoccurring under similar circumstances in the future.

Self-evaluation and reflection can also be recorded in more detail in the form of a personal development plan (PDP). A PDP is used to effectively look at the following on a personal basis:

- Professionally, where am I now?
- What qualifications, knowledge and special interests helped me to achieve this position?
- What learning needs do I have, if any?
- Do I wish to acquire new knowledge or skills?
- What is preventing me? – Carry out a **SWOT analysis**
- What can be done to overcome any obstacles identified?
- Collate all the information to develop a personal learning/development plan, with achievable time scales if possible
- Evaluate the PDP at least annually, to determine whether the development needs that were identified have been met, and to what extent

- Summarise the progress made, and use it to determine the desired future learning and development needs
- Keep a written record of all CPD events for each year, both verifiable and non-verifiable (this is a GDC requirement)
- Analyse the events attended not only to ensure that the core subjects are covered, but also to determine the necessity and relevance of the others to your learning and development needs

A SWOT analysis is an excellent method of determining whether the obstacles to future learning and development are identified as being of a personal nature, or involve external pressures. It is used as shown in Figure 3.2.

Once the relevant points have been identified and recorded, efforts can be made to determine how to overcome the obstacles to future development. In some instances, this may be as dramatic as determining that an unsupportive employer is holding you back, and that a change of work environment is required.

Strengths
These are personal to the individual, and may include previous achievements as well as points such as reliability or ambition

Weaknesses
These are personal, and may include a personal lack of ambition, or home circumstances that make studying difficult

Opportunities
These are beneficial external factors which will influence success, and may include a supportive employer who encourages and funds further training

Threats
These are harmful external factors, or obstacles to future success, and may include an unsupportive employer, or lack of training opportunities

---

Figure 3.2 SWOT analysis.

Staff appraisals

Private reflection carried out using diaries, portfolios, or personal development plans can be distorted, however, because by definition they record our own perception of ourselves. Consequently, a system of staff appraisal is also used in the workplace, where the employer or a senior colleague reviews the performance of the staff member in the workplace, to achieve the following:

- Identifying the strengths and weaknesses of the staff member
- Identifying the strengths and weaknesses of the running of the workplace, to give valuable information for good workplace development
- Disclosing any barriers to the efficient working of the dental team

■ Improving communication in the dental team
■ Encouraging problem solving
■ Reducing any negative tensions between staff members
■ Improving practice morale

Several areas of appraisal can be carried out at one time during an annual review, or just one area can be highlighted. Common areas to consider are:

■ **Personal** – hygiene, attitude, punctuality, dress code
■ **Administrative** – policies and protocols, regulations, filing, knowledge of paperwork
■ **Clinical** – infection control, mixing techniques, nursing skills, patient management
■ **Team work** – ability to function as a team member, acceptance of authority, ability to take responsibility
■ **Communication** – inter-personal, telephone manner, patient management
■ **Development** – self-evaluation, self-study, attendance at courses, learning by experience

Once the relevant areas to be appraised have been selected, discussed and agreed upon, an appraisal sheet can be drawn up which gives the dental nurse the opportunity to self-evaluate their performance in these areas, before being compared with the workplace evaluation (Figure 3.3).

Differences can be explored and resolved, and then an action plan can be developed to determine future goals and aims. All details should be recorded on the appraisal sheet and then copied so that both the nurse and the practice can refer back to it to assess the level of success of that appraisal. The sheet should also serve as a record of the dental nurse's self-development and progression within the practice, and expose any areas which continue to cause problems in future appraisals.

The areas can be adjusted to suit individual practices as necessary. The frequency of appraisal will also differ between practices as well as for different staff members. Younger, less experienced staff members are likely to require more frequent appraisal while learning all the relevant practice policies and protocols, and how to put them into practice. More experienced staff will need to be supportive and non-judgemental during this period.

When run correctly, appraisals can be an invaluable tool for the development of the whole dental team, so that the end result is the best possible outcome for the patient. They should identify the strengths and weaknesses not only of the staff members, but also of the workplace environment itself, indicating routes that can be taken for good workplace development. By relying on feedback and constructive criticism, they should remove any inter-staff communication barriers and improve problem-solving techniques. Overall, appraisals should improve the workforce morale by providing an opportunity for discussion by all, without recrimination.

Areas of appraisal	Self-appraisal	Practice appraisal	Notes
Personal hygiene Dress Punctuality			
NHS procedures Rules/regulations Medico-legal knowledge			
Materials techniques Infection control Patient management X-ray procedures Equipment handling			
Courses of study Self-study Experiential learning Problem-based learning Peer group learning			
Teamwork experience Innovation Originality			
Communication skills Interpersonal skills Administrative accuracy Telephone manner Complaints handling			
APPRAISAL SUMMARY			
Signed......................	Signed......................	Date......................	

Figure 3.3 Example appraisal sheet.

Non-verifiable CPD

Verifiable CPD has already been discussed, but that termed non-verifiable is also of great value in the development of the dental nurse. Both types of CPD could include any of the following, and the greater variety will provide the better learning and development opportunities:

- Reading relevant articles in work-related journals
- Reading new textbooks
- Exploring relevant websites on the internet
- Diversifying your skill base by training in new areas of dental nursing
- Taking post-certificate qualifications
- Attending seminars, conferences and other work-related events
- Attending training events in other than the CPD core subjects
- Taking an active part in workplace events such as staff meetings, running of quality assurance systems, risk assessment analyses, etc.

The types of knowledge gained from these sources will fall into one of the three broad categories recognised by the profession, and a suitable combination of the three is essential to good dental nursing skills:

- **Scientific knowledge** – models and theories that can be scientifically tested against data gathered, and is therefore verifiable – it can be written down and learned by others
- **Experiential knowledge** – that gained over time by intuition and repetitive practice, including reflection and self-evaluation
- **Ethical knowledge** – that considered to be morally correct, although it is based on beliefs and values rather than facts

With reference to ethical knowledge, a good dental nurse will always follow the principles of 'best practice', irrespective of their own personal values and beliefs. This must always include the following points:

- Promote equality, diversity and anti-discriminatory practice at all times
- Respect the patients' rights at all times
- Promote, develop and maintain effective working relationships with other team members
- Never stray outside the legal limits of their qualifications
- Take an active part in continuing professional development
- Ensure that all changes to effective dental nursing are known and acted upon, so that the concept of 'best practice' is always attained

4 Unit 3: Provide Basic Life Support (CHS36)

Knowledge specifications

Basic medical knowledge

K1 – A working understanding of the anatomy of the respiratory system

K2 – A factual awareness of the priorities in life support

K3 – A factual awareness of the time frame within which assessment of individual needs should be carried out and the life support response initiated in order to maximise an individual's chance of survival

K4 – A factual awareness of the information which may need to be recorded following the application of basic life support

Basic airway management and respiration

K5 – A working understanding of clinical signs of airway obstruction

K6 – A working understanding of what to do in the event of foreign body obstruction of an individual's airway

K7 – A working understanding of the differences in techniques needed for ensuring an open airway on different types of individual

K8 – A factual awareness of the factors to be taken into account in determining the technique that will lead to the best possible outcome for the individual

K9 – A working understanding of why the head tilt techniques should not be used where neck or spinal injury is suspected

K10 – A working understanding of the different techniques used to ventilate an individual and when each should be used

K11 – A factual awareness of the ventilation ratio and rate for different types of individual and conditions

K12 – A working understanding of the importance to outcome of the positioning of the individual and the person applying basic life support, including the specific positioning needs of pregnant women in the third trimester

K13 – A working understanding of the observations to be carried out to identify adequate oxygenation in different types of individual

Applying external chest compressions

K14 – A factual awareness of the rate and depth of compressions needed for different types of individual
K15 – A factual awareness of the compression: ventilation ratio in different types of individual
K16 – A working understanding of the procedure to establish the correct hand/finger placement for applying external chest compression
K17 – A factual awareness of the differences between certification and diagnosis of death in accordance with best practice, and who is authorised to carry out these activities
K18 – A working understanding of personal safety as well as general health and safety, and the range of situations and responses
K19 – A working understanding of why a firm base is needed for chest compressions, and what action to take when one is not available
K20 – A working understanding of the different methods of chest thrusts and back slaps to use in the cases of children/young people and adults
K21 – A factual awareness of the compression: ventilation ratio in one and two person basic life support

Legislation, policy and good practice

K22 – A working understanding of the legislation regarding confidentiality and information sharing, the provision of services, the rights of the individual, protection issues, anti-discriminatory practice, informed consent, relevant mental health legislation and care programme approach
K23 – A working understanding of how to interpret and apply legislation to the work being undertaken
K24 – A working understanding of the ethics concerning consent and confidentiality, and the tensions which may exist between an individual's rights and the organisation's responsibility to individuals
K25 – A working understanding of the importance of gaining assent from individuals who lack capacity to consent

Basic biology

The basic unit of living organisms is the cell. Many cells specialise to perform certain roles within the body, and when these specialised cells group together they are called tissues. Groups of tissues performing different functions are organs, while those with related functions are systems.

There are four basic types of cell:

- **Muscle cell** – these generate forces and produce motion, they may be attached to bones to allow limb movement, or enclose hollow cavities so that their forces cause expulsion of the cavity contents (as in the digestive tract)
- **Nerve cell** – these can initiate and carry electrical impulses to distant areas of the body along their length (as in the brain and spinal cord)
- **Epithelial cell** – found on the surface of the body or organs, or lining hollow structures within, and act to compartmentalise areas of the body to prevent uncontrolled movements of micro-organisms throughout the whole (as in skin and mucous membranes)
- **Connective tissue cell** – these connect various parts of the body together by anchorage and support (as in the bony skeleton and ligaments)

The interaction of all the body systems to maintain life allows the continual production of energy by food digestion.

The energy is then used to:

- Maintain body temperature above that of the surroundings
- Produce movement to allow hunting for food, and the production of more energy
- Allow reproduction to occur, for the survival of the species

The human body has ten organ systems, each with various components and specific functions to allow the continuation of life.

(1) **Circulatory system**:

- composed of heart, blood vessels, blood
- functions to allow rapid bulk flow of blood around body tissues

(2) **Respiratory system**:

- composed of nose, throat, larynx, trachea, lungs
- functions to exchange oxygen and carbon dioxide

(3) **Digestive system**:

- composed of mouth, pharynx, oesophagus, stomach, intestines, pancreas, salivary glands, liver, gall bladder
- functions to digest, process and absorb nutrients, and excrete waste products

(4) **Urinary system**:

- composed of kidneys, ureter, bladder, urethra
- functions to regulate plasma, and excrete waste products

(5)   **Musculo-skeletal system**:

- composed of cartilage, bone, ligaments, tendons, joints, skeletal muscle
- functions to support and protect internal organs, and allow movement

(6)   **Immune system**:

- composed of white blood cells, lymph, spleen, bone marrow, thymus gland
- functions to defend against infection, and produce red and white blood cells

(7)   **Nervous system**:

- composed of brain, spinal cord, nerves, sensory organs
- functions to give consciousness, and regulate and co-ordinate body activities

(8)   **Endocrine system**:

- composed of all glands secreting hormones
- functions to regulate and co-ordinate body workings

(9)   **Reproductive system**:

- composed of male/female sex organs
- functions to allow reproduction and continuation of the species

(10)   **Integumentary system**:

- composed of skin
- functions to protect against injury and dehydration, and maintain temperature

To understand and be able to carry out successful basic life support (BLS), a background knowledge of both the circulatory and respiratory systems and the way they function together is required.

Circulatory system

The main component of this system is the heart, which is a muscular pumping organ situated in the thorax (chest cavity). The heart is connected by blood vessels to every tissue in the body, and acts to pump **oxygenated blood** from the lungs to the body tissue cells, and to collect **deoxygenated blood** from the body and transport it to the lungs for excretion.

The heart has four chambers, the upper ones are the atria and the lower ones are the ventricles, and the two chambers on either side of the heart (left and right) are separated by valves (Figure 4.1). The left and right sides of the heart have no connection between them as the right side holds only deoxygenated blood, and the left side holds only oxygenated blood.

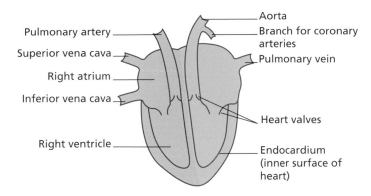

Figure 4.1 The heart. Source: *Levison's Textbook for Dental Nurses*, 10th edn, C. Hollins, 2008, Wiley-Blackwell.

Blood enters the two atria from large veins, the right side as deoxygenated blood from the body through the vena cava, and the left side as oxygenated blood from the lungs through the pulmonary vein (this is the only vein that carries oxygenated blood). As the heart beats, the blood is pumped from the atria into the ventricles and then from the ventricles out of the heart.

The right ventricle pumps the deoxygenated blood to the lungs through the pulmonary artery (this is the only artery to carry deoxygenated blood), and the left ventricle pumps oxygenated blood to the rest of the body through the aorta. The first arteries that branch off the aorta are the four coronary arteries, which supply the heart muscle itself.

After each heart beat, the blood is stopped from flowing backwards again by the valves within the heart which allow blood flow in one direction only, and once the blood has passed through the valves the pressure closes the flaps of the valve and prevents backflow.

The heart beat itself starts on the top surface of the right atrium in a group of specialised muscle cells called the 'pace-maker'. These cells receive stimulation from two sets of nerves from the brain, one set speeds up the rate of the heart beat and the other set slows it down. In this way the heart rate is regulated to allow both exercise and rest as necessary.

The whole circulatory system is connected together throughout the body, with oxygenated blood flowing from the left heart into large arteries, which become smaller arteries called arterioles and then into microscopic blood vessels only one cell thick, called capillaries. It is in the capillaries where the oxygen is released into the surrounding organs and tissues, and carbon dioxide is collected from them. This is called **internal respiration**. The blood has then become deoxygenated and it passes out of the capillaries into tiny veins called venules, which connect with the larger veins and take the deoxygenated blood back to the right side of the heart. This is the systemic circulatory system.

Once the deoxygenated blood arrives in the right side of the heart it is pumped to the lungs through the pulmonary artery to be reoxygenated, before passing back

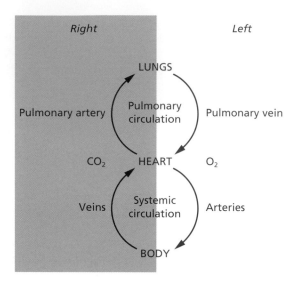

Figure 4.2 Circulation (deoxygenated blood shaded blue). Source: *Levison's Textbook for Dental Nurses*, 10th edn, C. Hollins, 2008, Wiley-Blackwell.

to the left side of the heart in the pulmonary vein ready to be pumped back around the body. This is the pulmonary circulatory system (Figure 4.2).

The pumping action of the heart produces pressure which drives the blood around both circulatory systems. The force is greatest in the large arteries close to the heart and gradually diminishes through the capillaries and veins. When a patient has their blood pressure measured, a reading is made of the blood pressure in the arteries when the heart contracts, and also when the heart relaxes. The average blood pressure of an adult at rest is therefore recorded as 120/80 mmHg (millimetres of mercury).

The arteries are elastic so that they can expand as a surge of blood passes through them following each heart beat, and then relax to their usual size again. Where the arteries lie over bone, this surge of blood can be felt as the pulse. In contrast, the veins are thinner walled and less elastic so that blood could flow in either direction if they did not contain one-way valves, like the heart.

The three basic blood cells are:

- **Erythrocytes** – red blood cells, which carry oxygen around the body
- **Leucocytes** – white blood cells, which defend against infection
- **Platelets** – which are portions of larger cells called thrombocytes, and help to prevent blood loss by forming clots at wound sites

Respiratory system

The main components are the lungs, which are situated in the thorax, the two main bronchi connecting them to the windpipe (trachea), which then connects them

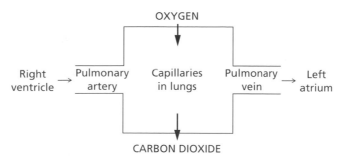

Figure 4.3 External respiration. Source: *Levison's Textbook for Dental Nurses*, 10th edn, C. Hollins, 2008, Wiley-Blackwell.

to the outside atmosphere. By the action of breathing in and out (inspiring and expiring), air, containing oxygen, is drawn into the lungs and is transferred into the circulatory system. At the same time, carbon dioxide passes out of the blood plasma into the lungs and is then expired. This is the waste product produced by the body tissues as they function to maintain life (Figure 4.3).

The exchange of oxygen and carbon dioxide occurs in the microscopic pouch-like end sacs of the lung tissue, called **alveoli**. These are just one-cell thick and allow the passage of oxygen from the lungs into the capillaries, and carbon dioxide from the capillaries into the lungs. This process is called **external respiration**.

The lining of the respiratory system before entering the lungs is covered in specialised cells that secrete mucus and have tiny hair-like projections called **cilia**. The sticky mucus helps to trap dust particles and bacteria before they reach and block the alveoli, and the cilia gently flick the trapped particles back towards the throat, so that they can be swallowed or coughed out.

The movement of air in and out of the lungs is caused by the movement of the ribs and a muscular sheet, which seals the bottom of the rib cage from the abdomen, called the diaphragm. On inhaling (breathing in) the ribs lift up and the diaphragm pulls down, and these two actions expand the size of the rib cage so that air is pulled into the lungs through the nose and mouth. External respiration occurs within the alveoli, then as the diaphragm and ribs relax the expired air is forced out of the lungs and into the atmosphere. This process of ventilation occurs approximately 16 times a minute in an adult at rest, exchanging about a half litre of air at each breath. The rate and depth of breathing increases dramatically during exercise.

Background medical knowledge

The aim of BLS is to maintain a flow of oxygenated blood to the individual until one of the following happens:

- They recover and begin to circulate oxygenated blood by breathing unassisted
- Their life support is handed over to specialists, usually paramedics

- The rescuer is too physically exhausted to continue
- Their death is confirmed by an authorised practitioner, such as a doctor at the scene

Oxygen is the atmospheric gas that is vital for life. It is breathed into the respiratory system through the nose and mouth, and then passes down the trachea to the two bronchi which enter the right or left lung. In the lungs the oxygen passes out into the circulatory system during external respiration, and is transported around the body in the arterial blood stream by the continual pumping action of the heart. Where required, the oxygen passes out of the blood vessel and into the body tissues during internal respiration, where it is used to provide energy for the cells to work.

The actions of the respiratory system in taking up oxygen from the atmosphere and absorbing it into the blood, and the circulatory system in transporting that oxygen around the body to the cells, are carefully controlled by the brain. If any one of these three vital organs fails, the other two will also fail shortly after.

Without oxygen, the cells and therefore the body, cannot function and death will occur. After only three to four minutes without oxygen, the brain cells can suffer irreversible damage, which if not fatal, will lead to some degree of permanent brain damage. The quicker the need for BLS is established and begun, the better the chances of survival for the individual – and ideally this should be within seconds of their own life support system failing.

So, the fundamental aims of BLS are to maintain the life of the individual (the casualty) by achieving the following:

- Providing oxygen to the lungs – by some form of **rescue breathing**
- Circulating the oxygen to the body tissues – by **external chest compressions** to mimic the pumping action of the heart

The death of an individual occurs when there is a permanent cessation of the function of the heart and lungs, and these are the criteria by which a medical doctor will diagnose and certify death. Other specialists, such as paramedics, are able to diagnose and determine that death has occurred by the absence of the following:

- Spontaneous breathing
- Heartbeat
- Pupillary response to light (pupils of the eyes remain dilated when exposed to light)

The lack of response to light by the pupils indicates brain death. However, only a medical doctor can certify that death has occurred and issue a Death Certificate, so all rescue attempts must continue until this has been established, or until any rescuers are too physically exhausted to continue in their efforts to resuscitate the individual.

If there is more than one rescuer able to provide BLS, it is important that the compression and ventilation role is regularly swapped between them, as chest compressions are physically tiring to perform and the rescuer will soon become exhausted.

Current BLS guidelines

In the UK, the general guidelines to be used for BLS are issued by the Resuscitation Council (UK) and should be followed nationally. Local protocol amendments may exist in some areas or in some workplaces (especially hospitals), and readers should ensure that they are aware of these. However, the current Resuscitation Council advice is that rescuers need to apply 30 chest compressions for each two rescue breaths given, no matter how many rescuers are present. This gives the current compression: ventilation algorithm of 30:2.

The two important signs that should be looked for when determining the need to provide BLS to an individual are:

- Unconsciousness
- Abnormal or absent breathing

Unconsciousness indicates that an individual is unresponsive to all stimuli, and that their heart may have stopped beating – they have gone into cardiac arrest. There is no instance where the heart can have stopped beating and a person remain conscious, as the body cells (especially the brain) will become starved of oxygen very quickly and will be unable to function.

Abnormal breathing, such as infrequent noisy gasps, indicates that there is a possible obstruction in the individual's respiratory system which is making normal breathing difficult. This will gradually reduce the oxygen supply to the body cells, and once breathing ceases completely the oxygen supply is cut off immediately. The individual's skin colour will change from pink, through pale to blue or grey as their body tissues become starved of oxygen.

This is more difficult to determine in those with darker skin tones, so the lips, nail beds and mucous membranes of the mouth may also be checked for signs indicating lack of oxygenation, or **hypoxia**.

The actions that may be required to help the casualty cannot be determined until the rescuer has fully assessed the situation, and although swift action is necessary to avoid brain damage or death, the following questions must be quickly considered:

- **Why has the individual become unconscious?** Are there any external causes such as trauma, electrocution, poisonous fumes, drowning?
- **How is unconsciousness established?** Are they alert or moving, are they responsive to noise or voices, are they responsive to pain, are they completely unresponsive?
- **Is their breathing abnormal?** Are they gasping, coughing or even clutching at their throat?

■ **Are there any breath sounds?** How is this established?
■ **What does the rescuer do next?** At what point should help be summoned, and what actions are required immediately?

The accepted order to follow when assessing an emergency situation and determining whether BLS is required can be summarised and easily remembered by the following code:

■ D for **Danger**
■ R for **Response**
■ S for **Shout for help**
■ A for **Airway**
■ B for **Breathing**
■ C for **Circulation**

This is best remembered as DRSABC (referred to as 'doctors – a – b – c').

Valuable time can be wasted during this assessment by attempting to open or remove clothing from the individual while trying to establish their condition, and should not be carried out by the rescuer. They may actually sustain further injury while clothing is being removed. In addition, many individuals would become very distressed at finding themselves partially clad and surrounded by strangers. The dignity and rights of decency and to privacy of the individual must be maintained at all times, by all rescuers.

DRSABC in detail

Danger

Check the immediate area for possible dangers, such as electric wires running through pooled water, punctured gas canisters, spilt chemicals giving off strong fumes, etc. If hazardous chemicals are suspected of being involved in the emergency situation, the workplace COSHH file (see Chapter 2) must be consulted at some point for information on first-aid actions that may be necessary. This action is best delegated to a spare rescuer, while BLS is being carried out by others.

If possible, any dangers should be made safe by the rescuer before approaching the individual, but not at the risk of endangering themselves in the process. Ideally, this should not involve moving the individual except in extreme circumstances, such as rising water levels that may cause drowning. This is to prevent any further injury being caused.

Response

The level of responsiveness will determine whether the individual is unconscious or not. Call loudly to them, asking if they can hear you or if they are alright, while gently shaking them. Their responsiveness can quickly be assessed and determined by a system referred to as the AVPU code:

- **Alert** – the casualty is fully conscious and able to communicate fully and spontaneously
- **Verbal** – the casualty is not fully conscious, but is able to respond to verbal commands and prompts
- **Painful** – the casualty is semi-conscious at best, but able to respond to painful stimuli such as a gentle pinch
- **Unresponsive** – the casualty shows no response to verbal prompts nor painful stimuli, they are unconscious and unable to be roused

If the individual shows no response whatsoever, then they are in need of help urgently.

Wherever possible, the level of responsiveness should be determined without moving the individual from the position in which they were found, to avoid any further injury.

Shout for help

If the individual is unresponsive and therefore unconscious, the rescuer will need help with any attempt at BLS if it is required, as well as to summon specialist help if necessary. If only one rescuer remains to aid the individual while help is being sought, they may need to continue BLS for a prolonged period of time, and ultimately this may result in their physical exhaustion. If attempts at BLS have to then be abandoned before specialist help arrives, the casualty is likely to die.

Shout very loudly to alert anyone else in the vicinity that an emergency situation has arisen. In the workplace, there may be internal communication systems in place for just such an event, such as intercoms, alarm bells or coded calls, and these must be known of and used appropriately by the rescuer.

Airway

The airway needs to be checked for any obstruction, such as vomit or debris or the tongue itself, which may have fallen back and blocked it. Any loose obstruction should be removed by rolling the casualty's head to the side to encourage it to drop out of the mouth. In the dental surgery there will also be electrically operated suction equipment available at the chairside, or a manually operated suction device within the emergency kit that all dental workplaces have to have on the premises (Figure 4.4). However, these must only be used by those rescuers who have been trained to do so, as they can push debris further down the airway or cause soft tissue injury if not used correctly.

The casualty's airway can then be opened to allow breathing to occur. This can be achieved by tilting the head back by placing the palm of one hand on the individual's forehead and lifting the chin with the fingers of the other hand at the same time (Figure 4.5). However, this technique must never be used when an individual has a suspected neck or spinal injury, as to do so would almost certainly cause further damage to the spinal cord. This could result in permanent paralysis of the individual. In such cases the airway can be opened by thrusting the lower jaw forward with both hands, without any head tilting occurring (Figure 4.6). This should avoid any further neck or spinal injury.

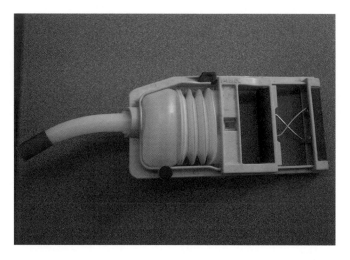

Figure 4.4 Portable suction unit.

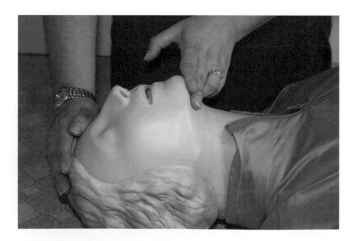

Figure 4.5 Head tilt to open airway.

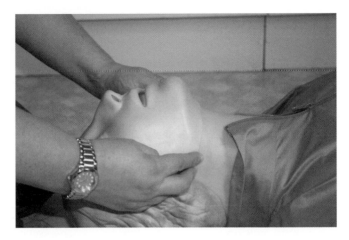

Figure 4.6 Jaw thrust to open airway.

Breathing

With the airway open, breathing is assessed quickly over a ten-second period (Figure 4.7). The rescuer needs to determine if any spontaneous breathing attempts are being made, and their quality, by checking for the following:

- **Look** to see if the chest is rising and falling
- **Listen** to any breathing sounds
- Are they regular or infrequent?
- Are they quiet or noisy?
- Are they normal or gasping in nature?
- **Feel** for air flow by placing the cheek close to the individual's mouth

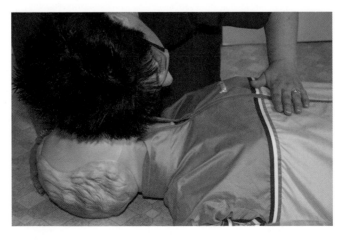

Figure 4.7 Look, listen, feel for breathing.

If breathing is absent or abnormal, the emergency services must be called as specialist help is required. Ideally a second person can be sent to do this, but if necessary the lone rescuer must leave the individual to call for emergency help.

If it is now decided that BLS is required to maintain the casualty's life until specialist help arrives, they may require moving to a position where this can be carried out effectively. This is usually achieved by very carefully rolling the individual onto their back with a firm surface beneath them, in a safe area and with enough room to manoeuvre as necessary, as BLS may need to be carried out correctly for a prolonged period until specialist help arrives.

Circulation

Any residual oxygenated blood within the casualty now needs to be quickly pumped around their body to the brain, and this is achieved by the rescuer carrying out chest compressions on the individual. These will only be effective if the heart is adequately compressed between the breastbone (sternum) and the spine, on a firm surface, and at a sufficient rate to actually cause the blood to flow through the circulatory system as required, rather than just swishing backwards and forwards.

If any spinal or neck injuries are suspected, it would be ideal not to move the casualty from the position in which they were found, to avoid further injury. However, this may not always be possible, especially if their position prevents successful BLS from being carried out. Ideally, several helpers should be used to very carefully roll the casualty onto their back on a hard surface, keeping their head in line with their spine at all times.

In the dental surgery, dental chairs are designed to be firm enough to carry out chest compressions without having to move the individual onto the floor. The correct point to apply the compressions is quickly located by:

(1) Kneeling at the side of the individual, or standing if they are still on the dental chair
(2) Run a finger along the lower border of the individual's ribcage, towards the midline
(3) Once in the midline the breastbone will be felt with the finger
(4) Place the heel of the other hand adjacent to the finger, towards the head of the individual
(5) Interlock the fingers of both hands over this compression point (Figure 4.8)
(6) Lean over the individual, keeping the arms straight and the elbows locked (Figure 4.9)

Thirty compressions can now be given at a rate of 100 per minute, by compressing the chest by 4–5 cm and then releasing to allow the heart to expand and refill with blood. Once the initial 30 compressions have been administered, two rescue breaths can be given by the lone rescuer, or ideally by a second rescuer.

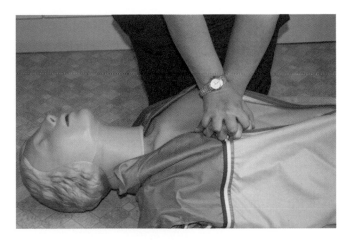

Figure 4.8 Hand lock for chest compressions.

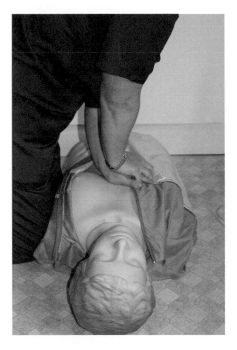

Figure 4.9 Arm lock for chest compressions.

Rescue breathing

Once the first 30 compressions have been administered, any residual oxygen in the blood will have been used up by the body tissues, and especially the brain. To maintain life, the oxygen now has to be regularly replaced before being distributed around the body again by the chest compressions, and this is achieved by artificial ventilation or rescue breathing.

The atmosphere contains 21% oxygen, but that expired (breathed out) only contains 16%, as our body tissues use up the 5% difference to produce energy for the cells to work. In an emergency situation, rescue breaths are usually given by breathing expired air into the individual in a mouth-to-mouth technique. If the individual has facial injuries affecting the mouth, it may be necessary to use a mouth-to-nose technique instead, and with small children or babies the rescuer will breathe into the individual's mouth and nose together.

The use of emergency oxygen supplies held by all dental practices will increase the amount of available oxygen for rescue breathing when given using masks, but the technique can only be successfully used by those trained to do so (Figure 4.10).

The airway will already have been cleared of obstructions during the DRSABC procedure, but will need to be held open now to administer rescue breaths, again using the head tilt – chin lift or jaw thrust technique. Two rescue breaths are then given as follows:

(1) Maintain the head tilt to keep the airway open
(2) Pinch the nostrils closed with the fingers of the hand being used to press onto the forehead
(3) Support the chin with the other hand while holding the mouth open
(4) Take a deep breath, then seal the mouth over that of the individual to ensure no air escapes (Figure 4.11)
(5) Breathe with normal force into their open mouth for about two seconds, watching from the corner of the eye to ensure that the chest rises
(6) With the airway still held open, move away from their mouth and watch the chest fall as the air comes out
(7) Repeat the rescue breath

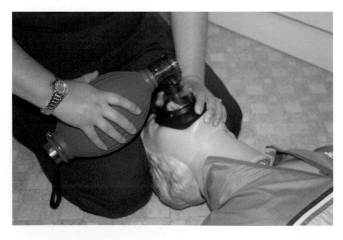

Figure 4.10 Use of the Ambu bag.

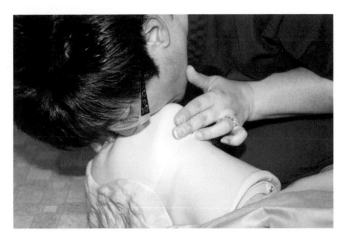

Figure 4.11 Rescue breathing.

(8)   If given successfully, follow with another 30 chest compressions as a BLS cycle

Sometimes problems will be experienced while attempting rescue breathing, the commonest one being that the chest does not rise. In the absence of an obstruction this is usually due to the airway not being fully opened, and the head tilt procedure should be repeated until successful. Otherwise, ensure that the nostrils are fully closed and that a good mouth-to-mouth seal is being achieved. If the abdomen is seen to rise while the breath is being given, air is being blown into the stomach by being too forceful or too prolonged. The rescue breath should stop once the chest stops rising, usually after just two seconds at a normal breath force.

BLS modifications

The BLS protocols described are to be used for adults and children over the age of 8 years. Babies and young children require less force to be used while carrying out both chest compressions and rescue breathing, to avoid injuring their bodies.

The weight of the fetus in a pregnant woman will also hinder BLS attempts if she is lying on her back, and the usual technique has to be modified for these casualties.

Babies and young children

Anatomically these age groups are different from adults in the following ways:

- They have narrower air passages in the respiratory system
- These air passages are more prone to blockages
- The trachea is more flexible, and so it is easily blocked if airway opening attempts are too severe

■ They have a relatively larger tongue than an adult, which is more likely to
   obstruct the airway when the baby or young child is unconscious

Cardiac arrest in these younger individuals is rarely due to heart problems, as in
an adult, but is far more likely to be caused by lack of oxygen to the brain due to
airway obstruction.

As the DRSABC code is being followed, it will soon become apparent if the
young casualty is unresponsive and having breathing difficulties or not breathing
at all, and it is imperative that rescue breathing is commenced **before** starting chest
compressions. This is because the likely cause of their collapse will be a shortage of
oxygen to their vital organs, and any reserves will have been quickly used up by
their young bodies and must be replenished as soon as possible.

So the full modified BLS sequence of events in cases involving a baby or a young
child is as follows:

■ **Danger** – check for dangers as usual
■ **Response** – less reliable in younger individuals, so merely determine whether
   they are unresponsive only
■ **Shout** – summon help from anyone in the vicinity, without leaving the individual
■ **Airway** – check the airway for obstruction, especially the tongue, then carefully open the airway, taking care not to overextend the head tilt and so block
   the trachea
■ **Breathing** – look, listen and feel for signs of spontaneous breathing for ten
   seconds, and if they are absent **give five rescue breaths using the mouth-to-
   mouth and nose technique**
■ **Circulation** – give 30 chest compressions, using two fingers for a baby or one
   hand for a young child, aiming to compress the chest by a third of its depth at a
   rate of 100 per minute
■ The lone rescuer must continue BLS for a full minute before going for specialist
   help

Pregnant women

Any pre-menopausal woman who collapses and requires BLS could potentially be
pregnant. In some cases it will be known or obvious that they are so, but otherwise
it should always be considered a possibility, especially if BLS attempts are failing
for no other obvious reason.

In a heavily pregnant woman lying on her back, the uterus (womb) tends to lie
over the major blood vessels (the inferior vena cava) that return blood from the
lower body to the right side of the heart. If this individual collapses and requires
BLS, the rescuer has the added difficulty of forcing blood through these con-
strained blood vessels during chest compressions, and the rescue attempt is likely
to fail.

Instead, the individual should be laid slightly on the left side with some form of
support under the right buttock so that these major blood vessels are not squashed

by the uterus. BLS can then be carried out in the normal way, while maintaining this angled position of the individual throughout.

Monitoring and evaluating BLS

Once the DRSABC code has been gone through correctly, the need for BLS established, and rescue attempts are under way, the situation and condition of the casualty must be carefully monitored by the rescuer, to determine if rescue efforts should continue or be stopped.

There are four instances where BLS attempts should be stopped:

- The individual recovers and is able to circulate oxygenated blood and breathe without assistance
- Their life support is handed over to specialists (paramedics)
- The rescuer is too physically exhausted to continue BLS
- The death of the individual is confirmed by an authorised practitioner (a doctor at the scene)

Recovery

It is unlikely that spontaneous recovery will occur, as once the heart has stopped beating it usually requires the specialist techniques of either drug administration or defibrillation to start functioning again. The purpose of BLS is to maintain an oxygenated blood flow to the brain to prevent death until specialist help arrives.

However in the rare event that the individual does regain airway and circulation control, the rescuer must be able to recognise their improved condition and act accordingly until specialist help arrives. In other emergency situations, the individual may have stopped breathing but still have a circulation, in which case chest compressions should not be attempted.

It is not advisable for the rescuer to waste valuable time attempting to find a pulse to determine if circulation has been re-established; it can be notoriously difficult to do so and should be left to specialists to determine. Indeed, a casualty can die through lack of BLS provision if a rescuer mistakenly identifies a non-existent pulse.

Other more obvious signs that indicate a functioning circulatory system are:

- Movement of the individual
- Coughing or signs of attempts to breathe
- Change in skin and lip colour, from grey or blue to pink, although this will be more difficult to determine in a casualty with darker skin tone

Once signs of a functioning circulation are recognised, the rescuer must continue giving rescue breaths until either the individual begins breathing again themselves, or specialist help arrives. The continuation of the circulation should be checked for after every ten rescue breaths.

Recovery position

If all airway obstructions have been cleared, the airway sufficiently opened, and rescue breathing carried out effectively by the rescuer, the individual may begin spontaneously breathing again. Once breathing has begun, or if an individual has been found unconscious but still breathing, their airway has to be maintained by the rescuer until specialist help arrives. If left lying on their back, the tongue may well fall back towards their throat and close off the airway, causing an obstruction to the oxygen flow in the respiratory system and precipitating a more serious emergency – an event that lay persons often refer to as 'swallowing the tongue'. To ensure that this does not happen, the rescuer must place the individual into the **recovery position** so that their tongue and any fluids (vomit or blood) can drain out of the mouth rather than obstructing the airway (Figure 4.12).

The recovery position involves rolling the individual onto their side and bending their limbs so that they are supported in that position, with the airway open and unobstructed. This can only be fully performed when the individual has no potential injuries to their spine or limbs, otherwise a modified position must be achieved.

For an individual lying on their back and breathing, with no injuries, the recovery position is achieved as follows:

(1)   Kneel at one side of the individual
(2)   Straighten out their arms and legs
(3)   Move their nearest arm out at a right angle and bend up at the elbow
(4)   Gently pull their other arm and furthest leg towards you, so that the individual begins to roll towards you
(5)   Place the furthest hand against the side of their face
(6)   Continue to roll them towards you by pulling the furthest leg, until their knee touches the ground

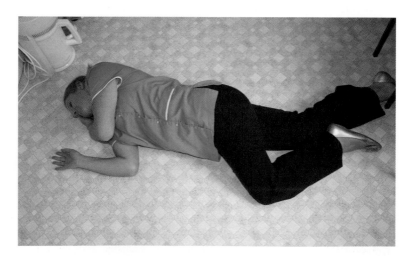

Figure 4.12 Recovery position.

(7)   Keep their hand against the face so that their head rolls onto it
(8)   Once the roll is completed, ensure the airway is open by tilting the head back as necessary
(9)   Adjust the bent leg to stabilise the recovery position

The technique is the same for all age groups except babies.

A baby will be unstable if placed in the conventional recovery position, and it is much easier to place them in a safe position while holding them. If breathing but unconscious, the baby should be picked up and held on their side, towards the rescuer, with one hand under the baby's head and the other under their side and bottom. They should be tilted down slightly so that the head is lower than their body, allowing the tongue and any fluids to fall forwards away from the airway.

Modified recovery position

If a spinal injury is suspected, such as if the individual has fallen onto their back from a height, performing the full recovery position manoeuvre may well cause permanent spinal injury and should not be attempted.

Ideally, the individual should be left in the position in which they were found until specialist help arrives, but this may not be advisable if there is a possibility that their airway could become obstructed. In this situation, the individual must be rolled onto their side and supported in that position using anything available, such as rolled up coats, or other rescuers. While rolling them, their head and spine must be kept in alignment at all times, so the manoeuvre can only be carried out when more than one rescuer is present. Similarly, if any limb injuries are suspected the individual must be rolled without pulling on their limbs, and supported by coats, etc. rather than by bending the limbs to achieve stability.

The most important point is that the airway is opened and remains unobstructed, so that life is preserved. The rescuer will need to monitor the breathing and ensure that it continues to be unobstructed until specialist help arrives.

Handing over to specialists

The likely first responders to an emergency call will be paramedics, complete with specialised equipment and drugs to take over the advanced life support of the individual. However, they will require an accurate report of the emergency from all rescuers present to determine how best to proceed. Specifically, the following points will require verification:

■   **What happened?** Did anyone witness the actual emergency event (trip and fall, road traffic accident, convulsion, heart attack, choking, etc.)
■   **What time?** How long ago did the event occur, and how quickly were rescuers on the scene
■   **Condition?** Was AVPU gone through by the rescuers, and if so what was the individual's initial level of responsiveness

- **BLS** – was BLS required, how long was it carried out for, were there any problems in maintaining life before the specialists arrived?
- **Background knowledge** – are any relatives or friends present with further information on the individual (including their name), are any Medic Alert identifiers present?
- **Personal items** – hand over all of the individual's personal items to the specialists, they will be able to check identity and medical status, and this is especially important in discovering if any medications are taken, such as an asthma inhaler
- **Remain at the scene** – do not leave until the specialists are happy that they have all the information they require, including your personal and contact details in case the individual dies, as a statement to the police may be required

After the emergency

If the emergency occurred in the workplace, it is highly likely that all other workplace activities will have been postponed. However, the area will be littered with various used items and equipment that may well have been abandoned while all minds focused on the rescue attempt.

The area must be cleaned and closed down in accordance with the local infection control policy, paying particular attention to the following:

- Wear full personal protective equipment
- All sharps should be carefully discarded in the usual sharps container
- All blood spillages should be covered with sodium hypochlorite (bleach) before being cleaned up
- All non-sharp items contaminated with body fluids should be disposed of in the hazardous waste sack
- All dental equipment should be wiped down and switched off as usual
- All dental instruments should be disposed of, or debrided and autoclaved in the usual manner
- Any opened and unused dental materials should be disposed of in the hazardous waste sack
- All work surfaces should be wiped down once cleared, with the usual disinfectant
- All records should be collated and filed in the usual place, those of the emergency individual having been written up in full beforehand

Choking

Choking in adults

One particular emergency that can occur in the dental practice setting is choking of an individual. It has particular relevance during dental treatment because of the following:

- Patients usually receive dental treatment while supine (lying flat)
- In this position their airway is particularly vulnerable to having foreign objects dropped into it
- Dental treatment often involves the use of small instruments and items that may be dropped while in the mouth
- Copious amounts of water are used in the patient's mouth while restorative dental treatment is being carried out
- Debris is produced in the mouth during many restorative procedures

Otherwise, the commonest cause of choking is a food item in a conscious individual. Again, this has particular dental relevance in that older individuals may have poor fitting dentures or very worn teeth that do not masticate food efficiently before being swallowed, making choking more likely.

As previously established, the tissues of the body and particularly the brain require oxygen to function. Any event that restricts or stops the oxygen flow will rapidly lead to brain damage or even death, and one such event is choking. Choking can occur in either a conscious or unconscious individual, but is obviously more immediately life-threatening in the latter case as the airway is unprotected and the individual is unable to try to clear the obstruction themselves. They are fully reliant on their rescuer to clear the obstruction and maintain their airway until they regain consciousness.

Signs of incomplete obstruction

In a conscious individual, a foreign body may only partially block the airway so that some oxygen is still able to pass and enter the lungs, and their choking episode may be classed as mild or severe. If **mild**, the individual will still be able to speak, breathe and cough effectively and remove the obstruction themselves.

If the choking episode is **severe**, the signs may include any of the following:

- Sudden coughing
- Wheezing or gurgling
- Lips or tongue change colour to blue or grey
- Intermittent laboured breathing
- Unable to speak

Assisting the patient

The individual should be encouraged to cough unassisted, as this is often enough to expel the foreign body and clear the airway. If they are supine while undergoing dental treatment, they will quickly sit upright to cough, and they may need support to do so.

If the foreign body is not quickly expelled, the condition of the individual may deteriorate rapidly and the rescuer should then assist them before consciousness is lost, by carrying out one of the following:

■   **Back slaps**
■   **Abdominal thrusts (Heimlich's manoeuvre)**

Back slaps

When an individual is conscious and choking, they tend to panic and the rescuer needs to keep them calm while trying to help. They should be encouraged to cough while leaning forwards to try to expel the obstruction themselves. If this is unsuccessful, the rescuer can administer back slaps.

(1)   Keep the individual leaning forwards
(2)   Support them in this position by placing one hand across their chest, respecting the individual's dignity and gaining consent as necessary, especially with females
(3)   Stand to one side and behind the individual
(4)   With the flat of the other hand give five sharp slaps between their shoulder blades (Figure 4.13)
(5)   If this fails to expel the obstruction, move on to abdominal thrusts

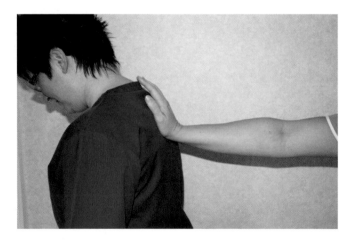

Figure 4.13 Back slaps.

Abdominal thrusts

This technique enables the rescuer to cause an artificial cough in the individual, which may be powerful enough to eject the foreign body causing the obstruction. As it involves giving sharp thrusts into the abdomen, it must **never** be used on a pregnant woman.

The technique is carried out as follows:

(1) Stand behind the choking individual, talking calmly to them and explaining what you are about to do
(2) Wrap your arms around them just below their ribcage
(3) Form a fist with one hand and grasp it with the other, positioning both over the individual's abdomen (Figure 4.14)
(4) Pull both hands inwards and upwards to administer sharp thrusts
(5) Air will whoosh out at each thrust, and if successful the obstruction will be dislodged
(6) If the individual is too large to span from behind, the thrusts can be given from the front while they stand with their back to a hard surface, such as a wall

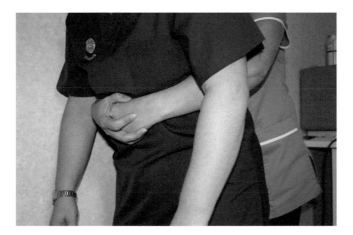

Figure 4.14 Abdominal thrusts.

If both methods fail, the casualty will eventually become unconscious as their body is starved of oxygen. They will collapse and the rescuer must continue trying to clear the obstruction and administer BLS as necessary.

Once collapsed, the individual's mouth should be checked for any signs of the obstruction and it can then be removed. Their airway should be opened in the usual manner, signs of breathing checked for, and if necessary two rescue breaths should be given while any helpers are sent to summon specialist help.

Chest compressions should now be given and these can be modified to chest thrusts in an attempt to clear the obstruction, as follows:

(1) Place the unconscious individual on their back
(2) Kneel to one side and give sharp chest compressions at a slower rate than for a collapsed individual with no circulation

(3)   Check their mouth for the obstruction at regular intervals
(4)   Continue rescue attempts until specialist help arrives, or the obstruction is cleared and the individual recovers
(5)   They should still be checked medically once recovered, as some of the obstruction may remain or there may be damage to the respiratory system

The chest thrust method can be modified for a conscious pregnant woman, or even for a large individual whose abdomen cannot be spanned by the rescuer's arms.

■   Have the individual stand or sit with their back against a firm surface, such as a wall
■   Push sharply against their chest with both hands, from the front
■   The rescuer should try to avoid being in line with the individual's mouth if possible, so that they are not hit by the expelled obstruction

Choking in young children

The signs and symptoms of choking in a young child will be as for an adult individual, and they are more likely to experience this emergency both due to their lack of awareness of danger, and their tendency to put objects into their mouths without realising the consequences.

The procedure to follow is very similar to that for an adult but with less force, and depends on whether the young child is conscious or not. The important point is that rescue breathing should only be carried out on an unconscious child, as their airway often becomes clear as their muscles relax during their loss of consciousness, and rescue breaths may not be necessary.

The procedure in a choking conscious child is as follows:

(1)   Keep calm and keep the casualty (and any attending parent) calm
(2)   Get the child to cough to try to expel the obstruction
(3)   If unsuccessful, give five back slaps and recheck their mouth
(4)   If unsuccessful, give five chest thrusts from behind against their breastbone, then recheck their mouth
(5)   If unsuccessful, send for help then repeat the back slaps and recheck their mouth
(6)   If unsuccessful, give up to five abdominal thrusts but with less force than that used for an adult, then recheck the mouth
(7)   Continue alternating all three techniques until the obstruction is cleared, the child loses consciousness, or specialist help arrives
(8)   If successful, have the child medically checked for any signs of respiratory system damage

If the choking episode is severe and prolonged, or the obstruction is complete, the child will collapse and become unconscious. The rescue procedure is as follows:

(1) Check the mouth for any obstruction and remove, then open the airway
(2) Try five times to give two rescue breaths, if the chest rises successfully then carry out chest compressions to circulate the oxygen around the body
(3) If the chest fails to rise, give five back slaps followed by five chest compressions if the child is still choking
(4) Recheck the mouth and open the airway, then give another five rescue breaths
(5) If unsuccessful give another five back slaps followed by five abdominal thrusts
(6) Continue the cycle until specialist help arrives or the obstruction is removed

Choking in babies

Babies are easier for the rescuer to handle during a choking episode, as they can be held face down for back slaps and carried towards help while still being aided, rather than having to be left. Obviously, the force used to attempt to dislodge an obstruction must be significantly less than that used for a young child. Also, under no circumstances should abdominal thrusts be attempted on a baby, as their internal organs would be easily damaged by this technique. Again, as with a young child, rescue breathing should not be attempted unless the baby is unconscious.

If the baby is conscious and choking, the procedure is as follows:

(1) Check the mouth for any obvious obstruction and remove it
(2) With the baby held face down along the rescuer's arm, give five back slaps (Figure 4.15)
(3) Turn the baby face up and remove any obstruction
(4) If unsuccessful, give five sharp chest compressions (as for BLS)
(5) If unsuccessful, call for specialist help and continue the cycle until the obstruction is removed or the baby becomes unconscious

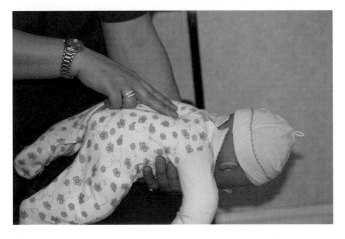

Figure 4.15 Baby back slaps.

If the baby becomes unconscious:

(1) Recheck the mouth and open the airway
(2) Try five times to give two rescue breaths
(3) If the chest rises, continue chest compressions to circulate the oxygen
(4) If not, give five back slaps followed by five chest compressions
(5) Recheck the mouth for any obstruction and open the airway, then repeat the cycle until specialist help arrives

Legislation

Dental professionals have a duty of care to their patients at all times, as laid out in the General Dental Council's 'Standards Guidance' documentation. While this is more relevant during the provision of dental treatment in the workplace, dental professionals as healthcare workers also have a duty of care to provide BLS in an emergency situation as necessary, and to update and maintain their skills in this area on a regular basis.

In particular, the principles of good practice laid out in the documentation can be broadly said to cover all aspects of the dental professional's working life, including the need to provide BLS, as follows:

- Put patients' interests first and act to protect them
- Respect patients' dignity and choices
- Protect the confidentiality of patients' information
- Co-operate with other healthcare workers in the interests of the patients
- Maintain your professional knowledge and competence
- Be trustworthy

In relation to the provision of BLS and all medical emergencies that may occur in the dental workplace, the necessary legislation can be interpreted and successfully followed by all dental professionals in the manner indicated below.

Put patients' interests first and act to protect them

As a healthcare professional, dental nurses have a duty of care to act in an emergency situation and try to maintain a casualty's life until specialist help arrives. There must never be any attempt to discriminate between casualty patients – the first to receive help in the form of BLS must always be the one whose life is at most risk. Their age, gender, race, etc is completely irrelevant.

Similarly, to make no attempt to help a casualty is only acceptable if to do so would put the rescuer's life at risk.

Respect patients' dignity and choices

While attending to a casualty and administering BLS, there is little need for all except outer clothing to be opened or removed. Identification of the correct point to administer chest compressions, for instance, will be made easier if a heavy coat is opened, but it would not be necessary to remove further garments. Indeed, to do so is likely to waste valuable resuscitation time.

It is also good practice to talk calmly to the casualty even though they may appear unconscious. The sense of hearing is usually the last to be lost when a casualty becomes unconscious, so they may actually be able to hear all that is going on around them while being unable to respond.

Talking to the casualty in these situations, and explaining in a 'running commentary' manner what actions are being carried out, makes the situation less fearful and embarrassing for them, as well as helping to focus the thoughts of the rescuer.

Protect the confidentiality of patients' information

The demise of a patient must never be openly discussed with anyone except those who have a right to know. These will include emergency services personnel (including the police), and authorities such as the Health and Safety Executive or environmental health officers.

The occurrence of an emergency situation should not be discussed as idle chatter among staff members, and especially not within earshot of other members of the public. The casualty has a right to have their privacy maintained, and their details kept confidential at all times.

Co-operate with other healthcare workers

During an emergency situation, it will be necessary for one rescuer to assume a lead role so that all rescue attempts can be co-ordinated correctly, to give the casualty their best chance of survival. All other rescuers must respect this senior person, and co-operate with them at all times in the best interests of the casualty. Otherwise, vital actions within DRSABC may be missed out, as one rescuer is unaware of another's actions – and this may cost the casualty their life.

Maintain your professional knowledge and competence

It is a compulsory GDC requirement that all dental staff must attend regular updates on medical emergencies and resuscitation techniques. Within a five-year cycle of continuing professional development (CPD), dental nurses must undergo a minimum of ten hours of verifiable training in these subjects – this means the training must be recorded as having been carried out, and certificated so that attendance can be proved if required.

Failure to comply with the GDC requirements could result in dental staff being removed from the register, and therefore be unable to work as health care professionals.

Be trustworthy

It goes without saying that the events surrounding a medical emergency must be clearly and accurately reported to the necessary specialists, even if mistakes occurred or the rescue attempts were not carried out correctly. Telling the truth in these instances may assist the specialists in the successful resuscitation of the casualty.

Similarly, the personal effects of the casualty may be strewn around and left behind as they are removed to hospital as necessary. The items should be collected together and handed over to someone in authority, so that they can be passed on to the casualty or their family.

5 Unit 4: Prepare and Maintain Environments, Instruments and Equipment for Clinical Dental Procedures (OH1)

Knowledge specifications

Infection and cross-infection

K1 – Apply factual knowledge of the principles and causes of infection and cross-infection

K2 – Apply factual knowledge of micro-organisms – the meaning and significance of the terms pathogenic and non-pathogenic

K3 – Apply factual knowledge of potentially infectious conditions (such as hepatitis B, HIV, herpes simplex, etc) – what they are, the appropriate action to take and why they should be reported

Cleaning methods and systems for limiting cross-infection

K4 – A factual knowledge of the scientific principles of and difference between sterilisation, asepsis, disinfection and social cleanliness, and how each relates to the patient, the setting, the procedure and equipment

K5 – A working knowledge of what is meant by standard precautions and how this is applied in the preparation of environments, including zoning and protective barriers

K6 – A working knowledge of when sterile, aseptic and disinfectant procedures may need to be carried out, and the possible consequences of not doing so

K7 – A working knowledge of good hygiene practice – what it is and methods of maintaining it

K8 – A working knowledge of effective hand cleansing – what it is and methods for achieving it

K9 – A working knowledge of the purpose of personal protective clothing and the different sorts which may be necessary

K10 – A working knowledge of the cleaning agents which are appropriate to different surface areas

K11 – A working knowledge of the nature of decontaminants, when and why they are used

K12 – A working knowledge of methods of cleaning different types of equipment, instruments and handpieces and the different activities which are appropriate to each

Sterilisation

K13 – A working knowledge of methods of sterilisation, the types of sterilisers which are used and their relationship to the different equipment/instruments (including pre-packed items) and the disposal of waste
K14 – A working knowledge of methods of testing to show that autoclaves and other equipment are functioning effectively
K15 – A working knowledge of the correct sequence and duration for different forms of sterilisation
K16 – A working knowledge of the different forms of packaging and storing sterilised instruments and handpieces and which methods are appropriate to which circumstances
K17 – A working knowledge of the potential long-term effects of using damaged or pre-used sterile goods
K18 – A working knowledge of methods of safe handling of items before, during, and after sterilisation and the reasons for this
K19 – A working knowledge of the actions which are appropriate to take when sterilisation equipment is not working to the optimum level

Preparation of environments for clinical dental procedures

K20 – A working knowledge of the purposes of maintaining the clinical environment as clear and clean as possible
K21 – A working knowledge of the reasons for keeping heating, lighting and ventilation appropriate to the treatment and the effects which they can have on infection and cross-infection
K22 – A working knowledge of safe and secure environments – what this means for treatment areas and the dangers which are inherent in them

Equipment, instruments, materials and medicaments

K23 – A working knowledge of the instruments, equipment, materials and medicaments which may be necessary for different treatments and correct methods of preparing these
K24 – A working knowledge of why shortfalls/failures in instruments, equipment, materials and medicaments should be reported
K25 – A working knowledge of the purpose and correct methods of preparing and handling the range of equipment, instruments, materials and medicaments used in dentistry
K26 – A working knowledge of the relationship of equipment, instruments, materials and medicaments to different treatments and the stages within them

K27 – A working knowledge of legal requirements and manufacturer's instructions relating to servicing of equipment including recording of maintenance and service intervals

Waste and spillage

K28 – A working knowledge of the different types of waste and spillage including those which may be of particular relevance to the procedure and setting
K29 – A working knowledge of methods of disposing of waste and spillage and the relationship of this to the different types
K30 – A working knowledge of procedures for disposing of damaged sterile pre-packed items
K31 – A working knowledge of the dangers of not disposing of waste and spillage in the correct ways
K32 – A working knowledge of why waste and spillage should be disposed of promptly
K33 – A working knowledge of why it is necessary to report damaged disposal containers
K34 – A working knowledge of why equipment, etc must be placed in the correct locations for storage, sterilisation or transportation

Legislation and work role

K35 – A working knowledge of health and safety regulations: the Health and Safety at Work Act and the Control of Substances Hazardous to Health Regulations
K36 – A working knowledge of the legal and organisational policies relating to the disposal of waste and spillage from clinical treatments and investigations (such as the Environmental Protection Act, Controlled Waste Regulations)

For any clinical dental procedure to be carried out safely and effectively, the environment, instruments and equipment must all be properly prepared and maintained before, during and after each procedure. These preparation and maintenance tasks are two of the main duties of a dental nurse working at the chairside.

Micro-organisms

The aim of the preparation procedure is to ensure that all of the instruments and equipment to be used are clean and free of all contamination by micro-organisms from a previous patient, or from dental staff. They can then be safely used in the prepared environment (the dental surgery) without the risk of passing on, or

cross-infecting, the next patient or staff. Similarly, the aim of the maintenance procedure is to ensure that all the instruments and equipment used are then disposed of safely, or cleaned to a high enough standard that they can be re-used without the risk of cross-infecting the next patient, and so on. Likewise, the environment must also be cleaned thoroughly so that it is safe to be re-used.

The risk that the micro-organisms pose is that they can spread disease and infection from one person to another, either directly from person to person, or indirectly via contaminated instruments or equipment. Those micro-organisms that are capable of causing disease are referred to as **pathogenic micro-organisms**, while those unable to cause disease are called **non-pathogenic micro-organisms**.

A full understanding of the principles of infection control involves an understanding of the basics in relation to microbiology and pathology, so that the actions of the micro-organisms and the way in which they cause disease, and the body's defence mechanisms against them, can be appreciated.

Background knowledge of micro-organisms

There are four main types of microscopic organisms involved in transmitting disease:

- Bacteria
- Viruses
- Fungi
- Protozoa

Protozoa have little clinical significance in dentistry.

Bacteria

- They are visible under a light microscope
- They are single-celled organisms
- Their rigid wall determines their shape, and therefore their name, so circular bacteria are called 'cocci', rod-shaped are called 'bacilli', and spiral shaped are 'spirochaetes' (Figure 5.1)
- They survive as spores in unfavourable environments
- Active bacteria are prevented from reproducing and multiplying by **bacteriostatic antibiotics**
- They can also be killed by **bactericidal antibiotics**
- Spores can only be killed by the process of **sterilisation**

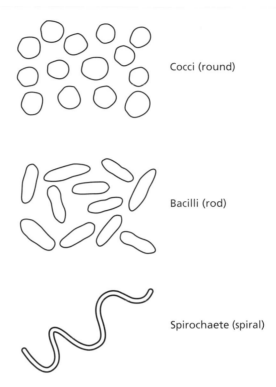

Cocci (round)

Bacilli (rod)

Spirochaete (spiral)

Figure 5.1 Bacteria shapes.

Viruses

- They are so small that they are only visible using an electron microscope (so their correct definition would be an ultra micro-organism)
- They must live within the cells of other organisms (host cells)
- They exist as a protein capsule containing the necessary chemicals to reproduce within the host cell (Figure 5.2)
- It is this protein capsule which causes our body to react against them, and it is unique for each virus
- They are unaffected by antibiotics, but some can be treated using **anti-viral drugs**
- **Vaccines** have been developed to provide immunity against some of the more serious viral infections (such as hepatitis, measles, mumps)

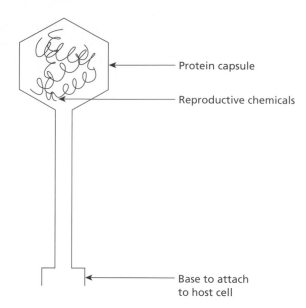

Protein capsule

Reproductive chemicals

Base to attach
to host cell

Figure 5.2 Structure of a virus. Source: *Levison's Textbook for Dental Nurses*, 10th edn, C. Hollins, 2008, Wiley-Blackwell.

Fungi

- They are larger than bacteria but still only visible with a microscope
- They are actually a type of microscopic plant which reproduce by budding or by spore production
- They grow by producing an extensive branching network across tissues (called hyphae)
- Only one fungus is clinically significant in dentistry, and that is the organism causing oral thrush – *Candida albicans*
- Oral thrush is unaffected by antibiotics but can be treated with **anti-fungal agents**

Infections caused by various micro-organisms that are of importance in dentistry include:

- **Dental caries** – bacterial infection of the hard tissues of the tooth, especially with *Streptococcus mutans*
- **Periodontitis** – bacterial infection of the periodontium, especially with *Porphyromonas gingivalis*
- **Cold sore** – viral infection of lip caused by **herpes simplex type I**
- **Oral thrush** – fungal infection of the oral soft tissues caused by *Candida albicans*
- **Hepatitis** – viral infection of liver caused by various organisms: **hepatitis A, B, C, E, or non-A–non-B**

- **Chicken pox** – viral infection of certain nerves caused by **herpes varicella**
- **Acquired immune deficiency syndrome (AIDS)** – viral infection of immune system caused by **human immunodeficiency virus (HIV)**
- **Shingles** – viral infection of certain nerves caused by **herpes zoster**
- **Meningitis** – bacterial infection of brain coverings caused by **meningococci**
- **Glandular fever** – viral infection of lymph glands caused by **Epstein–Barr virus**
- **Mumps** – viral infection of parotid salivary glands caused by **paramyxovirus**

More recently, **prions** have been discovered. These are not living micro-organisms, but are a type of special protein that is also capable of causing disease. Their associated diseases include 'mad cow disease' and the human variation of it, called **Creutzfeldt–Jakob disease (CJD)**. CJD affects the brain and spinal cord and has no known treatment or cure – it is a fatal illness.

The significance of prions to clinical dentistry is that they can be spread by cross-infection through nerve tissue, theoretically including that found within the root canals of teeth and referred to as 'the pulp'. Prions cannot be killed by the disinfection or sterilisation methods currently used in the dental surgery. For this reason, recent regulatory changes dictate that the dental instruments used to carry out root canal treatments (endodontics) must be regarded as single use, and safely disposed of between patients.

Infection, inflammation, immune response

Infection

Infection occurs when pathogenic micro-organisms gain entry to the body tissues. In the dental surgery environment, this can happen in a variety of ways:

- **Direct contact** with body fluids – blood, saliva or vomit
- **Airborne droplets** of blood or saliva – from sneezing or coughing
- **Aerosol spray** containing blood or saliva – created during the use of dental hand pieces and water sprays
- **Direct entry** through damaged skin or membranes – cuts, grazes, piercing the eye membrane
- **Inoculation injury** with a contaminated instrument – such as a 'needle stick' injury

Later in the text, the methods used in the dental surgery environment to reduce the risk of infection by a pathogenic micro-organism will be discussed in detail. However, exposure to these micro-organisms does not always result in an infection progressing to become a disease. The body has natural defence mechanisms in place to prevent the micro-organisms gaining entry in the first place, and to fight the invaders if they do manage to penetrate the body tissues.

Response of the body to infection

The body has three lines of natural defence against infection.

(1) An **intact skin and mucous membrane** to prevent the entry of the micro-organisms initially, with surface secretions to immobilise them – sweat, saliva, gastric juice produced in the stomach

(2) The **inflammatory response**, which is initiated if the skin or mucous membrane is breached

(3) The **immune response** – if infection takes hold, whereby the body's immune system is activated to fight the infection

Inflammatory response

If the micro-organisms do gain entry to the body, the tissues will be irritated and the five classic signs of inflammation will be seen:

- **Heat, redness, and swelling** – due to the increased blood flow to the area
- **Pain** – caused by the pressure of the increased blood flow on the surrounding nerve endings in the tissues affected
- **Loss of function of the affected tissue** – due to the pain and swelling present

When the inflammation and swelling occurs quickly and over a short period of time, the condition is very painful and is referred to as **acute inflammation**. A dental example is an acute alveolar abscess. When the swelling is less pronounced and occurs over a longer period, it tends to be far less painful or even painless, and is referred to as **chronic inflammation**. A dental example is chronic periodontitis.

In fit and healthy patients, the micro-organisms are usually overcome by the inflammatory response. The increased blood flow carries huge numbers of **leucocytes** (white blood cells) to the area, and these pass out of the capillaries and into the tissues at the site of the infection. They battle with the invading micro-organisms and **pus** is formed as the various cells die. In addition, **antitoxins** and **antibodies** may be carried to the area in the blood plasma and assist in the attack against the micro-organisms.

In the very young, the elderly, or those who are ill and debilitated, help is often required to stop the invasion. This is the role of antibiotics, anti-virals and anti-fungals. These drugs may also have to be prescribed when the micro-organisms involved are particularly nasty and strong, or **virulent**.

Immune response

Once the body has been exposed to an invasion by a micro-organism, our immune system develops **antibodies** to it and **antitoxins** to the poisons they produce. This ensures that the same micro-organism and its toxins are recognised in future, and this is referred to as **acquired immunity**.

Immunity can also be naturally received from our mother, or acquired by **vaccination** against an illness without actually suffering from that illness. This method tends to be used to give acquired immunity against more serious illnesses, such as hepatitis B. Unfortunately, vaccines have not yet been developed against other serious blood-borne diseases that pose a risk to dental staff, such as AIDS.

Infection control

Infection control is one of the most important parts of an effective risk management programme to improve the quality and safety of patient care, and the occupational health of staff. Control of cleanliness in the dental surgery environment is imperative because:

- All patients have hundreds of oral bacteria present, even in health
- When diseases are present, they may also have fungi or viruses too
- All instruments and equipment coming into contact with these micro-organisms could potentially become contaminated by them
- If the instruments and equipment are not cleaned thoroughly between patients, other patients and staff can easily be cross-infected
- The use of dental air turbines creates an aerosol, which falls onto the working surfaces and contaminates them
- Obviously, if staff are also not personally clean and are taking part in close dental procedures, they can contaminate patients

Basic principles of infection control

A system of **standard precautions** (previously referred to as 'universal precautions') has been adopted in healthcare work, which is designed to protect staff from inoculation and contamination risks, and to protect patients from being exposed to the risk of cross-infection.

The basic principle is to assume that any patient may be infected with any micro-organism at any time, and therefore they pose an infection risk to all dental staff and to other patients. A detailed medical history questionnaire, completed at the patient's initial attendance and updated at every appointment thereafter, will identify the majority of problems. However, a patient may be infected with a micro-organism without showing any signs of disease, and therefore be unaware of the risk they pose to others – these are called **carriers**. Also, a patient may choose not to disclose their full medical history to the dental staff, and would then be assumed to be 'safe' to treat.

So, if all patients are considered to be a possible source of infection and treated as such, the infection control techniques used in the dental environment will be good enough to reduce all cross-infection risks to a minimum. The other basic principles of infection control to be adopted are summarised below.

- Apply good basic personal hygiene with regular appropriate hand washing
- Cover existing wounds with waterproof dressings
- Do not undertake invasive procedures if suffering from chronic skin lesions on the hands
- Wear appropriate gloves at all times when assisting, and discard after single use
- Avoid contamination with body fluids by wearing appropriate protective clothing, safety spectacles and masks – referred to as 'personal protective equipment' (PPE)
- Institute approved procedures for decontamination of instruments and equipment
- Apply good basic environmental cleaning procedures
- Clear up blood and other body fluid spillages promptly
- Follow correct procedure for safe disposal of contaminated waste and sharps
- Ensure all staff are aware of, understand and follow infection control policies and procedures
- Ensure all staff are fully vaccinated against hepatitis B (this is now a legal requirement for all those who work in the clinical environment), and that all childhood immunisations are up to date

In the dental surgery environment, special methods of infection control are now routinely practised, as well as following the general points listed above. Best practice dictates that good infection control is achieved by the following:

- Correct cleaning of the hands
- Use of personal protective equipment
- Correct cleaning of the clinical environment
- Correct cleaning of dental equipment, hand pieces and instruments

The terms 'cleaning' and 'cleanliness' in a clinical context are quite different from a lay person's concept of them. The following are definitions of the relevant terms used here:

- **Social cleanliness** – clean to a socially acceptable standard, but not disinfected nor sterilised
- **Disinfection** – the destruction of bacteria and fungi, but not spores nor some viruses (the technique usually involves the use of chemicals)
- **Sterilisation** – the process of killing all micro-organisms and spores to produce asepsis (usually involves the use of high temperatures and pressure)
- **Asepsis** – the absence of all living pathogenic micro-organisms

Cleaning of the hands

Hand washing is the most important method of preventing cross-infection, and the technique used should be that stipulated by the Health and Safety Council.

Nails should be kept short and wounds covered with a water-proof dressing to reduce the number of areas for micro-organisms to contaminate. The minimum amount of jewellery should be worn by those working in a clinical environment, for the same reason.

The correct procedure for **clinical hand washing** is:

(1)   Turn on the tap using the foot or elbow control, to prevent contaminating the tap
(2)   Wet both hands under running water of a suitable temperature
(3)   Apply a suitable anti-bacterial liquid soap from the elbow operated dispenser, and wash all areas of both hands and wrists thoroughly – this should take at least 30 seconds to carry out thoroughly
(4)   Nail brushes are not advised unless they are autoclavable, as they can become contaminated with repeated use
(5)   Rinse both hands under running water, holding them so that the water does not flow back over the fingers
(6)   Dry the hands thoroughly, using disposable paper towels for single use

Heavy-duty gloves must be worn whenever the cleaning of dirty instruments is being carried out. Clinical gloves must be worn whenever patients are being treated, and discarded between patients.

Whenever a surgical clinical procedure is to be carried out, the hand washing procedure described above should be extended to include the forearms too, and should be carried out for a minimum of two minutes to be completed effectively. Special surgical grade handwash should be used, with a sterile, single-use scrubbing brush.

At the end of the cleaning, the hands should be held up during rinsing to allow the water to drain off the elbows, and then the hands and forearms should be dried with sterile paper towels. Sterile gloves should then be placed on both hands. This 'scrubbing-up' procedure is known as the **aseptic technique of hand washing**.

Social hand washing is that of a general level of cleanliness, and should be carried out before preparing food or eating, and especially after using the toilet facilities. It follows a similar technique to that used for clinical hand cleansing, but should not take as long as it need not include the wrists or forearms. Many suitable anti-bacterial handwash liquids are available for both the washroom area and the surgeries.

Use of personal protective equipment

PPE is worn to prevent staff from coming into contact with blood and other bodily fluids. It is a legal requirement for dental employers to provide the following protective clothing for their staff (Figure 5.3):

- Gloves of varying quality, as discussed above
- High temperature wash uniform, to be worn in the work area only

- Plastic apron to be worn over the uniform when soiling may occur during surgical procedures or while cleaning the surgery
- Safety glasses, goggles or visors, to prevent contaminated material entering the eyes
- Face masks of surgical quality should be worn whenever dental handpieces or ultrasonic equipment is in use, to prevent the inhalation of aerosol contamination and pieces of flying debris

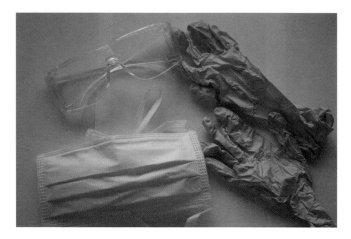

Figure 5.3 Personal protective equipment.

Cleaning of the clinical environment

The whole of the dental practice should be cleaned to a socially acceptable standard on a daily basis, and this is usually carried out by a domestic cleaner. In clinical areas, however, a far higher standard of cleaning is necessary because these are the areas where contamination of the environment by body fluids is greatest, and where cross-infection is most likely to occur.

The standard to be achieved in the clinical environment is that of **disinfection**. This involves the use of various chemicals to inhibit the growth of, or ideally kill, bacteria and fungi. However, most are not effective against bacterial spores or some viruses. Those in common use in the dental workplace include the following:

- **Bleach-based cleaners** – containing sodium hypochlorite and used to disinfect all non-metallic and non-textile surfaces, and to soak laboratory items
- **Aldehyde-based cleaners** – can be used on metallic surfaces and to soak laboratory items
- **Isopropyl alcohol wipes** – to disinfect items such as exposed x-ray film packets for safe handling during processing
- **Chlorhexidine gluconate** – as an irrigating disinfectant during root canal treatments, and as a skin cleanser

The practice as a whole should be kept clean, dry and well ventilated. Some workplaces have air conditioning installed, but care should be taken that the system operates without the risk of recirculating the contaminated surgery air.

A written protocol for surgery cleaning should be available in all dental workplaces, which lays out the correct procedure in a logical manner and details how each item should be dealt with. In general, it should include the following:

- All work surfaces should have the minimum items of equipment out for each procedure, and when these items are not in use they should be stored in drawers or cupboards to prevent aerosol contamination
- Ideally, all stored instruments should be kept in lidded trays or in sealed pouches while in the cupboards or drawers (Figure 5.4)
- Areas should be designated as 'clean' and 'dirty' so that dirty used instruments are not placed where clean items should be – this is called **zoning**
- Work surfaces should be cleaned after each session with a detergent solution or a suitable viricidal disinfectant
- Equipment likely to be contaminated such as chair and light controls, and headrests, should be covered with impervious plastic sheets (such as cling film) and changed between patients – this is called using **protective barriers**
- Dental aspirators that exhaust outside the surgery area will reduce the risk of aerosol contamination, they should be used routinely and flushed through daily with a recommended non-foaming disinfectant
- Clinical records and computer keyboards should not be handled while gloves are being worn
- All non-metallic equipment should be wiped down with a bleach-based preparation, which is particularly effective against viruses, at the end of each day
- Bleach-based disinfectants cannot be used on metallic items as they will corrode the metal
- All intra-oral radiographs should be wiped with an isopropyl alcohol wipe before being handled with clean gloves and taken for processing

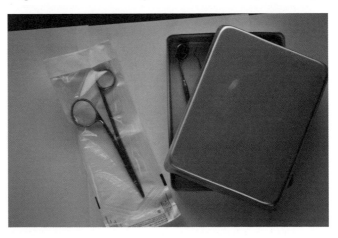

Figure 5.4 Lidded instrument tray and sterile pouch.

Cleaning of equipment, hand pieces and instruments

These are potentially the most infective of all items found in the clinical environment, as they are used in the patient's mouth where micro-organisms proliferate. Their potential to cause injury and disease by cross-infection to all dental staff should not be under estimated. All of these items should always be handled carefully and only while wearing the correct articles of PPE, to avoid direct contact to staff while transferring the items for disposal or cleaning.

The risk of cross-infection between patients can be eliminated by the use of **disposable items** which are safely discarded after a single use, rather than being cleaned and re-used. For expensive items, such as hand pieces and metal hand instruments, this is not feasible and so they must be **sterilised** to ensure that all micro-organisms and bacterial spores have been killed during the cleaning process.

Any items that are to be disposed of are classed as **hazardous waste** and treated accordingly (see Chapter 2). Other items are treated as follows:

- All items which are not disposable after a single use should be sterilised in an **autoclave**
- Before placing in an autoclave, all solid debris must be removed from the items, either by the use of an **ultrasonic bath** (Figure 5.5) or a **washer-disinfector**, with or without hand scrubbing
- Only then should these items be autoclaved, as residual solid debris will harbour micro-organisms and spores, and shield them from the sterilisation process
- Handpieces must not be placed in an ultrasonic bath, and the manufacturer's specific instructions should be consulted with regard to their advice on oiling after sterilisation
- Sterilised instruments should be stored in lidded trays in cupboards or drawers, or in sealed pouches until they are next used

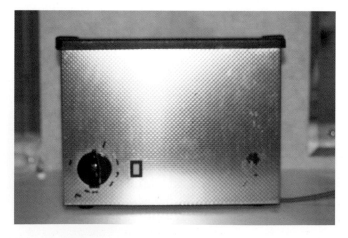

Figure 5.5 Ultrasonic bath.

Autoclaves

These are invaluable items of equipment in the clinical setting, where some non-disposable items can be sterilised to ensure all pathogenic micro-organisms and spores are killed. Two types are available for regular use in the dental environment. The difference between the two is that they can operate with or without vacuum and are referred to as 'S' type or 'N' type autoclave, respectively.

'N' type autoclaves have the following features:

- Heats the water to steam at 134°C and holds for three minutes, under 2.25 bar pressure
- This allows the steam to pass around and over all of the items within the chamber, killing the micro-organisms and spores as it does so
- The full cycle lasts for 15–20 minutes, depending on the make of autoclave
- They are suitable for unwrapped, solid instruments
- They can hold several trays of laid out instruments for each cycle
- There is no vacuum produced during the cycle (Figure 5.6)

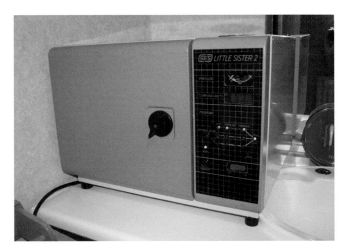

Figure 5.6 An autoclave. Source: *Levison's Textbook for Dental Nurses*, 10th edn, C. Hollins, 2008, Wiley-Blackwell.

'S' type autoclaves have the following features:

- Reach the same temperature and pressure as the 'N' type autoclave
- They work under vacuum, so the steam is actively sucked through and out of the chamber, taking all micro-organisms and spores with it
- They are therefore suitable for wrapped instruments and those with narrow lumens, as the vacuum sucks the steam through them

Neither type of autoclave will operate correctly unless all of the debris contamination has been removed from the items first, before they are put through the autoclave cycle.

Under current Health and Safety guidelines, the following tests must be carried out in all dental workplaces when using autoclaves.

■ A daily test run to be carried out during the first cycle of the day, where a log record is kept of the temperature, pressure and time intervals of the cycle
■ More modern autoclaves have an integral printer that will record these parameters as a printout which can be saved in the log book (Figure 5.7). Otherwise, a staff member must watch the cycle and record the necessary information manually
■ The sterility of the items in any cycle can also be checked by inserting a 'TST' indicator strip at the start – this will change colour (usually from yellow to purple) if the autoclave operated correctly (Figure 5.8)
■ If the cycle fails to reach the correct temperature or pressure, for the required length of time, or the indicator strip does not change colour, the matter should be reported to a senior staff member so that the autoclave can be removed from use and repaired

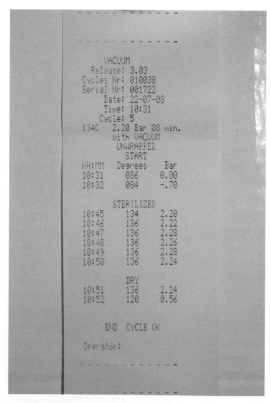

Figure 5.7 Cycle sterility printout.

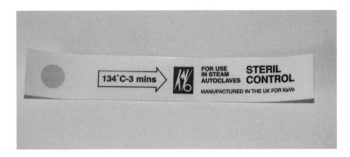

Figure 5.8 TST strip.

- Otherwise, all the items passing through that autoclave may not be sterilised during the procedure, and risk causing cross-infection to staff and other patients when re-used
- De-ionised water should be used in the autoclave (not tap water) and this must be drained from the reservoir chamber daily
- A weekly inspection of the door seal and the door safety devices must be carried out to determine that they operate correctly, and that the door cannot be opened during the cycle
- An annual test of the autoclave's correct operation must be carried out by an authorised person
- A periodic examination that the autoclave conforms to the Pressure Systems Safety Regulations must be carried out by an authorised organisation
- The dental workplace insurance policy should include third party liability cover for the use of autoclaves, as they are classed as pressure vessels

Other methods of sterilisation

In a dental environment within the hospital setting, it is likely that all items to be sterilised are collected and sent for decontamination and sterilisation **centrally**, along with any items from other departments and clinics. This is more efficient when large numbers of items are involved, than for each department to operate its own autoclave. The autoclaves used centrally tend to operate under high vacuum, and are much larger so that greater loads can be sterilised during each cycle.

Some items used in the dental environment are supplied in sterile, pre-packaged pouches by the manufacturers. They include scalpel blades and needles for local anaesthetic administration – items that are used to pierce a patient's tissues and which would easily transmit diseases if they were not guaranteed as sterile when used. They are sterilised **industrially** by exposure to **gamma radiation**, which kills all micro-organisms and bacterial spores. The effectiveness of the technique is checked for each batch of items, by carrying out microbiological tests on them before dispatch. All industrially sterilised items are considered as single-use and disposable, but any with faulty packaging should also be safely discarded, without being used.

Protection of staff by immunisation

With the close nature of dental treatment, staff members are likely to come into direct contact with several serious viral diseases, some of which can be fatal. It is therefore necessary that all staff are immunised (vaccinated) against the following viral infections, and that vaccine and booster records are kept and updated as necessary.

- **Diphtheria** – normally received during childhood
- **Pertussis** – whooping cough, normally received during infancy
- **Poliomyelitis** – normally received during childhood
- **MMR** – measles, mumps and rubella (German measles), normally received during infancy
- **Tetanus** – normally received during childhood, and can be boosted as required
- **Tuberculosis** – received routinely after a negative Heaf test, but may need a booster after 15 years
- **Hepatitis B** – received as an occupationally required vaccine before working in any clinical area; a blood test is required to prove seroconversion and ensure immunity; boosters are required every five years

Any staff not immunised against any of the above should not be working in clinical areas with patients. In addition, vaccination against meningitis is now carried out during childhood, and healthcare workers are also advised to receive immunisation against chickenpox and influenza as required.

Hazardous waste disposal

The safe disposal of hazardous and special waste has been fully covered in Unit 1 (see Chapter 2), so just the salient points will be reiterated here. All waste from the clinical area of the dental environment is classed as **hazardous waste**, as it is likely to be contaminated by a patient's body fluids – this is usually in the form of saliva or blood, but may include vomit. In addition, any sharp items (including used instruments) can cause an inoculation injury if great care is not taken while handling them.

All dental staff must wear the appropriate PPE while handling any hazardous waste, to avoid direct contact with any contamination. All non-sharp hazardous waste must be carefully gathered together and placed in the correct yellow/orange hazardous waste sacks. These must then be sealed correctly, and stored securely away from the public while awaiting collection from an authorised company. The sacks must be handled carefully and never over-filled, so that they do not split open and contaminate the surroundings with their contents. Any damaged sacks must be secured within new sacks immediately. The sacks should be stored in plastic bins for protection, and away from the public.

If a **blood spillage** occurs, the area should be sealed off to avoid its spread. Wearing full PPE, paper towels should be placed over and around the spillage, to soak the majority of the blood away. A solution of 50% sodium hypochlorite should then be used to disinfect the area thoroughly, placing all of the contaminated towels into the hazardous waste sack.

All laboratory items (both prosthetic and orthodontic) must be rinsed and then disinfected by immersion in a 10% sodium hypochlorite solution, before transferring between the laboratory and the surgery. An aldehyde solution may have to be used for some types of impression material and for chrome based prosthetic items. The hypochlorite solution has to be made up fresh each day, and the baths used must be clearly marked with their contents to avoid any injury, in accordance with COSHH regulations.

Sharp hazardous waste items must be carefully placed in the rigid, puncture-proof sharps containers, where they are unlikely to cause any inoculation injuries, especially if the guidelines below are followed.

- Ideally, the dentist using the sharp instrument should be responsible for its safe placement in a sharps bin
- Local anaesthetic needles should be re-sheathed using a needle holder
- All other needles should be left unsheathed and placed directly into the sharps bin
- Extracted teeth should also be treated as sharps, and placed in the sharps bin, except those containing amalgam fillings which have their own 'special waste' container (Figure 5.9)

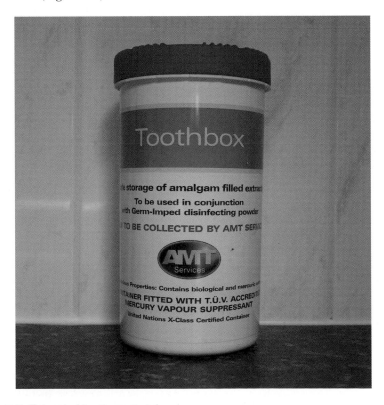

Figure 5.9 Extracted tooth waste tub.

■ Heavy-duty gloves and protective clothing should be worn when instruments are being handled and scrubbed prior to being autoclaved

Sharps injury procedure

If an inoculation injury does occur, the following actions must be carried out:

(1) Stop all treatment immediately and attend to the wound
(2) Squeeze the wound to encourage bleeding, but do not suck wound
(3) Wash the area with soap and running water, then dry and cover the wound with a waterproof dressing
(4) Note the name, address and contact details of the source patient if a contaminated item is involved, so that their medical history can be checked immediately
(5) Complete the accident book
(6) Report the incident to the senior dentist
(7) The consultant microbiologist at the local hospital must be contacted immediately if the source patient is a known or suspected HIV or hepatitis C carrier, as emergency anti-viral treatment must commence within 1 hour of the injury

Occupational hazards

The close nature of dental treatment exposes all surgery staff to a variety of micro-organisms. Those of particular concern are:

■ **HIV** – a viral infection that destroys the body's leucocytes, weakening the patient's immune system and leaving them unable to fight off diseases naturally. These patients eventually go on to develop AIDS, for which there is no current treatment or cure
■ **Hepatitis B** – a viral infection causing liver inflammation, which is often fatal. All dental staff must be immunised against the virus before working in the clinical environment
■ **Hepatitis C** – a similar virus to that causing hepatitis B, but much more likely to prove fatal. There is currently no vaccine against the virus
■ **Herpes simplex type I** – a viral infection affecting particularly the lips and oral cavity. It is not fatal, but is highly contagious when 'cold sore' lesions are present on the lips of the affected person

While always following 'standard precautions' to control infection within the clinical environment, it is good practice to take additional precautions when treating patients with any of these infections.

Any patient attending with an active cold sore should not be treated in the dental clinic except in an emergency. The lesion will diminish within ten days, so they can be rebooked as necessary. Any patient known to be a carrier or having any the other three diseases listed above should be treated as the last patient of a clinical session, so that time is available to strip down and re-equip the surgery before the next session begins.

All equipment except that actually required for the treatment should be removed from the room, to avoid aerosol contamination, and every item that remains in the surgery area should be covered with a protective barrier that can be removed and disposed off at the end of the session. Single-use disposable items should be used wherever possible, and other items such as burs and matrix bands should be disposed of in the sharps bin too.

If these patients require multiple extractions or minor oral surgery, they are best referred to a hospital dental department for the treatment.

6 Unit 5: Offer Information and Support to Individuals on the Protection of Their Oral Health (OH2)

Knowledge specifications

Oral disease and caries

K1 – A factual knowledge of the main types and causes of oral diseases (eg caries, gingivitis, and periodontal disease)

K2 – A factual knowledge of the development of dental plaque and methods for controlling it

K3 – A factual knowledge of the ways in which general health can affect oral health

K4 – A factual knowledge of the social, cultural, and environmental factors which contribute to health and illness

K5 – A factual knowledge of the diagnosis and management of facial pain of dental and non-dental origin

Oral health and diet

K6 – A factual knowledge of the effect of food and drink and nutritional values on oral and general health

K7 – A factual knowledge of the sugar content of a range of food and drink (both natural and manufactured) and the risks of high sugar content, frequency and timing

Fluoride

K8 – A factual knowledge of the role and mechanisms of fluoride in dental health, and its sources (topical, supplements, systemic)

K9 – A factual knowledge of the effects of ingesting too much toothpaste in terms of the amount of fluoride which is consumed

Promoting oral health

K10 – A factual knowledge of the behaviours which may benefit or endanger oral health (such as high sugar or acid content in diet, smoking and alcohol)

K11 – A factual knowledge of the reasons for ensuring that the information provided is accurate and consistent with that provided by other members of the oral health care team

Teaching and encouraging oral hygiene skills and demonstrating methods of maintenance

K12 – A working knowledge of methods of encouraging individuals to change their current practices and try new ways of doing things

K13 – A working knowledge of effective oral hygiene techniques for preventing or minimising oral disease (eg tooth brushing, use of interdental plaque removers) and techniques for effectively demonstrating their use to others (eg through the use of models)

K14 – A working knowledge of the different types of disclosing agents available

K15 – A working knowledge of the advantages and disadvantages of different types of toothbrush (size, material, texture, design)

K16 – A working knowledge of recommended frequency for tooth brushing and how this can be adapted to different individuals' lifestyles

K17 – A working knowledge of the areas of the teeth and gums that are most vulnerable to oral disease and how they can best be protected

K18 – A working knowledge of methods for caring for dentures and orthodontic appliances

Individuals' rights and choice

K19 – A factual knowledge of individual's rights in making choices regarding their health, and why it is important to respect them

Communication

K20 – A working knowledge of the methods and importance of communicating information clearly and effectively

K21 – A working knowledge of methods of modifying information and communication methods for different individuals, including patients from different social and ethnic backgrounds, children (including those with special needs), and the elderly

Work role

K22 – A working knowledge of the reasons for, and circumstances in which, individuals should be referred to another team member

To understand what oral health is, and the main types and causes of oral diseases that compromise it, necessitates an understanding of the anatomy of the oral tissues that may be affected.

The main types of oral disease are those that affect the teeth – **dental caries** – and those that affect the supporting structures of the teeth – **gingivitis** and **periodontitis**.

Anatomy of the teeth

The oral cavity contains the teeth, which have the following functions:

- To support the oral soft tissues to enable clear speech
- To cut up and masticate food into a suitable size before swallowing; by doing this, they expose the food surfaces to enzymes to allow digestion

All teeth are composed of a crown – the portion present in the mouth, and either one, two or three roots which anchor the tooth in the alveolar bone. There are four types of teeth:

- Incisors
- Canines
- Premolars
- Molars

The structure of all teeth is the same, but their shapes and the number of their roots (this is called their morphology) varies depending on their function (Figure 6.1). Microscopically, the structure of each tooth is composed throughout of a layer of

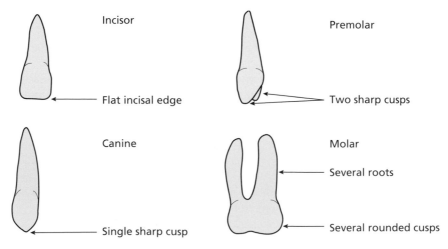

Figure 6.1 Types of teeth.

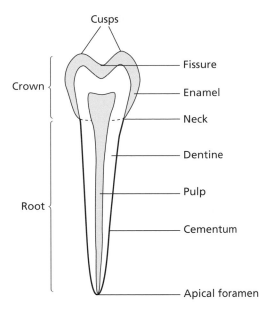

Figure 6.2 Tooth anatomy. Source: *Levison's Textbook for Dental Nurses*, 10th edn, C. Hollins, 2008, Wiley-Blackwell.

dentine, which surrounds the pulp chamber. The dentine is covered by enamel over the crown of the tooth, and by cementum over the root of the tooth (Figure 6.2). The details of each tissue are given below.

Enamel

Enamel is the outer layer of the crown.

- It is harder than bone
- It is made up of **96% inorganic** (mineral) crystals arranged as **prisms** in an organic matrix
- The main mineral crystals are **hydroxyapatite**
- The prisms lie at 90 degrees to the junction with the underlying layer of dentine
- The junction is called the **amelodentinal junction** (ADJ)
- Enamel contains no nerves nor blood vessels and therefore cannot experience sensitivity
- It is a non-living tissue which cannot grow and repair itself, but it can **remineralise** after an acid attack
- Enamel can exchange minerals between itself and the oral cavity, especially fluoride, to form **fluorapatite crystals**, which make the enamel surface harder still and more resistant to acid attack

- Enamel is formed before tooth eruption by **ameloblast cells**, which lie at the amelodentinal junction
- Enamel lies at its thickest at the occlusal (biting) surface of the tooth, and at its thinnest at the cervical margin (neck of the tooth)
- It is translucent in appearance

Dentine

The dentine is the layer beneath the enamel in the crown and cementum in the root, and forms the bulk of the tooth.

- It is up to **80% inorganic** in structure
- It is composed of **hollow tubules** containing **fibrils,** which are the sensory endings from the cells forming the dentine
- Dentine is therefore a living tissue, and can transmit sensitivity
- It is formed by **odontoblast cells**, which lie at the edge of the pulp chamber
- It can repair itself by producing **'secondary dentine'**
- Secondary dentine also forms within the tooth as part of the natural ageing process
- Dentine is yellowish and gives individual teeth their colour, and it is also slightly elastic
- Dental caries (tooth decay) progresses more rapidly through dentine because of its hollow nature, than it does through enamel

Pulp

This is the soft tissue within the centre of the tooth structure, enclosed by the dentine layer.

- The pulp contains sensory nerves and blood vessels
- It allows the tooth to feel hot, cold, touch and pain by stimulation of the fibrils in dentine
- The blood vessels and nerves enter the tooth through the apical foramen, at the end of each root apex
- These tissues are enclosed within the pulp chamber of the tooth
- The pulp chamber is lined by odontoblast cells
- The gradual formation of secondary dentine with age causes the pulp chamber to decrease in size and become narrower, making endodontic treatment more difficult
- The pulp chamber can also become blocked with pulp stones, which are lumps of calcified tissue similar to gall stones

Cementum

The cementum is the outer layer covering the dentine of the tooth root.

- It normally lies beneath the gingivae
- It allows the attachment of the tooth to the supporting structure of the peri-odontal ligament

Anatomy of the supporting structures

The supporting structures are those found around the roots of the teeth and hold the teeth in their sockets (Figure 6.3). The hold is not rigid, and this allows the teeth to 'bounce' in their sockets during chewing, etc. This shock absorber effect helps to protect teeth from fracture during normal usage. The details of each tissue is given below.

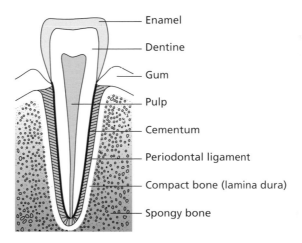

Figure 6.3 Anatomy of supporting structures. Source: *Levison's Textbook for Dental Nurses*, 10th edn, C. Hollins, 2008, Wiley-Blackwell.

Alveolar bone

Alveolar bone is present as the bony extensions of the maxilla and mandible, where the teeth are formed and from where they erupt into the mouth.

- It is a special bone found only in the jaws
- Its sole purpose is to support the teeth during their lifetime
- When teeth are extracted, the alveolar bone gradually resorbs away and disappears
- The outer layer of the alveolar bone is made up of hard compact bone, with the surface being called the **lamina dura**
- The inner layer is made up of cancellous bone, which is sponge-like in appear-ance to allow blood vessels and nerves to run through it

- The alveolar bone is covered in a specialised **alveolar mucosa** (soft tissue) to form the **gingivae** (gums) around the necks of the teeth
- Destruction of the alveolar bone can occur during periodontal disease

Periodontal ligament

The periodontal ligament is a specialised fibrous tissue which attaches the teeth to the alveolar bone and the surrounding gingivae.

- The fibres are made up of a protein called **collagen**
- They run in several different directions from the cementum to the alveolar bone and gingivae, and from the neck of one tooth to that of its neighbour
- The ligament acts as a shock absorber when the tooth undergoes normal chewing movements, allowing the tooth to 'bounce' a little in its socket and avoid its fracture
- Destruction of the periodontal ligament occurs during periodontal disease

Gingivae

Gingivae is the scientific term for the gums.

- In health, they are **light pink** in colour with a **stippled** (orange peel) surface, although variations will occur in different ethnic groups of patients
- They form a 2 mm crevice (**gingival crevice**) around the necks of each tooth, above the periodontal ligament
- **Gingivitis** occurs when the gingivae become inflamed
- Inflamed gingivae are **red** and shiny, with a **swollen** appearance

With the anatomical details of the teeth and their supporting structures in mind, the main types of oral disease that affect them can be considered in relation to the oral and general health of the patient.

Dental caries

Dental caries (tooth decay) is a **bacterial disease** of the mineralised tissues of the tooth, where the strong mineral components of the enamel are **demineralised** (dissolved) and the softer organic components of the dentine are broken down to form **cavities**.

Many different types of bacteria are normally present in the mouth, and the main ones associated with dental caries are:

- *Streptococcus mutans*
- *Streptococcus sanguis*
- Some lactobacilli

These bacteria use foods taken into the mouth as a source for their own nutrition. They digest food debris and produce **weak organic acids** as a by-product (for example, lactic acid). The acids are responsible for attacking the mineral structure of the teeth and causing their **demineralisation**. This can be summarised by the acidogenic theory of caries, which was first described in 1882:

Bacteria plus food → weak organic acids → demineralisation → cavities

Not all the foods that are eaten can be broken down by the bacteria into the weak organic acids involved in dental caries, the main food type required being **carbo-hydrates**. Foods that consist of fats and proteins are not relevant to the onset of caries.

The relevant factors that must be present to allow a cavity to form in a tooth are:

- The presence of certain types of bacteria
- Carbohydrate foods
- The production of the weak organic acids from the food, by the bacteria
- Adequate time for the acids to attack the tooth structure and cause demineralisation; this may also occur when carbohydrate meals are eaten very frequently

Effect of the diet on caries

Certain foods produce more acids than others, the most productive being some types of carbohydrates that are processed during food preparation by the food manufacturers. These tend to contain **non-milk extrinsic sugars** (NMES), which are sugars not naturally present in the food but are added during the preparation, manufacture or processing of food, for consumption by the public. The commonest NMES used in food production are **sucrose**, **glucose** and **dextrose**. Other types of sugars available, and which are relatively harmless include:

- Intrinsic sugars which occur naturally in foods, such as **fructose** in fruit
- Milk extrinsic sugars, especially **lactose**

Unfortunately, carbohydrates tend to be the cheapest food source of readily available energy, and are therefore consumed in great quantities in the majority of households. The higher the processed carbohydrate content of the diet, the greater the tendency to develop dental caries. Acidic drinks, especially pure fruit juices and carbonated 'pops', are the other source of acids and/or NMES that are associated with dental caries.

Role of dental plaque

The bacteria involved in the onset of dental caries are not freely floating around the oral cavity, but have become attached to the tooth surfaces by incorporating themselves into a sticky protein-containing film called **dental plaque**. This appears on the teeth as a creamy deposit, often very difficult to detect by the untrained eye, but easily made visible by the use of **disclosing agents** (Figure 6.4).

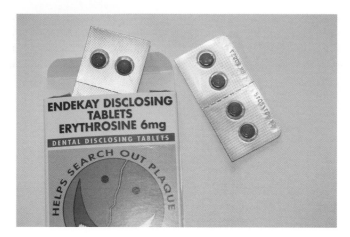

Figure 6.4 Disclosing tablets.

Disclosing agents are presented as a tablet or liquid form of a vegetable dye, usually red, blue or purple, which can be chewed and swilled around the mouth by the patient. They stain all the bacterial plaque present, making it easily visible to the patient and greatly assisting them to remove it effectively using oral hygiene techniques. Unexpected stagnation areas are shown up as deeply stained zones, indicating that special oral hygiene efforts are required to clean them sufficiently (Figure 6.5). Suitable patients should be encouraged to use these products at home, on a regular basis.

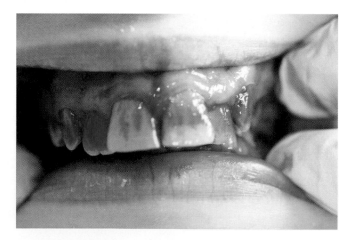

Figure 6.5 Use of disclosing agent to stain plaque. Source: *Basic Guide to Dental Procedures*, C. Hollins, 2008, Wiley-Blackwell, Oxford.

The dental plaque forms all over the tooth surface, but is easily dislodged from the smooth surfaces of the teeth by normal tongue and oral soft tissue movements. Other areas of the tooth surface will afford the bacteria some protection from dislodgement, such as in the gingival crevice around the necks of the teeth, and on the rough margins of fillings and other restorations. These are called **stagnation areas**, and the bacterial plaque forms within them after just two hours of being removed previously (such as by toothbrushing).

The bacteria produce sticky sugars (polysaccharides) themselves during food debris digestion, which are also a source of weak organic acids. However, the process of acid production increases considerably when carbohydrate foods containing NMES are eaten, such that acids are produced within minutes by the plaque bacteria and remain at their maximum strength for about the following 20 minutes, causing demineralisation of the tooth enamel. At this point, the acids tend to be neutralised by the **saliva** present in the patient's mouth, and the demineralisation process ends.

Process of tooth demineralisation

The oral cavity is bathed in saliva, which helps to create an environment that is neither acidic nor alkaline. This can be measured as a **pH value**, where neutral is measured as 7, acidic conditions range from 6 down to 1, and alkaline conditions from 8 up to 14. The process of tooth demineralisation occurs as follows.

(1)   The oral cavity is normally pH 7
(2)   The pH drops as the action of the plaque bacteria produces weak organic acids
(3)   This occurs within minutes of carbohydrates being ingested
(4)   The critical pH is 5.5, as at this point conditions within the oral cavity are acidic enough to allow tooth demineralisation to occur
(5)   It then takes up to 2 hours for the pH to rise to 7 again
(6)   This occurs as the minerals contained in saliva act to neutralise the acids
(7)   So, the more frequent the carbohydrate consumption occurs, the longer the periods of lowered pH will be, and the more chance that cavities will be formed
(8)   Any areas where plaque accumulates and is not removed by the normal self-cleansing actions of saliva and the oral soft tissues are more prone to prolonged acid attack. These areas are the stagnation areas, and include occlusal pits and fissures, interproximal areas, and ledges on poor dental restorations

Method of cavity formation

Microscopically, the process of demineralisation and cavity formation within the tooth structure occurs as follows (Figure 6.6):

(1)   Following the action of the plaque bacteria on food debris, weak organic acids are produced which attack the enamel surface and appear as '**white spots**'

(2)   The acid attack follows the prism structure of the enamel, and also any exposed cementum

(3)   Demineralisation occurs, and if prolonged or frequent enough to prevent the enamel undergoing **remineralisation** and repair, the mineral structure is eventually destroyed

(4)   Areas of remineralisation and repair are often seen as **brown marks** at contact points, following the extraction or loss of a neighbouring tooth

(5)   Otherwise, caries progresses deeper in the enamel and reaches the amelodentinal junction (ADJ), the point where the dentine layer of the tooth begins

(6)   Odontoblast cells at the ADJ react to the advancing bacterial attack by forming '**secondary dentine**' in an attempt to protect the underlying pulp of the tooth

(7)   However, once the caries reaches dentine, it progresses more rapidly due to the hollow tubular nature of this tissue

(8)   The lower mineral content of dentine also makes it **less resistant** to acid attack

(9)   The nerve fibrils lying in the dentinal tubules become stimulated, the pulp becomes inflamed and **reversible pulpitis** develops

(10) The patient will experience temperature sensitivity and pain associated with chewing

(11) At this point, the caries can still be removed and the tooth restored to full function by placing a filling in the cavity. If not, then the progressing caries front causes the dentine to shrink in on itself, and the overlying enamel becomes brittle and weak as it loses its support

(12) Normal occlusal forces are often enough to fracture pieces off, and a **cavity** is formed, which exposes more dentine to the oral cavity

(13) Secondary dentine production becomes outstripped now by the speed of the carious attack towards the pulp

(14) The patient will experience more pain and eventually lose the function of the tooth

(15) The pulpitis becomes **irreversible** once the caries penetrates close to the pulp chamber, the pain becomes constant and tends to disturb the patient's sleep with its severity

(16) Once the pulp chamber is breached, a **carious exposure** of the contents occurs

(17) The tooth can now only be treated by endodontics or extraction

(18) As the pulp contents become infected and die, necrotic tissue and bacteria flow out of the apical foramen into the surrounding periapical tissue

(19) They become trapped here and develop quickly into an **acute periapical abscess**, with consequent swelling, severe pain and malaise, or develop slowly into a painless chronic abscess

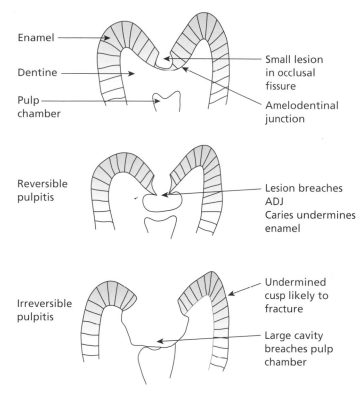

Figure 6.6 Cavity formation. Source: *Levison's Textbook for Dental Nurses*, 10th edn, C. Hollins, 2008, Wiley-Blackwell.

The role of saliva in oral health

The oral soft tissues in health are constantly bathed in saliva, a watery secretion from the three pairs of major salivary glands, and also from numerous minor salivary glands present in the cheeks and lips.

Saliva consists of:

- Water as a transport agent
- Inorganic ions such as calcium and phosphate
- Digestive enzyme, ptyalin (salivary amylase)
- Antibodies (called immunoglobulins)
- White blood cells

These constituents have the following functions:

- The ions are released as required to act as buffering agents to help control the pH of the oral environment by neutralising acids

- High ion contents produce thick, stringy saliva which gives teeth good caries protection but allows much calculus formation to occur
- Low ion contents produce watery saliva and low calculus formation, but gives poor protection against caries
- The watery nature of the saliva helps the mouth to self-cleanse by dislodging food debris from around the teeth before being swallowed
- It also moistens food and the oral soft tissues, allowing speech and swallowing (deglutition) to occur
- It also allows food ingredients to be dissolved so that they are able to be tasted, as the taste buds on the tongue are only stimulated by dissolved substances
- Both antibodies and white blood cells are present for defence purposes, as they are released to help fight oral infections

Reduced salivary flow

This has important consequences for the oral health team, for the following reasons:

- Reduced self-cleansing and buffering increases the risk of caries and periodontal disease
- Poor lubrication will cause difficulty in swallowing and speaking
- Reduced flow will affect taste capabilities
- Poor self-cleansing will leave food debris in the mouth and cause **halitosis** (bad breath)
- Reduced flow will hinder the natural retention of dentures

Reduced salivary flow produces the condition **xerostomia**, or dry mouth. It can be caused by:

- Normal age-related changes to the salivary glands
- Dehydration
- Some autoimmune disorders, especially Sjögren's syndrome
- Several drugs, including diuretics, some anti-depressants and beta blockers

The opposite condition to reduced salivary flow, that of excessive saliva production, is called **ptyalism**, and is often seen in patients with periodontal disease. It can also occur during pregnancy and in patients with Parkinson's disease.

Periodontal disease

The term periodontal disease actually covers a group of diseases which affect the supporting structures of the teeth, known as the periodontium:

- The gingivae (gums)
- The periodontal ligament (sometimes known as membrane)
- The alveolar bone

Periodontal disease is the main cause of tooth loss in adults. Like dental caries, it occurs due to the presence of bacterial dental plaque on the teeth, but specifically at the necks of the teeth where the periodontal tissues begin.

The bacterial production of weak organic acids has no relevance to periodontal disease, rather it is the irritation of the bacteria and the poisons they produce on the periodontium that causes inflammation and soft tissue destruction. In addition, the hardening of the original plaque into dental calculus (tartar) allows the bacteria to remain in position and cause more inflammation and destruction.

As the initial plaque bacteria cause gingival inflammation and swelling, specialised bacteria begin to colonise the area too, in particular:

■ *Actinomyces* species
■ *Porphyromonas* species

These specialised bacteria are capable of surviving in an environment low in oxygen, such as occurs down the sides of the tooth roots under the inflamed gingivae – they are referred to as **anaerobic bacteria**.

The relevant factors that must be present to allow periodontal disease to develop are:

■ The presence of bacterial plaque at the gingival crevice
■ Adequate time to allow the bacteria to produce toxins (poisons)
■ The presence of specialised anaerobic bacteria that can survive with little oxygen

When the bacterial plaque accumulation is recent and affects only the gingival tissues, it causes inflammation of the gingivae – this is called **gingivitis**. When the plaque accumulation is longer standing, gingivitis has been present for some time and the deeper periodontal tissues become inflamed, a more serious condition develops – this is called **periodontitis**.

Periodontium in health

When all of the periodontal tissues are healthy, the overall appearance of the periodontium is as follows (Figure 6.7):

■ Each tooth sits in a socket of alveolar bone, which surrounds each root of the tooth
■ The tooth is attached to the bone by the fibres of the periodontal ligament, which run from the bone to the cementum overlying the root dentine
■ The bone and periodontal ligament are covered by the mucous membrane of the gingivae lining the alveolar ridges
■ The gingivae is attached to the neck of each tooth at a specialised site called the junctional epithelium
■ In health, a gingival crevice no deeper than 2 mm exists, to form a 'gutter' around each tooth
■ Other periodontal ligament fibres run from the alveolar bone crest to the neck of the tooth, and from the neck of the tooth into the gingival papilla

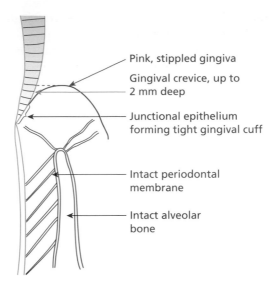

Figure 6.7 Periodontium in health.

The appearance of a healthy periodontium is summarised as:

- Pink colour (different ethnic variations will occur), often stippled like orange peel
- Tight gingival cuff around the tooth
- Gingival crevice present, no deeper than 2 mm
- No bleeding occurs when the crevice is gently probed during dental examination
- Knife-edge papillae present between the teeth
- Subgingivally, the periodontal ligament and alveolar bone are intact

The initial phase of periodontal disease is gingivitis, and it is fully reversible by carrying out effective oral hygiene techniques on a regular basis.

Sequence of events leading to gingivitis

In the absence of effective oral hygiene methods, gingivitis will develop, as follows:

(1) Poor oral hygiene methods allow the build up of bacterial dental plaque, particularly at the gingival crevice region of the teeth
(2) The bacteria within the plaque use food debris to nourish themselves and allow the colony to increase in size
(3) The bacteria produce **toxic (poisonous) by-products** as they digest the food debris
(4) These by-products irritate the gingivae in direct contact with them, and cause inflammation – this is called **chronic gingivitis**

(5) The inflamed gingivae swell and become reddened, and form **false pockets** around the necks of the teeth

(6) False pockets allow more plaque to develop as self-cleansing becomes impossible, and the plaque then extends below the gingival margin

(7) The continued action of saliva on plaque allows inorganic ions to be incorporated into the plaque structure, and **dental calculus (tartar)** forms

(8) Calculus formation can occur above the gingival margin, and is called **supragingival calculus** which is yellow in colour. It can also occur below the gingival margin, and is then called **subgingival calculus**, which is brown/black in colour due to the incorporation of blood pigments

(9) The calculus has a rough surface, allowing more plaque to form over it, and also irritating the gingivae further

(10) The abrasion of the calculus and the chemical action of the toxins causes painless **micro-ulceration** of the gingivae, and they will then bleed on touching or dental probing

The visible appearance and bleeding on probing of the gingivae are the classic diagnostic signs of chronic gingivitis (Figure 6.8).

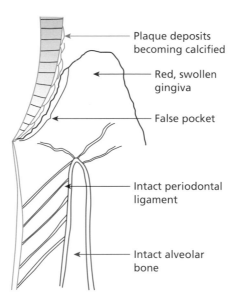

Plaque deposits becoming calcified

Red, swollen gingiva

False pocket

Intact periodontal ligament

Intact alveolar bone

Figure 6.8 Chronic gingivitis.

Sequence of events leading to periodontitis

If efficient oral hygiene measures are not carried out by the patient to remove the plaque, and by the dental team to remove any calculus present, the deeper periodontal tissues become affected and periodontitis develops, as follows:

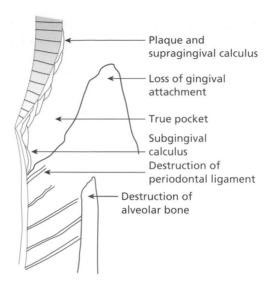

Figure 6.9 Chronic periodontitis.

(1) Non-treatment of chronic gingivitis allows the toxins to build up, and eventually enter the underlying gingival tissues through the micro-ulcerated areas
(2) The toxins then gradually destroy the periodontal ligament so that a **true pocket** forms, as the periodontal attachment to the tooth is lost from the neck of the tooth and down the side of the root (Figure 6.9)
(3) Further plaque develops and becomes mineralised, causing further irritation and more toxin infiltration
(4) The toxins eventually begin destroying the alveolar bone, and the tooth loosens in its socket and is eventually lost

Gingivitis can begin in childhood, but periodontitis can take many years to result in tooth loss. It is usually painless and therefore can be present undetected for years by the patient, unless it is diagnosed by a dentist. Periodontal disease also tends to have active phases, where much tissue destruction occurs, and quiescent phases with little destructive activity.

Plaque retention factors

Dental plaque forms in all mouths within hours of the teeth being cleaned. Periodontal disease is caused by plaque action on the periodontium, but its accumulation can be exacerbated by several factors:

- **Poor oral hygiene** on a regular basis, by the patient
- **Mal-aligned teeth** causing stagnation areas
- **Mouth breathing** or an incompetent lip seal, allowing drying of the oral soft tissues and any plaque already present on the teeth

■ **Small oral aperture**, making adequate toothbrushing difficult
■ **Poor dentistry**, with overhanging restorations and inadequate contact points creating stagnation areas
■ **Poorly designed** orthodontic or prosthetic appliances, causing stagnation areas

Once present, the extent of the periodontal disease can become worse due to any of the following factors:

■ **Smoking** – this reduces blood flow in the gingival tissues and masks the presence of the inflammation
■ **Hormonal imbalances** – such as those that occur during pregnancy and puberty
■ **Medical conditions** – which compromise a patient's immune response so that they are unable to fight the inflammation sufficiently, such as:
    – Diabetes
    – Vitamin C deficiency
    – Leukaemia
    – Blood disorders
    – Stress
■ **Drugs** that cause overgrowth of the gingival tissues (**gingival hyperplasia**), such as:
    – Phenytoin (used for the control of epilepsy)
    – Nifedipine (used for the control of hypertension)
    – Cyclosporin (used for the prevention of organ transplant rejection)

Other periodontal conditions

Other periodontal conditions that can occur, besides gingivitis and periodontitis, are summarised below. They are all related to poor oral hygiene in one way or another.

Acute necrotising ulcerative gingivitis

This is a condition that often occurs in teenagers and young adults.

■ It is directly related to poor oral hygiene
■ It has a sudden onset
■ The patient experiences **very painful gingivitis**
■ **Ulceration** of the gingival papillae occurs
■ The patient has halitosis
■ It is a specific infection with either *Treponema vincentii* or *Bacillus fusiformis*
■ It is treated with the antibiotic **metronidazole** followed by a thorough **scaling** and **oral hygiene instruction**
■ The patient also has a short course of chlorhexidine mouthwash (such as 'Corsodyl')

Lateral periodontal abscess

This is **acute abscess** formation in an existing periodontal pocket.

■ The condition occurs on the side of the root, that is **laterally**, of a vital tooth
■ It is treated by **draining** the pus present followed by thorough **scaling** of the area and local administration of **metronidazole** into the periodontal pocket
■ The patient is given oral hygiene instruction

Sub-acute pericoronitis

This is an infection of the **operculum** (gum flap) of a partially erupted tooth.

■ The condition especially occurs around the **lower third molars**
■ It is due to poor oral hygiene of the operculum, often coupled with trauma from the opposing tooth
■ It is treated by **irrigating** all food debris from under operculum followed by oral hygiene instruction and advice on the use of mouthwashes
■ Broad spectrum antibiotics are given if the patient has a raised temperature (pyrexia)
■ An **operculectomy** is carried out if the condition reoccurs (surgical removal of operculum) or extraction of the opposing tooth to prevent further soft tissue trauma

Oral cancer

The final condition that may affect the oral health of a patient is oral cancer, and all dentists carry out checks for any suspicious lesions within the oral cavity whenever they carry out a dental examination. Cancer can occur in the soft tissues of the mouth, in the salivary glands, or in the bones associated with the oral cavity. However, 90% of oral cancers affect the soft tissues of the mouth, predominantly as **squamous cell carcinoma** (SCC).

The suggested causative factors of SCC are:

■ **Tobacco habits**, as all contain chemicals which can cause cancer (carcinogens)
■ **High alcohol consumption**, as alcohol acts as a solvent for the carcinogens and allows easier entry into the tissues
■ Smoking and alcohol together are the highest risk factors possible
■ Excessive exposure to **sunlight** in fair-skinned people can cause cancer of the lower lip
■ Research is ongoing into the effects of diet on oral cancer, especially in relation to low vitamin A intake, high fat and red meat intake, and low iron intake
■ Some patients have a genetic predisposition to cancer

The effects of smoking on general health are well known, and include increased risk of several types of cancer, as well as heart disease and respiratory problems, but the effects on oral health are not so well advertised.

These are as follows:

- More than 4600 new cases of oral cancer per year in the UK
- Development of oral white patches (leukoplakia), which are capable of becoming malignant
- Periodontal disease and tooth loss
- Impaired oral wound healing
- Tendency to post-extraction infections ('dry socket')
- Stained teeth
- Halitosis (bad breath)

Smoking causes 20% of all deaths in the UK (Department of Health, 1998), and there is evidence to suggest that more women and more teenagers are starting to smoke nowadays too. Some ethnic groups also chew tobacco *paan* and betel nuts, both habits having a known link to oral cancer.

The signs and symptoms of SCC that the dentist looks out for when examining a patient are:

- A painless ulcer or lump in the mouth which fails to heal within three to six weeks
- This is usually associated with the tongue or the floor of the mouth
- Alternatively, a white or red patch on the buccal mucosa or tongue

A blue dye is being developed which stains cancerous lesions and should prove invaluable for detecting early lesions, which are often invisible to the naked eye. Early detection and referral for treatment increases the survival rate, but even then there is only around a 55% survival rate for five years. Thus, as with all cancers, prevention is better than cure and the dental team has an important role in the education of high-risk patients.

With an understanding of how the main oral diseases occur, the methods available to the patient and the dental team in preventing or controlling them can now be considered. The role of the dental team in offering support and information to patients on the protection of their oral health is of great importance, and can have a 'knock-on' effect on the improvement of their general health too.

Prevention of dental caries

As identified previously, caries occurs due to a combination of certain types of bacteria being present within dental plaque that use NMES to produce acids that cause enamel demineralisation, There are therefore three main areas of prevention available to the patient and the dental team.

■ **Increase the tooth resistance to acid attack** – by incorporating fluoride into the enamel structure
■ **Modification of the diet** – to include fewer cariogenic foods and drinks, and to reduce their frequency of intake
■ **Control the build up of bacterial plaque** – to practise its regular removal by using good oral hygiene techniques

Fluoride

This is the single most important salt in strengthening teeth and making them less susceptible to acid attack and damage by dental caries. It occurs naturally in the water in some areas, and is added artificially to water supplies in other areas during the process of water fluoridation, as an oral health measure to aid in the reduction of caries incidence.

Fluoride can be taken into the enamel structure by the direct application of various oral health products onto the teeth (this is called **topical fluoride application**), or by being taken internally with food and drink products (this is called **systemic fluoride application**). It acts in the following ways.

■ It can be taken into the crystalline structure of enamel to form **fluorapatite crystals**. These replace the normal hydroxyapatite crystal structure of the enamel with fluorapatite crystals
■ Fluorapatite can resist acid attack to a greater degree than hydroxyapatite, and thereby reduce the solubility of the enamel in acid
■ Fluoride also has an inhibitory effect on the **feeding rate** of oral bacteria. This effect produces less weak acids and polysaccharides to initiate the carious attack

The protective effect of fluoride on the teeth is at its best after they have formed and erupted into the oral cavity. Many oral hygiene products are now available which contain fluoride to allow their regular use by the general public.

Topical fluorides

These are administered externally to the tooth surface, either by the patient or the dental team, to provide a continual source of fluoride directly onto the enamel.

(1) For use by the patient:
■ **Fluoride toothpastes** containing the current recommended dose for all patients of 1000 parts per million (ppm), up to 1500 ppm for use by adults at high risk of developing caries
■ A minimum of twice daily brushing is advised to achieve maximum benefits
■ Patients should be advised **not to rinse out** after brushing, as it washes the fluoride away and is less effective
■ **Fluoride mouthwashes** for regular use by those with a high caries risk, and for those undergoing orthodontic treatment

- **Dental floss** and tape impregnated with fluoride, for delivery to the interproximal areas

(2) For use by the dental team:

- **Fluoride gels** applied in trays over all of the teeth for several minutes, they are administered at each examination appointment and are especially useful for patients with special needs and a high caries risk
- **Fluoride varnish** applied to individual teeth showing areas of previous acid attack

Systemic fluorides

These are usually provided as a public health measure to reduce the incidence of dental caries in a population. Whatever their form of delivery, the fluoride is ingested and then taken from the digestive tract to be incorporated into the enamel structure.

- **Fluoridated water** supplies by the addition of the optimum concentration of **1 ppm** to drinking water
- Naturally occurring fluoridated water supplies, in some parts of the world
- Addition of fluoride to table salt, but not in the UK
- **Fluoride drops and tablets**, available on prescription for children, to be taken daily during the period of tooth development (up to 13 years), the doses required vary with age and the amount of fluoride in the water supply
- Usually reserved for those with medical or physical conditions which would make dental treatment difficult, or for those whose general health would suffer if caries occurred

Enamel fluorosis

Enamel fluorosis is a condition which occurs when excessive fluoride is ingested during enamel formation. The teeth erupt with mottled white areas in the enamel surface which vary in severity but can be quite unsightly. Restorative techniques are available to mask the areas but the condition is prevented by ensuring that parents receive the correct advice regarding fluoride.

- Children below 8 years should have toothbrushing supervised by an adult, to prevent ingestion of the toothpaste
- The amount of toothpaste should be kept to a minimum and allowed just twice daily
- The parents must ensure that children spit the toothpaste out after use, not swallow it
- All fluoride supplements should only be prescribed as necessary, and at the correct dosage dependent on the local water fluoridation levels
- The dental team must have knowledge of any local water fluoridation levels

In addition, the dentist, therapist or hygienist can carry out the technique of **fissure sealing** the occlusal pits and fissures of the posterior teeth of children, soon after these teeth have erupted. A resin-based material is used to seal these naturally occurring stagnation areas, therefore preventing damage from acid attacks and avoiding the onset of dental caries.

Modification of the diet

The required modification of the diet is in particular reference to NMES and acidic drinks: their amount and frequency of consumption. Obviously, the greater the amount of potentially cariogenic products eaten and drunk, the more likely it is that the patient will experience dental caries. Each episode of NMES ingestion will lower the pH of the oral environment as the plaque bacteria produce their weak organic acids, and the tooth enamel will be at risk of demineralisation until the pH balance is restored.

If much of the diet is made up of these types of food and drink, or if they are consumed on a frequent basis throughout the day, the pH balance will not be restored often enough to prevent tooth damage from occurring. When giving dietary advice to patients, it helps if they are made aware of which food and drink products are safe or harmful, in relation to dental caries. This is especially important with what are known as 'hidden sugars' in foods – where NMES have been artificially added during the manufacturing and processing of foods for taste and preservation purposes, very often in foods that patients would not expect to be harmful to their teeth. A simple list of 'good' and 'bad' foods and drinks can then be developed.

Good snacks:

- Non-citrus fruit, such as apples, pears, peaches
- Vegetables such as carrots and celery, which act as 'detergent foods' by cleaning plaque off the teeth during chewing
- Plain crisps, although the amount of salt present must also be considered for the overall health of the patient
- Low fat cheese
- Unsweetened yoghurt

Bad snacks:

- Sweets and other confectionery
- Biscuits and cakes
- Carbonated drinks
- Pure citrus fruit juices
- Tea and coffee with sugar
- Citrus fruits such as oranges, clementines, lemons, satsumas, and limes

Those foods containing 'hidden sugars' can be identified by reading the contents label of each product. These include:

- Cooking sauces, especially those with a tomato base
- Table sauces, including ketchup
- Flavoured crisps
- Fruits tinned in syrup
- Some tinned vegetables, including baked beans and the like
- Some breakfast cereals
- Jams, marmalades and chutneys
- Some low fat products, as sugar is added to improve their taste
- Tinned fish and meat in tomato sauce
- Soups
- Savoury crackers and biscuits
- Some processed ready meals

Although the incidence of caries is gradually reducing in this country, it remains a major health problem. It is most prevalent in younger age groups, so parental support is imperative if oral health messages are to be successful. The following dietary advice should be given:

- Eat a healthy diet with foods of low cariogenic (caries-causing) potential
- Follow the 'good snacks' list given previously
- Limit any cariogenic foods to mealtimes, so that they can be neutralised by the increased flow of saliva that occurs while chewing
- Avoid carbonated drinks and confine fruit juices to mealtimes only
- Use diet sheets to determine if any hidden sugars are being taken
- Advise mothers on the damage caused by using cariogenic drinks in baby feeders
- Parents should be encouraged to request sugar-free medicines for their children whenever possible

Control of bacterial plaque

Plaque forms within hours on newly cleaned tooth surfaces, due to the action of oral bacteria on foods. Unless removed, the plaque will allow dental caries to develop, and that formed around the gingival crevice will be involved in the onset of gingivitis and eventually periodontitis.

Controlling bacterial plaque on a daily basis is the main method available to patients to assist themselves in the protection of their oral health. It is the role of the dental team to ensure that the patients are taught the correct oral hygiene methods suitable to them, and that they carry them out on a frequent enough basis to avoid damage to their oral health. In addition, the dental team will remove any calculus that has formed by scaling the patients' teeth, and ensure that all plaque retention factors are reduced to a minimum.

Plaque can be easily and regularly removed by the patient at home, by tooth brushing, interdental cleaning and using mouthwashes.

This is carried out to remove plaque that has formed on the smooth surfaces of the teeth, and in the gingival crevice at the necks of the teeth. The advice to be given to patients is as follows:

■ They should carry out either manual or electric tooth brushing on a **twice daily basis**, to remove plaque accumulations at the gingival margins, and on the easily accessible smooth surfaces of the teeth

■ Many different makes of toothbrush are available, with various bristle designs and intended actions for each (Figure 6.10)

■ Several methods of tooth brushing are recommended, but the technique is irrelevant as long as it achieves the aim of plaque removal, without being so vigorous that gingival or tooth damage occurs (such as **toothbrush abrasion**)

■ Several makes of **re-chargeable electric toothbrush** are currently available, and these are of great value to those with physical disabilities or with difficult to reach oral areas (Figure 6.11)

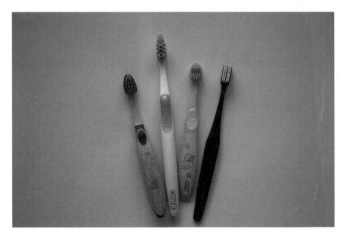

Figure 6.10 Types of toothbrush.

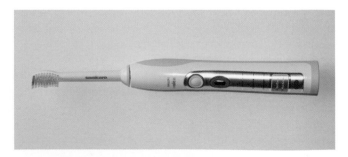

Figure 6.11 Sonicare® toothbrush.

- Different **head sizes** are available, and obviously children require smaller headed toothbrushes than adults
- Several **interdental toothbrushes** are also available and invaluable for cleaning plaque from necessary stagnation areas, such as fixed orthodontic appliances, but on the whole they are too bulky for actual interproximal cleaning unless the patient's teeth are spaced
- Parents will need to **supervise** or carry out effective tooth brushing for children under 8 years of age, by standing behind them and brushing all areas of the mouth thoroughly, while allowing the child to watch in a mirror if possible (Figure 6.12)

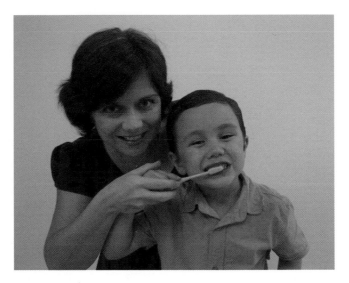

Figure 6.12 Supervising toothbrushing of child. © Joon Chai Yeoh. Reproduced with permission. Source: *Levison's Textbook for Dental Nurses*, 10th edn, C. Hollins, 2008, Wiley-Blackwell.

Toothpastes

A huge variety of toothpastes are available nowadays, from shops' own brands to specialised ones with ingredients to fight against all aspects of common oral disease. Individual recommendations should be given for any patient requesting advice from the dental team (Figure 6.13).

- Over 95% of toothpastes available in the UK contain **fluoride**, as *sodium monofluorophosphate* and *sodium fluoride* at 1000 ppm
- **High fluoride** toothpastes containing 2800 ppm, for use by adult patients with an existing high caries rate or an excessive risk to develop caries
- Several other toothpastes contain ingredients specifically to slow down **calculus** formation

- Many now contain the substance *triclosan* combined with zinc, which acts as an **antiseptic plaque suppressant**
- Some toothpastes are specifically formulated to help **relieve sensitivity**, and contain *stannous fluoride*
- Others are advertised as '**whitening toothpastes**' and act to remove surface tooth staining by the use of abrasives, or more recently with biological enzyme systems
- More recent developments have included toothpastes designed to help protect teeth against **acid erosion**

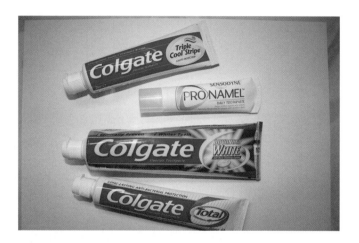

Figure 6.13 Types of toothpaste.

Interdental cleaning

Several oral health aids are available to assist patients to remove plaque that has formed between the teeth, or interdentally, as these areas cannot usually be accessed by ordinary tooth brushing alone.

- **Dental floss** and **dental tape** are widely used by many patients to achieve interdental plaque removal, however, correct usage depends to some extent on manual dexterity and on sound oral health instruction (Figure 6.14)
- '**Flossette-style**' handles, which hold pieces of floss in place for the patient so that they can floss with one hand, make the procedure less difficult, especially for posterior teeth where access is difficult for the majority of patients (Figure 6.15)
- '**Bottlebrush style**' interdental brushes are available for cleaning in larger interdental areas, as well as around the individual brackets of fixed orthodontic appliances (Figure 6.16)
- Woodsticks are also available to dislodge food debris from interproximal areas, as well as to massage the gingivae in these areas. Their use should

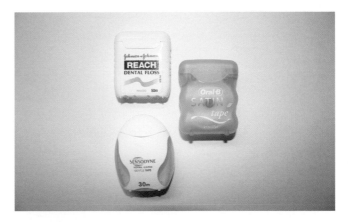

Figure 6.14 Dental flosses and tapes.

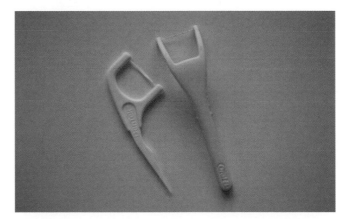

Figure 6.15 Flossettes®.

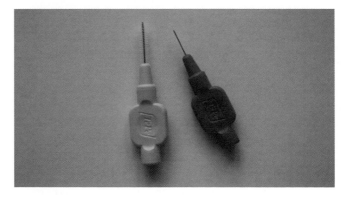

Figure 6.16 Interdental brushes.

be restricted to competent adults whenever possible, as they can easily get stuck into the gingivae and cause problems if used incorrectly or by the inexperienced

Mouthwashes

As with toothpastes, there are a vast number of mouthwashes available for home use, from shops' own brands to more specialised types with specific oral health roles (Figure 6.17).

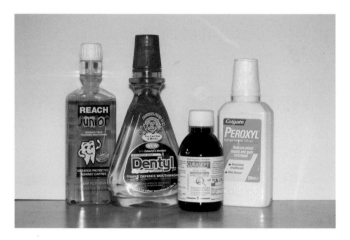

Figure 6.17 Types of mouthwash.

- General use mouthwashes contain various ingredients to promote good oral hygiene, including *sodium fluoride* and *triclosan*
- Others are specialised for use on sensitive teeth
- Some are used specifically in the presence of oral soft tissue inflammation as a first aid measure, and contain **hydrogen peroxide**
- Specialised mouthwashes are also available for patients with both acute and chronic periodontal infections, and contain *chlorhexidine* which is an **antiseptic plaque suppressant**

Prevention of periodontal disease

As indicated previously, the main cause of periodontal disease is consistently poor oral hygiene, along with contributory factors such as smoking, and in some cases an unfortunate genetic predisposition to periodontal problems. The prevention of periodontal disease can be achieved in most patients, whereas the disease can only be controlled in others:

- **Control the build-up of bacterial plaque** – using good oral hygiene tech-niques, as discussed previously
- **Modify the contributory factors** – by giving advice on smoking cessation, for instance
- **Control the host response** – in patients predisposed to periodontal problems, by more frequent dental attendance for monitoring and evaluation, and inter-vention where necessary

Control of bacterial plaque

The control of bacterial plaque by good oral hygiene measures has been discussed previously in relation to preventing dental caries, and the same information and advice is relevant in the prevention of periodontal disease.

Specific instruction by the dental team on effective tooth brushing of the gin-gival crevice area of the teeth may be required, as well as advice on the use of oral health products that contain active ingredients to reduce calculus build-up in susceptible patients.

Modifying the contributory factors

Modification of the contributory factors may not always be possible, especially where the contributory factor is a medical condition such as diabetes. However, in those cases the dental team can at least advise the patient on the increased import-ance of maintaining a good level of oral hygiene.

- All **plaque retention factors** must be removed if possible, and this may involve replacing restorations and appliances, or aligning teeth orthodontically
- Give advice on the importance of **smoking cessation** and **control of alcohol consumption**, including information on their link to periodontal disease and oral cancer
- Provide more regular oral hygiene reinforcement sessions for patients experi-encing hormonal and stress-related problems
- Be aware of existing medical conditions that may exacerbate periodontal prob-lems, and provide a more intensive oral hygiene regimen if necessary

Controlling the host response

Some patients are unfortunate enough to be prone to periodontal problems, often for genetic reasons. No matter how thorough their oral hygiene efforts become with help and support from the dental team, and even in the absence of any contributory factors, they may still go on to develop periodontal disease. These patients may require interventional dental treatment on a regular basis.

- Any calculus that has built up must be removed by **scaling** and **subgingival debridement**, by a suitable member of the dental team (see Unit 8 (Chapter 9))

- Advice should be given on suitable oral health products that act specifically to control calculus formation
- Patients taking drugs that cause **gingival hyperplasia** may require the overgrown tissue to be surgically removed, thereby eliminating plaque retention areas
- Areas of persistent periodontal infection that fail to respond to treatment may require the **extraction** of the teeth involved, to remove the associated periodontal pockets as a source of the anaerobic bacteria
- Patients who require a high level of periodontal maintenance are best referred to a **periodontal specialist** for their treatment

The effect of general health on oral health

It is essential that patients understand that the condition of their oral health is not a separate issue from that of their general health, the two are very much linked together. The dietary and lifestyle advice that the dental team give to ensure good oral health will also be relevant to maintaining an overall high level of general health, if the patient chooses to follow that advice. There are numerous examples of the links between oral health and general health, as illustrated below:

- Several chronic diseases have the **same risk factors** as oral diseases:
    - The association of **smoking** and other tobacco habits with heart and respiratory disease, periodontal disease, and cancers such as oral cancer
    - Diets high in **NMES** and those containing many processed meals are linked to dental caries, obesity, and an increased risk of heart disease
    - **Excessive alcohol consumption** is associated with liver disease, periodontal disease, dental trauma, and several cancers including oral cancer
    - **Eating disorders**, such as anorexia nervosa and bulimia, are associated with general ill health and acid erosion of the enamel of teeth
    - **Diabetic patients** experience poor wound healing generally, which also affects the oral soft tissues
- **Physical disabilities** – such as rheumatoid arthritis and those caused by drugs (for example, thalidomide), will prevent adequate tooth brushing and exacerbate periodontal disease
- **Mental disabilities** – will make oral health messages difficult to teach and to be interpreted by some patients
- **Low socio-economic groups** – several chronic illnesses generally occur more among people from low socio-economic groups and they also experience more dental caries and periodontal disease – this is linked to association with poor housing, unemployment, stress, poorer nutrition and less social support

    Certain commonly prescribed drugs **reduce saliva flow**:

- Some anti-hypertensives
- Some anti-depressants

Some **medical conditions** also reduce saliva flow, with similar results (such as Sjögren's syndrome).

Some drugs cause **gingival hyperplasia**:

- **Phenytoin** – used for epilepsy
- **Nifedipine** – used for heart problems
- **Ciclosporin** – used to combat transplanted organ rejection

The effects of ageing on the oral tissues also have to be taken into consideration by the dental team. A greater proportion of the population is being made up of those over the age of 65 years. Dentally, as oral health has become understood and methods of maintaining good oral health have been developed, these patients are also keeping their natural teeth for longer, but because of age-related changes to the oral tissues, the dental treatment for these patients is different in some aspects, and is classed separately as 'gerodontology'.

The changes to the oral tissues with age, and their relevance to dentistry, are summarised below.

Skin

- Has less underlying fat and elasticity
- This gives increased tissue fragility and the likelihood of soft tissue trauma and bruising post-operatively

Bone

- Tend to be more brittle, especially in post-menopausal women
- The jaw bones are therefore at increased risk of fracture during extraction

Oral mucosa

- Is thinner and less elastic
- It is therefore easier to traumatise during treatment
- The ridge areas are less tolerant of bearing dentures, with discomfort and ulceration more likely

Salivary glands

- Undergo an alteration of the salivary components and volume, especially with certain drugs
- More likely to have a dry mouth (xerostomia)
- This leads to an increased caries rate, as the self-cleansing action of saliva is reduced
- It may also cause problems with swallowing, speech and denture retention

Teeth

- Undergo a gradual darkening in colour
- This leads to difficulties with colour-matched restorations
- Narrowing of the pulp chamber leads to difficulties in gaining access to the root canals during endodontic treatment
- Have reduced sensitivity

Armed with all of this information, the dental team can proceed in their key role of offering information and support to patients on an individual basis, for the protection of their oral health. Each patient must be assessed for the following:

- Evaluation – of their knowledge of oral health, the level of their skill in carrying out oral hygiene tasks, and their motivation towards improving their oral health
- Support and development – of these skills, to improve their oral hygiene efforts and to improve their motivation
- Review – the progress of the patient at future appointments, and reinforce the oral health and general health messages as necessary

Evaluation of knowledge, skills and motivation

Each patient's knowledge and skills in relation to oral health are evaluated by adequate communication with them, and the aim is to identify what the actual problems are for each individual – what is preventing them from achieving and maintaining good oral health? All of the following points need to be considered and taken into account:

- Do they just need direct advice, help and support to adequately achieve good oral health, such as one-to-one oral hygiene instruction with a member of the dental team?
- Are factors involved which prevent them from achieving good oral health, such as a disability or a diet- or habit-related problem?
- Are they simply disinterested in their oral health, or are they unaware that they have a problem?
- Are general health factors involved which either exacerbate or actually cause the oral health problem?
- Is a serious general health problem present – which overrides their oral health problems?

Following the evaluation of each patient, their individual problems will have been identified and help can then be given by the dental team to aid the patient in achieving a better standard of oral health.

Any risk factors identified during the evaluation need to be discussed with the patient. These risk factors will vary, depending on the age group of the patient involved, and tend to be influenced by complex social attitudes and outside pressures.

Adults

- Smoking and drinking habits should be discussed in relation to oral health, but in a non-judgemental manner. Information should be given on the links between these risk factors and both the general and oral health problems associated with them, especially periodontal disease and oral cancer
- Some patients may require referral to their dental or medical practitioner for individual advice on aids to stop smoking, such as nicotine patches and substitutes, and this is easier to arrange nowadays with the National Health Service (NHS) smoking cessation schemes
- Similarly, excessive alcohol intake should be discussed, but it is the patient's choice whether to act on the advice given, or not
- Diet should be discussed in detail, using accurate diet sheets filled in by the patient to identify any hidden dietary problems if necessary, such as a high NMES intake, or frequent snacking episodes
- The patient's diet should be assessed in relation to any general health effects too

Young people

This group of patients will require a quite different approach to support and motivation in relation to their oral health, for the following reasons:

- They have a different outlook on life and different priorities in their lives than adults, events that are important to adults are often of less concern to young people, and *vice versa*
- They are likely to have little, if any, experience of long-term oral and general health problems and will therefore require convincing that a problem actually exists
- They are likely to require evidence for the existence of a problem from the dental team, rather than just accepting it, so the use of disclosing agents to stain bacterial plaque on their own teeth is often an invaluable aid
- Some young people may already be experimenting with alcohol and tobacco usage because of peer pressure, and this may already be having an effect on their oral health
- Some may not wish to accept responsibility for maintaining their own oral health yet, and prefer to rely on their parents for this
- Parental influence will be greater for some young people than for others
- Similarly, parental support will differ, but is of great importance – well-motivated parents tend to instil their attitudes and beliefs into their youngsters

Children

The oral health of this group depends very much on their parental influence and support, especially for the younger patients of the group. Parents who have little interest in their own oral and general health are unlikely to instil their children with high levels of interest and motivation, although exceptions do occur. The following points are relevant:

■ Wherever possible, parents should be included in their child's oral health education, and their support should be gained
■ The oral health messages given by the dental team can then be reinforced at home by the parent, and will usually revolve around brushing techniques and dietary advice
■ A suitable vocabulary should be established for each child; if it is aimed too high they are unlikely to understand, but if too low they will be insulted by being treated childishly
■ A friendly, non-threatening approach is required so that their trust is gained
■ The patient should also feel comfortable when asking questions, so the oral health team should develop an open, frank manner with each child
■ Oral health messages need to be fun so that the interest of the child is maintained
■ Consequently, the use of games, drawings and competitions should be considered wherever possible
■ Again, the use of disclosing agents (either tablets or liquids) should be encouraged, both by the dental team and at home, to stain the bacterial plaque and make its removal easier

Motivation can be thought of as the act of persuading people to do something for their own benefit. When there is a lack of motivation by patients to take an interest in their oral health, it needs to be established as to whether this is due to lack of knowledge, disinterest, or because of the presence of previously unrealised risk factors. Once these points have been understood, priorities and goals can be set out for each patient and the role of the dental team can be established.

Support the development of the skills and abilities, and improve patients' motivation

Having established the different groups requiring oral health advice, and the factors that can affect both oral and general health, the various methods available now need to be considered in detail, especially in relation to caries and periodontal disease.

The necessary oral health message can be communicated to **adults** in various ways:

■ By use of specific oral health leaflets from dental suppliers
■ One-to-one discussions of relevant oral health issues with a member of the dental team, in a non-patronising manner
■ The non-use of dental jargon unless it is appropriate, but without condescension
■ The adoption of an attentive manner, so that the patient's own difficulties and problems relating to their oral health maintenance are listened to and understood

- Any queries raised need answering at a level that the patient will understand, and may require referral to another member of the dental team
- Eye contact should be maintained with the patient during the discussions
- Reflective replies to their queries and concerns should be given, which relate to the patient's individual experiences

The more mature **young people** can be approached in a similar fashion, but less mature patients will require an individual approach aimed at their level of understanding. Pubescent teenagers may even take offence at the implication that they have a 'dirty' mouth, and act quite negatively during this time. This tends to be especially so for male teenagers.

A young person with a 'rebellious' nature will be determined not to make efforts to improve their oral health, enjoying the 'shock tactic' approach on both the dental team and their parents. Thankfully, most tend to grow out of this phase as they mature.

Oral health messages can be communicated to this group as follows:

- The use of relevant leaflets and dental literature, many of which are specifically aimed at this age group
- Definitely a one-to-one approach to give oral health messages for those members of this age group who are easily embarrassed
- Some will tend to react better in small groups, especially with similarly aged siblings or friends
- Authority and control of the situation need to be maintained by the dental team throughout, but in a friendly manner
- The dental team should never lose patience with these individuals, no matter how obstreperous they become
- Good patient management by the dental team at this age should produce attentive and responsible adults in the future

Children tend to respond best to a group approach when learning new information, but their interest in a subject can soon be lost, or they can be easily distracted. Consequently, short and interactive sessions are best, with plenty of opportunities for individual involvement by the children:

- The use of disclosing tablets to show the presence and position of bacterial plaque
- Supervise individual attempts at tooth brushing, to determine how to improve plaque removal
- Develop relevant games to play, especially any involving current television or film characters
- Encourage parental involvement in the oral health sessions wherever possible, as the parents need to maintain and promote the oral health messages discussed at home

Having received all of the available oral health advice given by the dental team, the patient should now be able to determine whether they are motivated and willing to improve their oral health. A gentle reminder of the reasons why good oral health should be required by the patient should be given at this stage:

■ To avoid the embarrassment of having halitosis (bad breath)
■ To avoid the embarrassment and pain of having carious teeth
■ To avoid tooth loss due to periodontal disease or caries
■ To avoid the need for fixed or removable prostheses, and their expense

Review the patients' progress towards promoting good oral health

The patient will need to be seen on a regular basis to determine whether progress on the level of their oral hygiene has been made or not. The success or failure by the dental team of promoting and maintaining oral health depends on an understanding of the determinants of oral health:

■ Social factors
■ Environmental factors
■ Economic factors
■ Patient's knowledge
■ Patient's skills

Oral health education should aim to modify any damaging behaviour, rather than unrealistically trying to reverse this behaviour, and oral health educators need to have an understanding of why the damaging behaviour occurs. For example, people from lower socio-economic groups tend to use sweets for their children as treats, or even bribes, because sweets are often cheaper to buy than books, toys or other presents. The finances of these families cannot be changed, so it would be totally unrealistic to try to stop the parents buying sweets for their children under these circumstances, and the oral health promotion would fail. It would be more sensible to educate the parents to restrict sweets consumption to mealtimes, so that the frequency of acid attacks on their children's teeth is minimised, and hopefully their caries experience will be reduced or even eradicated.

Similarly, it would be unrealistic to expect older smokers to give up without lots of encouragement and support from a smoking cessation scheme, as nicotine is addictive and the longer the patient has smoked, usually the harder they will find it to stop. Advice about current aids to help to stop smoking, such as nicotine patches or chewing gum, can be given, or a referral made to the local cessation scheme. Teenage smokers may be easier to re-educate, as they often only smoke to appear socially acceptable or because of peer pressure. Advice regarding the overall damage to health caused by smoking, given in an informed but friendly manner, is often the first step in their re-education.

Bearing these points in mind, the dental team is able to consider and decide on what each patient's outcome has been at their review appointment:

- Has progress been made, resulting in a higher standard of oral hygiene?
- Has the original oral hygiene status been maintained, but with no improvement?
- Has the oral hygiene status deteriorated, such that more damage has occurred?

When the first event has occurred, the patient should be congratulated and encouraged to maintain this raised standard of oral hygiene. Children can be given stickers, badges or certificates – all of which are available from oral hygiene product distributors. Many computer programmes are also available that can be used to design and print out certificates exclusive to the dental practice.

It should be remembered that oral health promotion is a long-term process, so regular monitoring will still be required for some time, although if the higher standard of oral hygiene becomes consistent, then review appointment intervals can be gradually lengthened.

Dental examination recall intervals depend on several factors for each patient:

- Caries experience
- Periodontal experience
- State of general health
- Any controllable risk factors, such as smoking, alcohol consumption, sugar intake
- Medical risk factors
- Social risk factors, such as finances, peer pressure, lifestyle
- Children with developing dentition

These will cause variations in the frequency of dental attendance for each patient, and recent guidelines issued by the National Institute for Health and Clinical Excellence (NICE) will help to determine what is appropriate in each case (Figure 6.18).

When the second event has occurred, the patient should still be congratulated on the fact that their oral hygiene status has not relapsed, and encouraged to try harder. These patients tend to have considered the financial and emotional costs and benefits to themselves of changing their oral hygiene status, and decided that the costs outweigh the benefits at the present time. All is not lost, as this decision may be transitory, due say to a particularly stressful period in their lives at the current time, so they feel unable or unwilling to attempt change now. Once this period is over however, they may be receptive to further attempts by the dental team to promote oral health.

For these patients, the goals set by the dental team are not achievable, or are felt to be unrealistic for now. They should be reviewed regularly and supported until they feel able to try again.

The patients who have undergone deterioration in their oral health may need referral to the dentist or hygienist for specialist input and reinforcement. However, reflection still needs to determine whether the goals set were completely unrealistic and unachievable for that particular patient. If so, then new ones will need to be discussed and agreed on with the dental team.

NHS

National Institute for Clinical Excellence

Issue date: **October 2004**

Quick reference guide

Dental recall

Recall interval between routine dental examinations

Guidance

- The recommended interval between oral health reviews should be determined specifically for each patient, and tailored to meet his or her needs, on the basis of an assessment of disease levels and risk of or from dental disease.
- This assessment should integrate the evidence presented in this guideline with the clinical judgement and expertise of the dental team, and should be discussed with the patient (see pages 2 and 3).
- During an oral health review, the dental team (led by the dentist) should ensure that comprehensive histories are taken, examinations are conducted and initial preventive advice is given. This will allow the dental team and the patient (and/or his or her parent, guardian or carer) to discuss, where appropriate:
  - the effects of oral hygiene, diet, fluoride use, tobacco and alcohol on oral health
  - the risk factors (see the checklist on page 2) that may influence the patient's oral health, and their implications for deciding the appropriate recall interval
  - the outcome of previous care episodes and the suitability of previously recommended intervals
  - the patient's ability or desire to visit the dentist at the recommended interval
  - the financial costs to the patient of having the oral health review and any subsequent treatments.
- The interval before the next oral health review should be chosen, either at the end of an oral health review if no further treatment is indicated, or on completion of a specific treatment journey.
- The recommended shortest and longest intervals between oral health reviews are as follows.
  - The shortest interval between oral health reviews for all patients should be 3 months.
  - The longest interval between oral health reviews for patients younger than 18 years should be 12 months.
  - The longest interval between oral health reviews for patients aged 18 years and older should be 24 months.
- For practical reasons, the patient should be assigned a recall interval of 3, 6, 9 or 12 months if he or she is younger than 18 years, or 3, 6, 9, 12, 15, 18, 21 or 24 months if he or she is aged 18 years or older.
- The dentist should discuss the recommended recall interval with the patient and record this interval, and the patient's agreement or disagreement with it, in the current record-keeping system.
- The recall interval should be reviewed again at the next oral health review, in order to learn from the patient's responses to the oral care provided and the health outcomes achieved. This feedback and the findings of the oral health review should be used to adjust the next recall interval chosen. Patients should be informed that their recommended recall interval may vary over time.

Clinical Guideline 19

Developed by the National Collaborating Centre for Acute Care

Figure 6.18 NICE guidelines for dental recall.

Checklist of modifying factors						
Name:		**Date of birth:**				
Oral health review date:						
Medical history	Yes	No	Yes	No	Yes	No
Conditions where dental disease could put the patient's general health at increased risk (such as cardiovascular disease, bleeding disorders, immunosuppression)	☐	☐	☐	☐	☐	☐
Conditions that increase a patient's risk of developing dental disease (such as diabetes, xerostomia)	☐	☐	☐	☐	☐	☐
Conditions that may complicate dental treatment or the patient's ability to maintain their oral health (such as special needs, anxious/nervous/phobic conditions)	☐	☐	☐	☐	☐	☐
Social history						
High caries in mother and siblings	☐	☐	☐	☐	☐	☐
Tobacco use	☐	☐	☐	☐	☐	☐
Excessive alcohol use	☐	☐	☐	☐	☐	☐
Family history of chronic or aggressive (early onset/juvenile) periodontitis	☐	☐	☐	☐	☐	☐
Dietary habits						
High and/or frequent sugar intake	☐	☐	☐	☐	☐	☐
High and/or frequent dietary acid intake	☐	☐	☐	☐	☐	☐
Exposure to fluoride						
Use of fluoride toothpaste	☐	☐	☐	☐	☐	☐
Other sources of fluoride (for example, the patient lives in a water-fluoridated area)	☐	☐	☐	☐	☐	☐
Clinical evidence and dental history						
Recent and previous caries experience						
New lesions since last check-up	☐	☐	☐	☐	☐	☐
Anterior caries or restorations	☐	☐	☐	☐	☐	☐
Premature extractions because of caries	☐	☐	☐	☐	☐	☐
Past root caries or large number of exposed roots	☐	☐	☐	☐	☐	☐
Heavily restored dentition	☐	☐	☐	☐	☐	☐
Recent and previous periodontal disease experience						
Previous history of periodontal disease	☐	☐	☐	☐	☐	☐
Evidence of gingivitis	☐	☐	☐	☐	☐	☐
Presence of periodontal pockets (BPE code 3 or 4) and/or bleeding on probing	☐	☐	☐	☐	☐	☐
Presence of furcation involvements or advanced attachment loss (BPE code *)	☐	☐	☐	☐	☐	☐
Mucosal lesions						
Mucosal lesion present	☐	☐	☐	☐	☐	☐
Plaque						
Poor level of oral hygiene	☐	☐	☐	☐	☐	☐
Plaque-retaining factors (such as orthodontic appliances)	☐	☐	☐	☐	☐	☐
Saliva						
Low saliva flow rate	☐	☐	☐	☐	☐	☐
Erosion and tooth surface loss						
Clinical evidence of tooth wear	☐	☐	☐	☐	☐	☐
Recommended recall interval for next oral health review:	months		months		months	
Does patient agree with recommended interval? If 'No', record reason for disagreement in notes	Yes	No	Yes	No	Yes	No

BPE code * is used when attachment loss is ≥7mm and/or furcation involvements are present

2

Figure 6.18 (*Continued*)

Frustrating though it is, some patients simply do not wish to change their lifestyle, nor do they accept the consequences to their oral health that may occur, as indicated by the dental team. Regular monitoring and review is all that the dental team can hope to achieve for these patients, although they should stay alert to any indication by the patient that they are willing to try again at any time. The patient's right to choose not to accept the oral health advice given by the dental team should be respected and accepted by all.

Communication skills

The final skills that the dental team need to develop, to be able to assist the oral and general health efforts of their patients, involve those of good communication. There are various ways in which to communicate with patients and with other members of the dental team, both verbally and non-verbally, and misinterpretation of information being given can have poor consequences for all.

Communicating means 'to give or exchange information', and in the dental setting full communication is the only way in which patients can give informed consent for their dental treatment. If they are not given all the necessary information say, regarding endodontic treatment, either deliberately by exclusion or accidentally by misinterpretation, then they cannot understand all the pros and cons of the treatment and therefore cannot give informed consent.

Methods of communicating are:

- Talking
- Written explanations
- Information leaflets and posters
- Body language
- Eye contact and facial expressions
- Body position, such as sitting or standing
- Touching, to reinforce points

Ethnic groups

In our modern, multiracial society there are bound to be patients whose first language is not English, and who will then be at an obvious disadvantage with regard to interpreting information. In these situations, patients should be encouraged to bring a responsible interpreter to their dental appointments, so that full communication occurs and the patient is fully aware of the state of their oral health, and fully informed of all risks and benefits before undergoing any dental procedure. The NHS issues patient information leaflets in various languages nowadays, and it would be advisable for practices with a large ethnic minority patient base to have them to hand as required.

Dental staff should also be aware of any cultural differences between ethnic groups, and accept and deal with them in an appropriate manner. Religious beliefs may prevent oral examination and dental treatment occurring at certain times, and these facts should be accommodated and handled sympathetically as far as possible, rather than being seen as an unnecessary hindrance to the running of the practice.

Religion probably plays the most important role in the differences encountered among many ethnic groups, both in their culture and in their daily lives, including their diet and eating habits. Several points of interest for dental staff are summarised below.

Hindus

- Many are vegetarian, some are vegan, and they do not eat beef
- Fasting days for religious reasons are common
- Their diet tends to be very high in saturated fats, and is often expensive

Sikhs

- They eat more dairy products than other ethnic groups
- They are often vegetarian
- If meats are eaten, they tend to avoid beef and pork

Muslims

- They have strict food laws, even including the methods used for animal slaughter
- They avoid both alcohol and pork
- They abide by Ramadan – a period of fasting during daylight for one month per year
- They tend to eat a diet rich in fish if possible

All Asian groups tend to breastfeed their babies for up to two years, and sugar is routinely added to feeds, especially as milk-based additions that are therefore cariogenic and have low nutritional value.

All of these issues are of relevance to both the oral health and the general health of these patient groups, but are unlikely to be altered because of their religious bases. The dental team must accept this and respect the wishes of each patient.

Socio-economic groups

Similarly, there is a wide diversity of socio-economic classes in most dental practice areas, and assumptions should never be made about a patient and the role that they wish to take with regard to their own oral health. Studies indicate that patients in lower socio-economic groups tend to have poorer general and oral health overall, and advice given by the dental team must be sympathetic to this, as it is often related to the financial situation of these patients in particular.

A common, and often erroneous, belief made by the dental team is that those patients in the lower social classes are unable to afford expensive dental treatments, so that full information regarding proposed treatment is denied to them. The same information must be given to all patients, regardless of their perceived status, otherwise they cannot give valid consent for any treatment.

Non-verbal communication

Non-verbal communication is just as important to ensure that patients are kept fully informed. Staff who have a defensive style of body language, such as standing with their arms folded when talking to patients, give the impression that they are unapproachable and likely to refuse help to the patient if asked. Failure to make eye contact when addressing a patient gives the impression of disinterest, as well as being rude.

Obvious differences in patient management between males versus females, and able-bodied versus disabled is blatantly discriminatory, and must be avoided at all costs. Some patients also find that close proximity between themselves and staff during discussions of their oral health is intimidating, and that they are being pressurised into accepting treatment when they do not wish to proceed. Older patients may also find unnecessary physical contact between themselves and staff as offensive, especially between female patients and male staff. Many areas run courses on these subjects, and dental nurses may wish to attend them when available.

Patients with disabilities

Disability comes in many forms, and can be either mental or physical in its effect on the patient. Patients with mental disabilities range from those with minor learning disabilities, to older people with various forms of dementia and to those with congenital problems, such as Down's syndrome.

The dental care of these patients can be very demanding and time-consuming for the dental team, but also challenging and rewarding. Whatever the disability, the patient has the same rights as all others, including access to full dental care. Obviously the ability of some to be able to comprehend and accept more complicated forms of treatment may be limited, and carers and family should be kept fully involved by the dental team at all stages of oral health support and dental treatment. These patients do have special needs, but this should not mean that the standard of their dental care should suffer as a result.

Similarly, physically disabled patients range from those who are deaf or blind to those with limited body movements or who are even confined to a wheelchair. Again, they are patients with special needs who may require more time and delivery of dental treatment at a slower pace than those patients who are able-bodied, but the standard and extent of that care should be no different.

Effective oral hygiene measures may require adaptations to oral health products, such as adapting a toothbrush handle so that it can be gripped more firmly by an arthritic patient, for instance. The oral health of the patient may even be the responsibility of a carer, and it is vital that they attend the evaluation, support and review appointments with the dental team.

Angled toothbrushes, or even children's sizes rather than adult size, can make access to the teeth so much easier, either for the patient themselves or their carer. Good quality rechargeable electric toothbrushes, when used correctly, can ensure a good standard of oral hygiene, although battery-operated designs are not particularly recommended as they can lose their charge with time and become quite inefficient at plaque control. Several floss holders are now available to allow efficient interproximal cleaning, indeed even manually dextrous patients may find these less cumbersome than the traditional method of wrapping floss around the fingers.

Deaf patients will appreciate being spoken to by the dental team with no mask blocking their view of the lips, as many can lip read extremely well. Blind patients will appreciate being allowed to handle instruments before their use, and having clear and detailed explanations of the noises they will hear in the surgery so that they are not startled.

Many of these points will also apply to older patients too, especially those who are becoming infirm and unsteady. More of the population in Britain is composed of older people now than ever before, and their dental care raises new challenges for the dental team. More people are retaining their natural teeth for longer rather than having a dental clearance and full dentures, and the treatment of these patients has developed into a whole new speciality of dentistry called gerodontology.

Consent

The aim of good communication is to fully inform the patient of their proposed treatment needs, including the risks and possible complications of that treatment, so that they can give **valid** and **informed consent** to the dentist.

For the consent to be valid it must:

- Be given voluntarily
- Be fully informed and specific to the particular treatment for that patient
- Be either oral, written or implied consent (such as sitting in the dental chair)

Ideally, all oral discussions with regard to treatment are reinforced with a written consent agreement between the dentist and the patient. Include details of all costs, and agreement to pay these costs when requested to do so, whether NHS or private treatment is being provided. Be specific for any necessary changes to the original treatment plan.

By law, consent is deemed to be valid and informed if given by:

- Patients over 16 years old, of sound mind
- Patients under 16 years old who are deemed able to understand the information given ('Gillick competent')
- As the written consent of a parent or guardian for other under 16-year-olds

And also if:

- The patient understands the pros and cons of each option, and why the final choice of treatment is recommended by the dentist
- The patient can make an informed decision, once all the information has been given
- The patient understands and accepts any risks that may be involved
- The patient has realistic and achievable expectations of the treatment
- The patient has given consent directly to the dentist offering the treatment
- Written consent is given for extensive and costly courses of treatment

However, the law is equally specific on the following points:

- No person can give consent on behalf of an incompetent adult
- These patients must be assessed by the dentist as to whether any consent given is valid
- A second professional opinion may be necessary
- The dentist must always act in the best interests of the patient, after undertaking a risk versus benefit analysis
- Any actions taken by the dentist must be justified, if necessary

To summarise, good communication skills practised by all the dental team revolve around their ability to listen to the patient, to communicate at a level appropriate to each patient (which often means the avoidance of dental jargon), never to make incorrect assumptions about a patient, and always to be open and honest with them.

Confidentiality

Patients have a right to expect that their dental records will not be disclosed to a third party without their permission, and all dental staff are bound by this duty of confidentiality. Until the recent registration of all dental care professionals (DCPs) with the General Dental Council became compulsory, dentists had **vicarious liability** for all the acts and omissions of their staff – this means that the dentist was wholly responsible for any mistakes made by the staff, and it was therefore the dentist's responsibility to ensure that all staff were made aware of this fact and that they were all trained in correct practice protocols and procedures accordingly.

Since registration became compulsory, the professional standing that this gives all DCPs, including dental nurses, means that some acts and omissions on their part are now entirely their responsibility. This is why qualified and registered dental nurses must now have personal indemnity insurance cover in place, so that if an act or omission on their part results in a patient injury or complaint, they have financial insurance cover to defend themselves legally, or to have costs awarded against them without fearing personal bankruptcy.

The necessary training in patient confidentiality provided by the dental workplace should incorporate the seriousness of a breach of confidentiality, as the dentist or the DCP is likely to be accused of serious professional misconduct. The current regulations and legalities with regard to patient confidentiality are as described below.

Information about a patient can only be disclosed to a third party with the patient's written consent. However, there are some circumstances under which the dentist has a statutory obligation to disclose information, such as:

- To assist in the identification of a driver involved in a road traffic accident, under the Road Traffic Act 1988
- When requested to do so by the Business Service Authority (formerly known as the Dental Practice Board)
- To provide information about a child to their parent or legal guardian
- When it is in the public's interest, as with suspected criminals
- When requested by a Court Order from the police, under the Prevention of Terrorism Act 1974–1989, or the Police and Criminal Evidence Act 1984

General confidentiality in the dental practice should be observed at all times by all staff, including the secure storage of all patient records under the **Data Protection Act 1998**. The following points should also be borne in mind:

- Patients should not be discussed among staff within earshot of others
- All conversations with patients about personal matters should be done in private
- Even the fact that a patient has attended the practice on a certain day, or that they are a patient at the practice, is confidential. This means that schools and employers have no legal right to know whether a patient has attended at any time
- All written communications with patients, including their dental recall notification, should be sent in sealed envelopes
- All dental records have to be kept for 11 years or until the patient is 25 years old, whichever is the longer. Therefore, under no circumstances must a dental nurse destroy any portion of a patient's records

To ensure the security of the patient records held at the dental workplace, all of the following points must be considered and acted on as necessary:

- Written records must be stored away from public access areas
- All record storage cabinets must be lockable, and with a limited number of key holders having access
- All computerised records must be password protected, and with a limited number of staff having access
- Computer screens must be positioned to prevent their viewing by unauthorised persons
- Written records must never be left lying in the open and unattended by staff

- Written records must never be handed to the patient to be carried around the dental workplace
- The system used to record patient and treatment details must be **contemporaneous** (in date order), and **unalterable** once written, whether the information is held on paper or on a computer
- This means paper records must be written in ink, not pencil
- The computer software must not allow records to be altered without recording the date that the alterations were made, so that their authenticity is guaranteed
- Paper records must be destroyed only by **shredding** or **incineration**, so that they are unreadable, and only when they have been held for the required length of time
- Computer hard drives and all back-up discs must be correctly and fully **erased** before being disposed off, and only when their contents have been held for the required length of time

Patients have the right of access to their own written and computerised health records, under the **Access to Health Records Act 1990**, and the Data Protection Act 1998. The following conditions apply:

- Only the record holder (that is, the dentist) can approve access
- The patient has to make their request in writing
- The dentist must respond within 40 days
- The dentist must check the identity of the person making the disclosure request, prior to releasing the records
- The patient has the right to request amendments to their records, once viewed, if they believe that incorrect information has been recorded
- All disclosed data should be provided with an explanation of the dental terms or short hand notifications that have been used

The dentist can legally refuse to disclose some or all of the records if:

- Disclosure would cause serious harm to the patient
- Another person (other than healthcare workers) is mentioned in the records, and they have not given consent to be involved
- A deceased patient's records include notification that access is not to be granted after their death

7 Unit 6: Provide Chairside Support During the Assessment of Patients' Oral Health (OH3)

Knowledge specifications

Assessing oral and medical health

K1 – A working knowledge of the purpose of dental assessments and methods of explaining this clearly to patients

K2 – A working knowledge of the medical conditions which may affect oral health assessment and treatment

K3 – A factual knowledge of the types and purposes of orthodontic treatment available and your role in providing support during the assessment and treatment of a patient's occlusion

Regional and dental anatomy, physiology and dentition

K4 – A factual knowledge of primary and secondary dentition and the average dates of eruption

K5 – A factual knowledge of the structure and function of teeth and gingivae including the number of roots

K6 – A factual knowledge of regional (head and neck) and dental anatomy

K7 – A factual knowledge of common oral diseases, including both malignant and potentially malignant lesions, and methods for their diagnosis, prevention and management

K8 – A factual knowledge of the function and position of salivary glands, muscles of mastication and facial expression, and the types of diseases which may affect facial movements

K9 – A factual knowledge of the diagnosis and management of diseases of the oral mucosa, of other soft tissues, of the salivary glands and the facial bones and joints

K10 – A factual knowledge of oral manifestations of systemic diseases, and the diagnosis and management of facial pain of dental and non-dental origin

K11 – A factual knowledge of the effects of ageing upon the oral tissues and the particular needs of the elderly dental patient

Health, safety and infection control

K12 – A working knowledge of the purpose, method of use, and function of protective wear and the reason for their use during assessment

K13 – A working knowledge of standard precautions and quality standards of infection control and your role in maintaining them

Equipment, instruments, materials and medicaments

K14 – A working knowledge of safe methods of handling instruments and equipment

K15 – A working knowledge of the uses of the different materials used within dental assessment, including impression materials for study models

K16 – A working knowledge of methods of measuring pulp vitality and their advantages and disadvantages

K17 – A working knowledge of the main classes of drugs which are used in dentistry and the reasons for their use, ie analgesics, antibiotics, tranquillisers/hypnotics, emergency drugs, drugs which reverse the action of other drugs (such as anti-anaphylactics)

Dental and medical records and charts

K18 – A working knowledge of the different types of dental record and charts (including personal details, dental charts, radiographs/photographs and study models for assessment and treatment planning) which are used, and the functions of each

K19 – A working knowledge of the information required for a medical history, and the implications that relevant medical conditions have on dental treatment

K20 – A working knowledge of the terminology and charting notation/symbols for tooth surfaces, cavities and particular tooth problems related to the type of dental chart being used

K21 – A working knowledge of methods of dental charting (eg computer, manual)

K22 – A working knowledge of the reasons for taking radiographs and photographs (both for treatment and for the monitoring of dental practices)

K23 – A working knowledge of the measurements and records taken to record any malocclusion

K24 – A working knowledge of the classifications used in recording malocclusion

Providing support to patients

K25 – A working knowledge of methods of communicating clearly with the patient, especially when they might be in some discomfort or distress

K26 – A working knowledge of methods of modifying information and communication methods for different individuals, including patients from different social and ethnic backgrounds, children (including those with special needs), and the elderly

K27 – A working knowledge of methods of monitoring the physical characteristics of a patient, and the signs and symptoms to be aware of to recognise a potential emergency

Medical emergencies

K28 – A working knowledge of carrying out resuscitation techniques

K29 – A working knowledge of how to identify that a medical emergency has arisen, and provide support both for the individual with the emergency and to those providing immediate management of the emergency

K30 – A working knowledge of the principles of first aid

Work role and its relationship to others in the oral health care team

K31 – A working knowledge of methods of effective team working in oral health care

Legislation and policies

K32 – An in-depth understanding of why it is important that information relating to patients is treated as confidential, and what this means for the storage, recording and disclosure of patient information

K33 – A working knowledge of legislation and guidelines relating to patients' records and confidentiality (eg the Data Protection Act)

K34 – A working knowledge of informed consent and its application before any treatment is undertaken

The assessment of a patient's oral health involves checking and recording the findings made of all of the relevant areas around and within the oral cavity. To do so accurately requires knowledge of the anatomy of these areas, as well as the use of the correct dental terminology.

Information on the following areas will be included here:

- Anatomy of the skull
- Muscles of mastication and facial expression
- Nerve and blood supplies
- Salivary glands
- The tongue
- Tooth morphology

The anatomy of the teeth and their supporting structures is covered in Unit 5 (Chapter 6).

Anatomy of the skull

The skull is effectively what a patient would refer to as 'the head', and can be divided into three anatomical regions (Figure 7.1):

- **The cranium** – enclosing the brain, and forming the largest part of the skull
- **The face** – supporting the eyes and nose and their surrounding structures
- **The jaws** – supporting the teeth and the tongue, and providing openings for the respiratory and digestive tracts

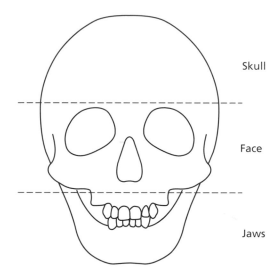

Figure 7.1 The three regions of the skull.

Like most bones in the body, the skull develops in the fetus as **cartilage**, which is gradually converted to bone as the body grows and develops. The outer layer of all bone is called **compact bone**, and it has some holes called **foramina** that allow the passage of blood vessels and nerves from structures outside the bone to within it, and vice versa. The inner layer is called **cancellous bone**, and is of a spongy appearance to reduce the overall weight of the bone, and to allow the progression of the nerve and blood vessels within.

The **cranium** is made up of six plates of bone:

- Frontal bone – forming the forehead region
- Two parietal bones – joined at the top midline of the skull, and forming its upper sides behind the forehead

- Two temporal bones – forming the lower sides of the skull in the region of the ears
- Occipital bone – forming the back of the skull

The six bony plates (Figure 7.2) interlock with each other at the coronal sutures, which is a type of joint between the plates. The sutures allow for growth and expansion of the brain during childhood.

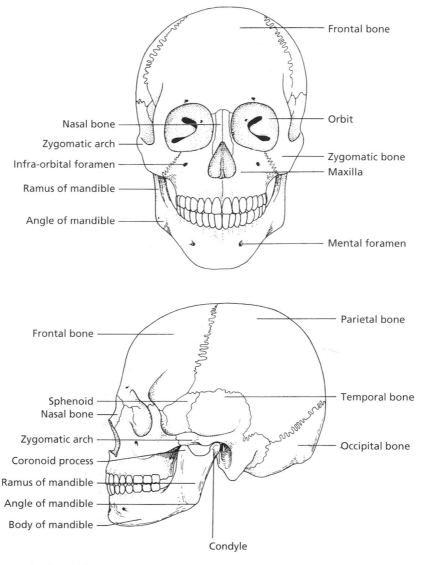

Figure 7.2 The skull in detail. Source: *Clinical Anatomy*, 11th edn, H. Ellis, 2006, Blackwell Publishing, Oxford.

The large foramen at the base of the skull through the occipital bone is called the **foramen magnum**, and this is where the brain stem becomes the spinal cord within the spinal column.

The **face** is composed of many bones; the six which are relevant to dentistry are:

- Two zygomatic bones – joining the upper jaw to the cranium
- Two zygomatic arches – forming the cheek bones
- Two nasal bones – forming the bony bridge of the nose

These six main bones (Figure 7.3) also form parts of the orbital cavities, enclosing the eyeballs, and the nasal cavity of the nose, containing the nasal septum and the turbinate bones.

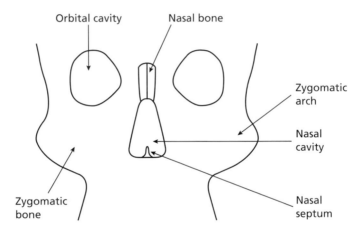

Figure 7.3 The face in detail.

There are two jaws: the upper (**maxilla**) and the lower (**mandible**) jaws. The maxilla is rigid and is joined to the zygomatic bones. The dentally relevant details are as follows (Figure 7.4).

- It is made up of two bones which join rigidly in the centre
- It supports the bony, horse shoe-shaped **alveolar process** which holds the upper teeth
- It forms the bony roof of the mouth, called the **hard palate**
- It also forms the floor of the nose
- The maxilla is hollow within, to reduce its weight, and the enclosed air spaces are called **sinuses**, or **antra**
- It has the **greater palatine foramina** posteriorly to allow the exit of the **greater palatine nerves**
- It has the **incisive foramina** anteriorly to allow the exit of the **nasopalatine nerves**
- The two ends of the alveolar process are called the **maxillary tuberosities**

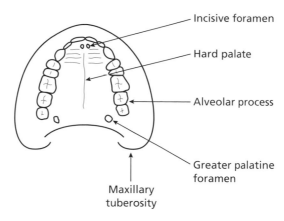

Figure 7.4 The maxilla.

The mandible is horse shoe shaped with a vertical strut at each end where it joins the cranium. The dentally relevant details are as follows (Figure 7.5):

- It is composed of two bones which join at the midline
- This junction is called the **mental symphysis**
- It connects with the cranium by two hinge joints – **temporomandibular joints**

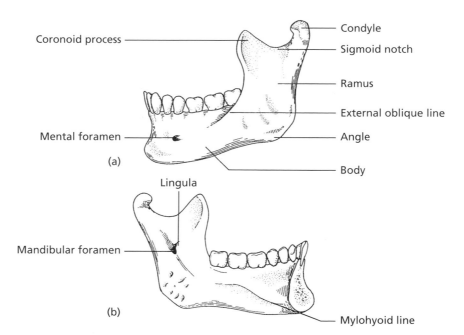

Figure 7.5 The mandible. (a) Outer side; (b) inner side. Source: *Clinical Anatomy*, 11th edn, H. Ellis, 2006, Blackwell Publishing, Oxford.

- It supports the bony alveolar process which holds the lower teeth
- The ridge of bone running along the inner surface is the **mylohyoid ridge**
- This supports the mylohyoid muscle which forms the floor of the mouth
- It has the **mandibular foramina** opening on the inner surfaces of the ramus, to admit the **inferior dental nerves**
- It has the **mental foramina** opening between the lower premolars for the exit of the inferior dental nerves

Temporomandibular joint (TMJ)

These are the hinge joints on either side of the skull, formed between the underside of the cranium and the heads of the condyle of the mandible, which allow the mouth to open and close. The head of the mandibular condyle lies in a groove of the temporal bone called the **glenoid fossa**, and the articulation of the two bones at this point forms the TMJ. The front edge of the fossa is raised into a ridge called the **articular eminence**, and this stops the condylar head from slipping out of the joint and dislocating. The two bones are separated by a pad of cartilage (**the meniscus**) so that they do not grate against each other (Figure 7.6).

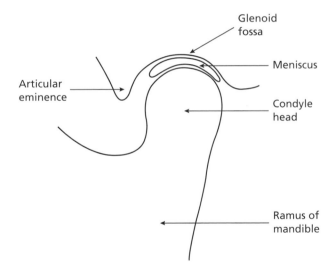

Figure 7.6 Temporomandibular joint.

Muscles of mastication and facial expression

There are three groups of muscles around the face and jaws (Figure 7.7):

- **Suprahyoid muscles** – those running from the chin to the hyoid bone in the throat, and they act to open the mouth

- **Muscles of mastication** – those running from the cranium to the mandible, and they act to close the mouth and effect chewing movements
- **Muscles of facial expression** – those running in the soft tissues surrounding the mouth, nose and eyes

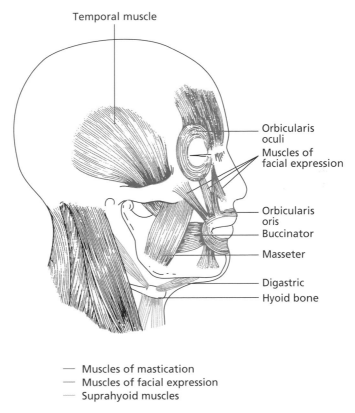

Figure 7.7 Oral musculature. Source: *Levison's Textbook for Dental Nurses*, 10th edn, C. Hollins, 2008, Wiley-Blackwell.

The muscles of mastication are arranged as four pairs connecting the mandible to either the cranium or the face. The four muscles are:

- **Temporalis**
- **Masseter**
- **Lateral pterygoid**
- **Medial pterygoid**

When the muscles contract their length shortens, and this causes various movements of the mandible – jaw closing, clenching and chewing movements. The point at which each set of muscles is connected to the cranium or the face is called their **point of origin** and the other end is connected to the mandible at their **point of insertion**. The origin, insertion and actions of the each of the muscles are summarised below.

Temporalis

- Point of origin – **temporal bone** of the cranium
- Point of insertion – **coronoid process** of the mandible, passing under the zygomatic arch
- Action – pulls the mandible backwards to close the mouth

Masseter

- Point of origin – outer surface of zygomatic arch
- Point of insertion – outer surface of mandibular ramus and angle
- Action – closes the mouth

Lateral pterygoid

- Point of origin – **lateral pterygoid plate** at the base of the cranium
- Point of insertion – **head of the mandibular condyle** and into the TMJ meniscus
- Action – both contracting brings the mandible **forwards**, to a tip to tip position of the teeth, one contracting pulls the mandible **to the opposite side**

Medial pterygoid

- Point of origin – **medial pterygoid plate** at the base of the cranium
- Point of insertion – inner surface of the mandibular ramus and angle
- Action – closes the mouth

Acute inflammatory conditions may result in the onset of protective spasms of the muscles of mastication, a condition called **trismus**, which results in limited mouth opening. It occurs in cases of pericoronitis around erupting third molars, following the surgical removal of these teeth, and in cases of mumps, a viral infection of the parotid salivary glands. In addition, excessive or habitual clenching and grinding of the teeth (**bruxing**) causes overuse of these muscles, resulting in a variety of symptoms ranging from TMJ pain, clicking or locking of the joint on opening or closing, or even arthritis of the joint. Treatment can involve any of the following:

- Advice and relaxation techniques
- Use of tranquillisers
- Physiotherapy
- Use of occlusal guards and splints
- Joint surgery

The muscles of facial expression are those lying within the soft tissues of the face, and are responsible for the production of facial movements and expressions, such as smiling, frowning, winking, and lip pursing. They are found in three areas of the face:

- Muscles around the eyes – in particular **orbicularis oculi**
- Muscles around the mouth – in particular **orbicularis oris**
- Cheek muscles – **buccinator** which is attached above and below to the alveolar processes of the jaws

Nerve supply to the oral cavity

All nerves supplying the oral cavity run directly from the brain as **cranial nerves**, whereas those supplying the rest of the body run from the spinal cord, as systemic nerves. The cranial nerves are either **sensory** (carrying sensory stimuli to the brain), **motor** (carrying electrical stimulation from the brain to the muscles), or a **combination** of the two. Twelve pairs of cranial nerves leave the brain, of which the following four pairs are relevant to dentistry:

- **Trigeminal nerve** – cranial nerve V, supplying the teeth and soft tissues of the oral cavity, and the muscles of mastication
- **Facial nerve** – cranial nerve VII, supplying some salivary glands, the muscles of facial expression, and parts of the tongue
- **Glossopharyngeal nerve** – cranial nerve IX, supplying other salivary glands, the throat, and parts of the tongue
- **Hypoglossal nerve** – cranial nerve XII, supplying the tongue

Trigeminal nerve (Figure 7.8)

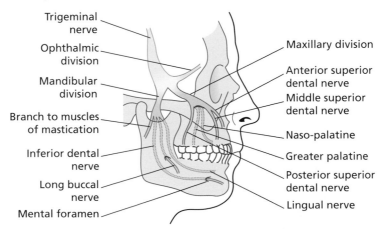

Figure 7.8 Trigeminal nerve distribution. Source: *Levison's Textbook for Dental Nurses*, 10th edn, C. Hollins, 2008, Wiley-Blackwell.

This is so called because it splits into three divisions, each of which has several branches:

(1) **Ophthalmic division** – this supplies the soft tissues around the eye and upper face
(2) **Maxillary division** – this provides the sensory supply of upper teeth, maxilla and middle face; it has five branches:
  - Anterior superior dental nerve
  - Middle superior dental nerve
  - Posterior superior dental nerve
  - Greater palatine nerve
  - Nasopalatine nerve
(3) **Mandibular division** – this provides sensory supply to the lower teeth, mandible and lower face, and motor supply to muscles of mastication; it has four branches:
  - Inferior dental nerve
  - Lingual nerve
  - Long buccal nerve
  - Motor branch to muscles of mastication

Maxillary division

- **Anterior superior dental nerve** supplies incisor and canine teeth and their labial gingivae
- **Middle superior dental nerve** supplies premolars and mesial half of first molar teeth and their buccal gingivae
- **Posterior superior dental nerve** supplies distal half of first molar and second and third molar teeth and their buccal gingivae
- **Greater palatine nerve** supplies palatal gingivae of molars, premolars and half of canine teeth
- **Nasopalatine nerve** supplies palatal gingivae of incisors and half of canine teeth

Mandibular division

- **Inferior dental nerve** supplies all lower teeth, the labial/buccal gingivae of the premolar, canine and incisor teeth, and the soft tissues of the lower lip and chin
- **Lingual nerve** supplies the lingual gingivae of all the lower teeth, the floor of the mouth, and all but taste sensation from the anterior two-thirds of the tongue
- **Long buccal nerve** supplies the buccal gingivae of the molar teeth
- **Motor branch** supplies stimulation to the muscles of mastication

Facial nerve

This nerve has both sensory and motor components:

■ The **motor component** supplies the muscles of facial expression to create the variety of facial expressions mentioned earlier
■ The **sensory component** supplies taste sensation from the anterior two thirds of the tongue to the brain, where they are recognised as sweet and salty sensations
■ It also supplies the submandibular and sublingual salivary glands so that these glands can secrete saliva into the mouth

A condition of temporary paralysis of this nerve leads to the condition known as **Bell's palsy**.

Glossopharyngeal nerve

Again, this nerve has both sensory and motor components:

■ The **motor component** supplies the muscles of the pharynx (back of the mouth) so that actions such as swallowing can be achieved
■ The **sensory component** supplies taste and sensation from the posterior third of the tongue to the brain, where they are recognised as sour and bitter
■ It also supplies the parotid salivary glands, so that their salivary contents can be secreted into the mouth

Hypoglossal nerve

It has a **motor component** only, which supplies the muscles of the tongue and effects its movements during speech, chewing, and swallowing.

Blood supply to the teeth and gingivae

All these areas are supplied by branches of the **external carotid artery**, which runs from the aorta to the head region through the neck. All the blood vessels run as neurovascular bundles with the nerves supplying the area. The veins draining the area will eventually join the **superior vena cava** and enter the right side of the heart, where the deoxygenated blood will pass to the lungs for reoxygenation.

Salivary glands

There are many small salivary glands within the cheeks and lips, and three pairs of principal salivary glands situated around the oral cavity. Their main function is to secrete saliva into the mouth. The three principal pairs of salivary glands (Figure 7.9) are:

- **Parotid glands**
- **Submandibular glands**
- **Sublingual glands**

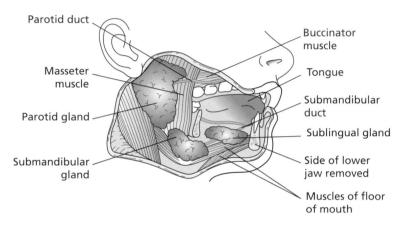

Figure 7.9 Salivary glands. Source: *Levison's Textbook for Dental Nurses,* 10th edn, C. Hollins, 2008, Wiley-Blackwell.

Parotid glands

- These are the largest of the three principal salivary glands
- They lie around each ramus of the mandible, in front of the ears
- They are connected to the oral cavity via Stensen's ducts, which open into the mouth against the upper first and second molar teeth
- They are the only salivary glands affected by the viral infection **mumps**
- They are the commonest salivary glands to be associated with benign and malignant tumours
- They are activated to release their saliva contents by the **glossopharyngeal nerve**

Submandibular glands

- They lie within the horseshoe shape of the body of the mandible, posteriorly and partly **below** the mylohyoid muscle
- They connect to the oral cavity via the Wharton's ducts, which open beneath the tongue
- They are the likeliest ducts to become blocked by **salivary stones** (calculi) because of their length
- They are activated to release their saliva contents by the **facial nerve**

Sublingual glands

- They lie beneath the tongue, **above** the mylohyoid muscle
- They have several ducts opening under the tongue into the oral cavity, against the lingual surfaces of the lower incisor teeth
- They are activated to release their saliva contents by the **facial nerve**

Tongue

The tongue is a muscular organ lying in the floor of the mouth and attached to it by the **lingual frenum**. When this attachment is excessive, the patient is said to be 'short tongued' or 'tongue tied', and usually they speak with a lisp.

The tongue is composed of many bands of fibres which run in all directions to allow the organ its wide range of movements. The top surface, called the **dorsum**, is covered by a variety of taste buds which allow the patient to taste all items put into the mouth. The functions of the tongue are:

- **Speech** – by moving to various points in the mouth to allow vocal sounds to be made
- **Taste** – by detecting sweet, sour, salt and bitter tastes through the taste buds
- Aids **mastication** – by packaging food particles ready for swallowing
- Aids **swallowing** – by guiding the food to the back of the mouth
- Aids **cleansing** of the oral cavity – by moving around the oral cavity and dislodging plaque from the teeth

The muscular movements of the tongue are controlled by the **hypoglossal nerve**, while taste sensations are detected by both the **facial nerve** and the **glossopharyngeal nerve**.

Tooth morphology

All people have two sets of teeth – the first, or **deciduous teeth**, and the second, or **permanent teeth**. Teeth have different shapes and their appearance differs from each other, both between sets and within each set, and this is how they can be identified. This method of identification is called **tooth morphology**.

Deciduous teeth

These are also called primary teeth, baby teeth or milk teeth.

- They make up a total set of 20, ten in each jaw
- They begin developing in the fetus
- They begin erupting approximately eight months after birth

- They are referred to in dentistry by letter – A, B, C, D, E, starting from the midline
- They are smaller than permanent teeth, and whiter in colour
- Their roots are often partially or completely **resorbed** during the eruption of the underlying permanent teeth
- They have larger pulp chambers than permanent teeth, with thinner enamel
- The roots of deciduous molars are widely **divergent** because the permanent premolar teeth crowns develop between them

Deciduous teeth are known as (Figure 7.10):

- **A = central incisor**
- **B = lateral incisor**
- **C = canine**
- **D = first molar**
- **E = second molar**

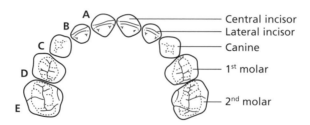

Figure 7.10 Deciduous teeth. Source: *Levison's Textbook for Dental Nurses*, 10th edn, C. Hollins, 2008, Wiley-Blackwell.

Lower As tend to erupt first, and upper Es are usually the last, at around 29 months.

Permanent teeth

These are also called adult teeth or second teeth.

- They make up a total set of 32, 16 in each jaw – if the third molars (wisdom teeth) are present
- It is relatively common to have some adult teeth congenitally missing (called **hypodontia**), especially the third molars
- They are referred to in dentistry by number – 1, 2, 3, 4, 5, 6, 7, 8 starting from the midline
- They begin developing around birth, and start erupting at age 6 years

■ Three permanent molar teeth develop behind the deciduous teeth in the space that becomes available as the jaws grow and lengthen

■ So deciduous **molar** teeth are succeeded by permanent **premolar** teeth

Permanent teeth are known as (Figure 7.11):

■ **1 = central incisor**
■ **2 = lateral incisor**
■ **3 = canine**
■ **4 = first premolar**
■ **5 = second premolar**
■ **6 = first molar**
■ **7 = second molar**
■ **8 = third molar (wisdom tooth)**

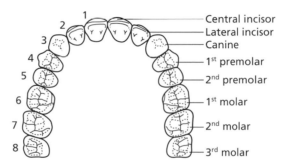

Figure 7.11 Permanent teeth. Source: *Levison's Textbook for Dental Nurses,* 10th edn, C. Hollins, 2008, Wiley-Blackwell.

Lower 1s and all 6s erupt first, and 8s erupt last – at anything from 18 to 25 years normally, but they can erupt even later.

Tooth surface nomenclature

All surfaces of the teeth are named from the midline backwards, and from the inner to the outer areas of the oral cavity (Figure 7.12):

■ Surfaces towards the midline are **mesial**
■ Surfaces furthest from the midline are **distal**
■ Lower inner surfaces (against the tongue) are **lingual**
■ Upper inner surfaces (against roof of mouth) are **palatal**
■ Outer surfaces of front teeth (against the lips) are **labial**
■ Outer surfaces of back teeth (against the cheeks) are **buccal**

Uppers

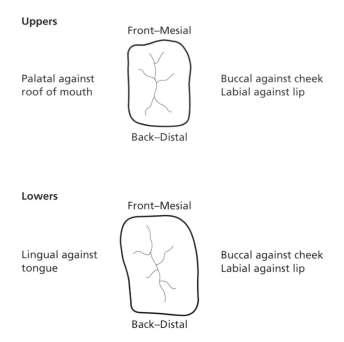

Front–Mesial

Palatal against
roof of mouth

Buccal against cheek
Labial against lip

Back–Distal

Lowers

Front–Mesial

Lingual against
tongue

Buccal against cheek
Labial against lip

Back–Distal

Figure 7.12 Tooth surface nomenclature.

Front teeth are incisors and canines, referred to as the **anterior teeth**, and they have incisal edges, while back teeth are premolars and molars, referred to as the **posterior teeth**, and they have cusps.

Identification of permanent teeth (Figure 7.13)

Incisors

- These teeth have a flattened crown with one root
- The central incisors are larger than the lateral incisors
- Their incisal edges are used to cut food
- The palatal or lingual surface of all the incisors has an enamel plateau called the cingulum
- The upper central incisor is the largest of all the incisors

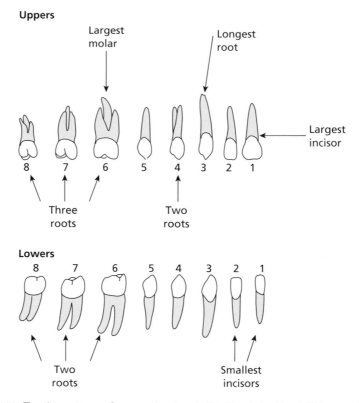

Figure 7.13 Tooth anatomy. Source: *Levison's Textbook for Dental Nurses,* 10th edn, C. Hollins, 2008, Wiley-Blackwell.

Canines

- They have a **large conical crown** with a pointed incisal edge and **one long root**
- They are used to cut and tear food
- The upper canines are larger than the lowers
- The upper canines have the longest of all roots

Premolars

- They all have **two cusps,** which are of equal size in the uppers, but with a smaller lingual cusp in the lowers
- The upper first premolar has **two roots** (buccal and palatal), all the others have **one root**
- They are used for tearing and chewing food

Molars

- They all have a large **occlusal surface** for grinding and chewing food
- All the upper molars have **three roots** (palatal, mesiobuccal and distobuccal)
- All the lower molars have **two roots** (mesial and distal)
- The upper first molar has five cusps, the fifth one is called the **cusp of Carabelli**
- The lower first molar has **five cusps**, three buccal and two lingual
- All other molars have **four cusps**
- The roots of third molars vary in number, with the uppers often being fused together

In a normal mouth, all incisal edges and cusps of upper and lower teeth interlock, to give a stable bite (occlusion). The upper arch is usually wider so that the lower teeth bite into the middle of the upper molars and premolars and the cingulum of the incisors and canines.

Occlusal classification

Tooth occlusion is assessed and problems diagnosed in the speciality of **orthodontics**. Orthodontics includes the study of the size and position discrepancies which occur between the teeth and the jaws, and the treatment carried out to resolve these discrepancies.

With the mouth closed and the teeth touching together, the teeth are said to be in occlusion, and the occlusion is determined by the position of the first molars and the canines to each other. This is known as **Angle's classification**.

More recently, a similar classification based on the position of the incisors has been developed and is commonly used by dentists in the UK.

Class I – ideal occlusion (Figure 7.14)

Ideal occlusion is denoted as **Class I**, where the mesiobuccal cusp of the upper first molar lies in the buccal groove of the lower first molar. The tips of the upper central incisors project forward from the labial surface of the lower central incisors by between 2 mm and 4 mm – this is called the **overjet**. The upper central incisors cover the labial surface of the lower central incisors by 50% – this is called the **overbite**.

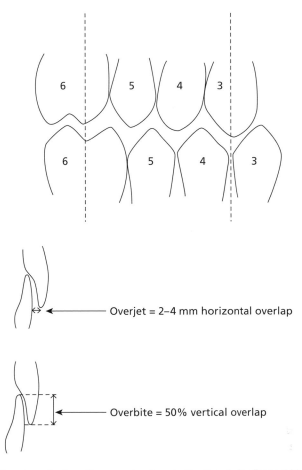

Figure 7.14 Class I occlusion. Source: *Levison's Textbook for Dental Nurses,* 10th edn, C. Hollins, 2008, Wiley-Blackwell.

Class II occlusion

When the lower jaw develops further back than normal, the relationship of the first molars to each other will be incorrect, so that the upper mesiobuccal cusp lies in front of its normal position. This is called **Class II** malocclusion.

If the upper central incisors escape the confines of the lower lip as they erupt, they will tend to develop sticking out, or **proclined**, and the overjet will measure more than 4 mm – this is called **Class II division 1** (Figure 7.15). If the upper central incisors remain inside the lower lip as they erupt, they tend to be tipped upright or even backwards by the strong muscular force of the lower lip, and appear **retroclined**. This tends to allow the lower incisors to erupt past their normal position onto the cingulum of the upper incisors, and the overbite will be greater than 50% – this is called **Class II division 2** (Figure 7.16).

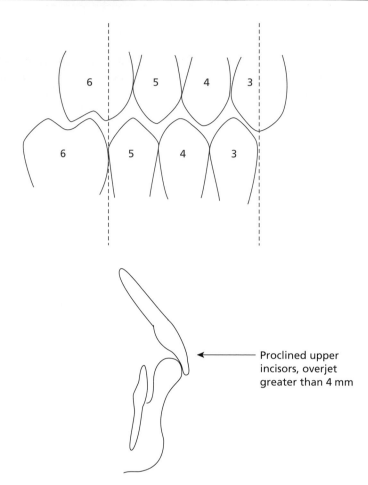

Figure 7.15 Class II division 1 malocclusion. Source: *Levison's Textbook for Dental Nurses,* 10th edn, C. Hollins, 2008, Wiley-Blackwell.

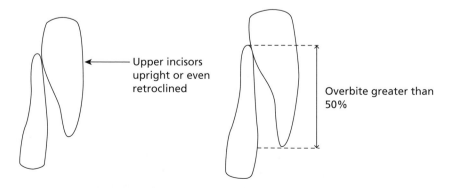

Figure 7.16 Class II division 2 malocclusion. Source: *Levison's Textbook for Dental Nurses,* 10th edn, C. Hollins, 2008, Wiley-Blackwell.

Class III occlusion

When the lower jaw develops further forwards than normal, the relationship of the first molars will again be incorrect, with the mesiobuccal cusp of the upper being behind the buccal groove of the lower. This is called **Class III** malocclusion.

The upper central incisors may develop with a reduced overjet, or bite edge to edge, or there may even be a reverse overjet because the upper central incisors are behind the lower central incisors – this is called a **negative overjet** (Figure 7.17). The overbite tends to be less than 50%, or zero if the incisors bite edge to edge, or they may not even meet – this is called an **anterior open bite**.

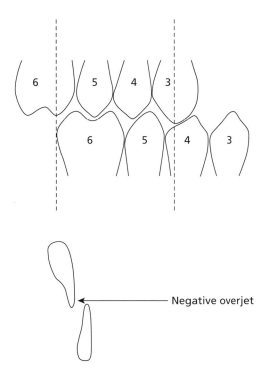

Figure 7.17 Class III malocclusion. Source: *Levison's Textbook for Dental Nurses*, 10th edn, C. Hollins, 2008, Wiley-Blackwell.

Dental clinical assessments

Clinical assessments are carried out each time a patient attends the dental practice. Some patients attend more frequently than others by choice, and some require more frequent attendance than others, in the dentist's professional opinion. The dentist's opinion is based on the known risk factors of oral disease, and the patient's frequency of exposure to these risk factors. Assessment of oral health is carried out in the following areas:

- Extra-oral soft tissues
- Intra-oral soft tissues
- Deciduous and mixed dentition of children
- Permanent dentition
- Periodontal tissues
- Occlusion

The main purpose of carrying out the dental clinical assessment is to promote the prevention of oral diseases by regular examination, and education in the prevention of disease to the patient.

If disease is already present, regular oral assessment will detect it at an earlier stage and allow full recovery to be more likely. If serious disease is present, such as oral cancer, regular inspection will identify it earlier and allow the patient to be referred for specialist care, with a better chance of successful treatment and recovery.

Extra-oral soft tissue assessment

The following are examined and assessed for any abnormality:

- **External facial signs** – checking for skin colour, facial symmetry, the presence of any blemishes, especially moles
- **The lips** – checking for any change in colour, and felt for any abnormalities, and the presence of any blemishes
- **The lymph nodes** – lying under the mandible and in the neck, these are palpated to detect any swellings or abnormalities

Variations in skin colour do occur, especially among different ethnic groups. Some patients are naturally pale and others are naturally ruddy. However, an unusual facial appearance can sometimes indicate problems, such as nervous patients becoming pale and clammy as they are about to faint, or the unnatural ruddiness of a patient with hypertension.

Facial asymmetry (where one side of the face is shaped differently from the other) could indicate the presence of swelling, or problems with nerve supply or muscular control, all of which require further investigation. The sudden appearance of unusual skin blemishes, especially moles, may indicate the presence of an early skin cancer (**melanoma**), which will need urgent treatment.

Similarly, the lips are examined and details recorded of blemishes, such as the presence of a **cold sore** indicating infection with the herpes simplex type 1 virus, or the presence of minor salivary gland cysts (mucoceles). Lips tinged bluish-purple indicates some degree of chronic heart failure, which needs noting before local anaesthesia and traumatic dental procedures are carried out.

Lymph nodes are part of the body's immune system, and any enlargement of these indicates that the body is fighting infection or some other disease process, and requires further investigation.

Intra-oral soft tissue assessment

This is carried out at each dental examination and in a systematic manner, so that no areas are not investigated:

■ **Labial, buccal and sulcus mucosa** – checked for their colour and texture, moisture level noted
■ **Palatal mucosa** – both the hard and soft palates, the oropharynx, and the tonsils (if present)
■ **Tongue** – checked for colour and texture, symmetry of shape and movement, level of mobility, all surfaces especially beneath the tongue, as this is one of the commonest sites for oral carcinoma to develop
■ **Floor of mouth** – checked for colour and texture, and the presence of any swellings

Low moisture levels in the mouth can indicate salivary gland problems, especially in older people and those taking certain medications. Saliva has important functions with regard to defence, cleansing and dental disease initiation.

The commonest areas for oral cancers to develop are on the borders or beneath the tongue, and in the floor of the mouth, and these areas will be particularly well examined in patients with known risk factors. All findings can then be recorded on a suitable assessment sheet (Figure 7.18).

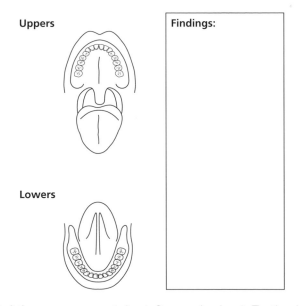

Figure 7.18 Soft tissue assessment sheet. Source: *Levison's Textbook for Dental Nurses*, 10th edn, C. Hollins, 2008, Wiley-Blackwell.

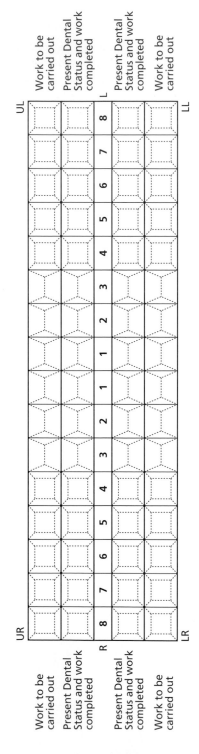

Figure 7.19 Forensic notation. Source: *Levison's Textbook for Dental Nurses*, 10th edn, C. Hollins, 2008, Wiley-Blackwell.

Tooth charting

For ease of recording, a system of charting of the teeth has been developed which is universally recognised by all those in the dental profession. It allows a speedy but accurate record of an individual's dentition to be produced, which can be clearly read and understood by other dental professionals.

The Palmer notation of tooth charting divides the mouth into quadrants:

- **Upper right**
- **Upper left**
- **Lower left**
- **Lower right**

Each anterior tooth has four surfaces and an incisal edge or canine cusp, and each posterior tooth has five surfaces. The shapes of the teeth can be simplified and drawn on the dental chart to show all of these surfaces with each tooth referred to as its corresponding number (for permanent teeth) or letter (for deciduous teeth) as shown in Figure 7.19. The teeth are recorded from the centreline backwards for both the deciduous and permanent dentition.

The condition of the teeth and the presence of any restorations can then be charted in a code form on the inner grid, and work to be carried out is recorded in the outer grid. Examples of some of the recognised charting notations are shown below, but readers are advised to consult the 'Charting Booklet' produced by the National Examining Board for Dental Nurses for the full range of definitive notations.

- UE – unerupted
- PE – partially erupted
- — – missing
- X – recently extracted
- → – space closed
- # – tooth fracture
- PJC – porcelain jacket crown
- FBC – full bonded crown
- FGC – full gold crown
- SSC – stainless steel crown
- AJC – acrylic jacket crown
- CV – composite veneer
- PV – porcelain veneer
- IMP – implant
- FS – fissure sealed
- FF – fissure filled
- GI – gold inlay
- CI – composite inlay
- PI – porcelain inlay
- RF – root filling

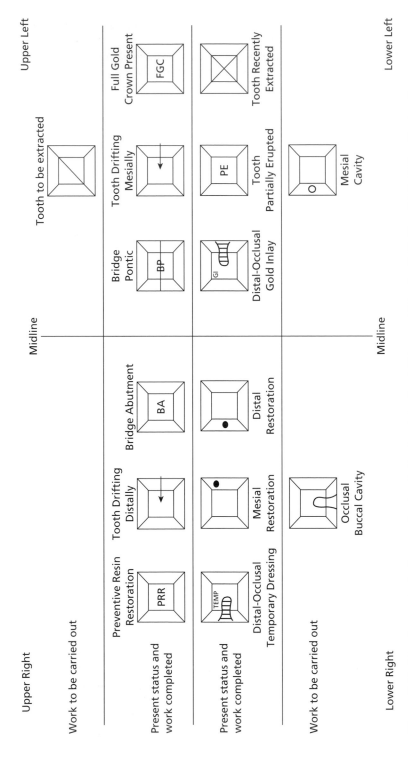

Figure 7.20 Charting symbols. Source: *Levison's Textbook for Dental Nurses*, 10th edn, C. Hollins, 2008, Wiley-Blackwell.

An example of a completed chart is shown in Figure 7.20. The problem with this system is that the growing use of computers in dental practice makes the accurate recording of these items more difficult as the notations are not present on a computer keyboard, and it varies with the computer software used too. A more modern approach is the two-digit FDI system (International Dental Federation) whereby each quadrant as well as each tooth is numbered (Figure 7.21).

Adult

Upper right quadrant 1	Upper left quadrant 2
Lower right quadrant 4	Lower left quadrant 3

Child

Upper right quadrant 5	Upper left quadrant 6
Lower right quadrant 8	Lower left quadrant 7

Figure 7.21 FDI charting.

- Upper right quadrant of adult is 1
- Upper left quadrant of adult is 2
- Lower left quadrant of adult is 3
- Lower right quadrant of adult is 4
- Upper right quadrant of child is 5
- Upper left quadrant of child is 6
- Lower left quadrant of child is 7
- Lower right quadrant of child is 8

The permanent teeth are numbered 1 to 8 from the midline and the deciduous teeth are then numbered 1 to 5, from the midline (Figure 7.22).

So tooth notations are recorded as:

- Upper right first molar is either UR6 or 16 (pronounced 1–6)
- Upper left second premolar is either UL5 or 25 (pronounced 2–5)
- Lower left deciduous canine is either LLC or 73 (pronounced 7–3)
- Lower right second deciduous molar is either LRE or 85 (pronounced 8–5)
- Lower left first premolar is either LL4 or 34 (pronounced 3–4)
- Lower right second molar is either LR7 or 47 (pronounced 4–7)

Adult

18	17	16	15	14	13	12	11	21	22	23	24	25	26	27	28
48	47	46	45	44	43	42	41	31	32	33	34	35	36	37	38

Child

55	54	53	52	51	61	62	63	64	65
85	84	83	82	81	71	72	73	74	75

Figure 7.22 FDI notation.

The instruments used to carry out the tooth charting assessment are:

- **Mouth mirrors** – to reflect light onto the tooth surface, to retract soft tissues for clear vision, and to protect the soft tissues
- **Angled probe** – to detect soft tooth surfaces, and to detect margins on existing restorations
- **Briault probe** (Figure 7.23) – specially angled to detect inter-proximal caries

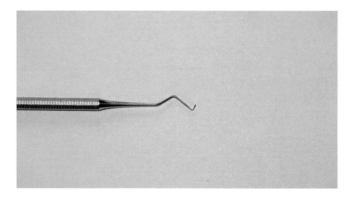

Figure 7.23 Briault probe.

Eruption dates of deciduous and permanent teeth

Each tooth has an age range during which it normally erupts into the mouth, and knowledge and recording of the teeth present at each oral assessment helps to determine whether younger patients are likely to require dental intervention during the 'mixed dentition' stage, when both deciduous and permanent teeth are present. For example, permanent teeth erupting later than normal can cause crowding problems.

Deciduous teeth begin erupting at around 6–8 months of age, and are usually all present by 29 months of age. Permanent teeth begin erupting at around 6 years of age, and are usually all present by 13 years of age, except the third molar, which tends to erupt any time after 18 years of age (see below).

Deciduous dentition

Tooth	Letter	Upper eruption date – months	Lower eruption date – months
Central incisor	A	10	8
Lateral incisor	B	11	13
Canine	C	19	20
First molar	D	16	16
Second molar	E	29	27

Permanent dentition

Tooth	Number	Upper eruption date – years	Lower eruption date – years
Central incisor	1	7–8	6–7
Lateral incisor	2	8–9	7–8
Canine	3	10–12	9–10
First premolar	4	9–11	9–11
Second premolar	5	10–11	9–11
First molar	6	6–7	6–7
Second molar	7	12–13	11–12
Third molar	8	18–25	18–25

Periodontal tissue assessment

The periodontal tissues are those acting as **supporting tissues** around the tooth – the gingivae, the periodontal ligament, and the underlying alveolar bone forming the tooth socket. These tissues can undergo disease processes to varying degrees, and in the worst case scenario, healthy teeth can be lost due to periodontal disease. Periodontal disease is often painless and can remain undetected for many years if thorough oral assessments are not carried out, as the patient is often unaware of its existence.

As with tooth charting, a system has been developed whereby the presence of periodontal disease can be quickly recorded during routine oral assessment, by dividing the mouth into sextants and recording the presence of any periodontal pockets down the side of the teeth. This is called a **Basic Periodontal Examination (BPE) assessment** and is recorded as shown in Figure 7.24. A special periodontal probe is used which has graduation marks so that the depth of the pocket in millimetres can be measured (Figure 7.25). This is then coded depending on the depth of the pocket.

Upper teeth

18–14	13–23	24–28
48–44	43–33	34–38

Lower teeth

Figure 7.24 BPE chart.

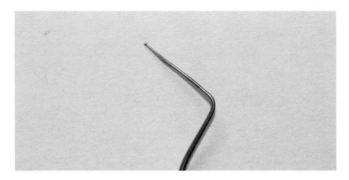

Figure 7.25 BPE probe.

- ▪ **Code 0** – healthy gingival tissues, no bleeding
- ▪ **Code 1** – coloured area of probe visible, no calculus or defective margins present, bleeding on probing (pocket less than 3.5 mm)
- ▪ **Code 2** – coloured area visible, plaque retention factors detected (pocket less than 3.5 mm)
- ▪ **Code 3** – coloured area partly visible (pocket less than 5.5 mm)
- ▪ **Code 4** – coloured area not visible (pocket more than 6 mm)
- ▪ **Code*** – furcation involvement, or recession and pocket depths 7 mm or more

Higher codes therefore indicate more serious periodontal problems in that sextant (Figure 7.26). Any patients with scores of code 3 maximum, or codes 4 or * anywhere, require individual pocket depths to be recorded in full on a periodontal

2	0	4
2	1	3

Figure 7.26 Completed BPE chart. Source: *Levison's Textbook for Dental Nurses*, 10th edn, C. Hollins, 2008, Wiley-Blackwell.

chart, so that intensive periodontal treatment can be initiated (Figure 7.27). The oral health status can also be noted during periodontal assessment, such as the presence and extent of dental plaque. The standard of oral hygiene can be graded as excellent, good, fair, or poor.

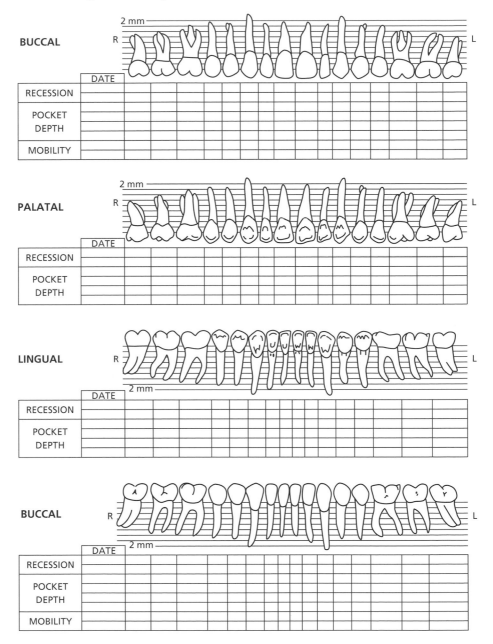

Figure 7.27 Periodontal disease chart. Source: *Levison's Textbook for Dental Nurses*, 10th edn, C. Hollins, 2008, Wiley-Blackwell.

Several different styles of full periodontal charts are available, and the example shown can also be used to record tooth mobility, and the presence of plaque or gingival bleeding.

Tooth mobility is graded as:

■   **Grade I** for side to side movement of less than 2 mm
■   **Grade II** for side to side movement of more than 2 mm
■   **Grade III** for vertical movement as well

Assessment of occlusion for orthodontics

A full orthodontic examination is carried out by the dental surgeon to record the following points:

■   Buccal and incisal classification of **malocclusion**
■   **Overjet** measurement
■   **Overbite** measurement
■   Presence in each arch of any **crowding**, its severity (mild, moderate, severe) and whether occurring labially or buccally
■   Presence of any **retained deciduous teeth**
■   Presence of any **tooth rotations**
■   Presence of unilateral or bilateral **crossbites**
■   Presence of upper or lower **centreline shifts**, and whether to the right or left of normal

The severity of any malocclusion can then be determined by taking the worst feature and scoring it in accordance with the Index of Treatment Need (IOTN) clinical score. It is not necessary for dental nurses to have an in-depth knowledge of the use of the IOTN. Suffice it to say that the higher the number scored from 1 to 5, and the closer the letter to 'a' in the alphabet, then the worse the malocclusion.

Study models

These are accurate models of both arches produced by taking alginate impressions and a wax bite of the patient (see Unit 9 (Chapter 10) for details of impression materials and mixing techniques). They are cast in dental stone, and articulated by hand and trimmed so that the malocclusion present is correctly reproduced (Figure 7.28). Their use allows the dentist to study the malocclusion from all angles, at leisure.

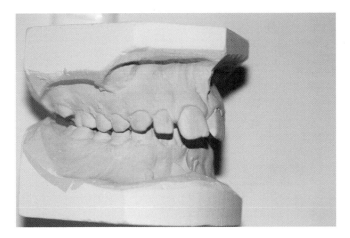

Figure 7.28 Orthodontic study models.

Radiographs

The basic radiographic view required is ideally an orthopantomograph (OPT), or bilateral oblique views (see Unit 7 (Chapter 8) for details). These should show all of the following:

- Presence or absence of any **unerupted teeth**
- Positions of unerupted teeth
- Presence of any **supernumerary teeth**
- Presence of any **pathological lesions**, such as cysts, caries, periodontal disease
- Presence or absence of **third molar teeth**, and their positions

Often, a naso-occlusal or maxillary occlusal view is also taken to show the following:

- Shape of incisor roots
- Any pathology associated with the incisor roots
- Presence of any supernumeraries, and their relationship to the incisors
- Presence and extent of any root resorption of incisors

The two radiographs together can then be used to determine the position of any unerupted and impacted teeth, and are especially useful when determining the position of unerupted upper canine teeth.

Methods used to carry out assessments

The main methods available to carry out dental clinical assessments are:

- **Visual inspection** to detect visible problems
- **Manual inspection** to feel abnormalities
- Use of **mouth mirrors** for intra-oral and tooth assessments
- Use of various **probes** for tooth inspections
- Use of **periodontal probe** for periodontal assessment
- Use of various **radiograph** views, and **photographs**
- Use of **study models**
- Use of **trans-illumination** of anterior teeth to detect interproximal cavities (bright light such as that from the curing lamp is shone through the tooth, and cavities show as dark lesions)

Vitality tests

These are sometimes necessary, to aid in determining whether a tooth is vital (alive) or non-vital (dead), and the tests available are:

- Cold stimulus with **ethyl chloride**
- Hot stimulus with warmed **gutta percha**
- Electrical test with **electric pulp tester**

The first two techniques are used to diagnose toothache where the symptoms include pain with cold or heat, whereas electric pulp testers are more accurate in determining the 'degree' of vitality of a tooth, as follows:

- Normal response – healthy pulp
- Increased response – early pulpitis present
- Reduced response – pulp is dying, or tooth has heavily lined deep restoration present so the voltage cannot be adequately transmitted to the pulp
- No response – pulp tissue is dead

Patients will vary in their response to electric pulp testers, so it is always advisable to test several apparently healthy teeth to establish what their 'normal' response is, before testing the suspect tooth.

Electric pulp testers are either battery operated or mains operated, and they work by sending an increasing voltage into the tooth until the patient is aware of a sensation. The point at which the patient indicates a sensation is recorded numerically on a scale, so that the 'degree' of vitality can be determined in relation to 'test' teeth.

Study models

In some situations, it is necessary for the dentist to consider the patient's occlusion before being able to decide on any treatment necessary, for example when provide partial dentures or orthodontic treatment (see above). Impressions are taken of both dental arches using alginate impression material and then cast up to produce a set of study models.

Study models are useful in the following cases:

- Occlusal analysis in complicated crown or bridge cases
- Orthodontic cases, to determine if extractions are required and which type of appliance is necessary
- Occlusal analysis where full mouth treatment may be necessary, to determine the functioning of the dentition
- Where tooth surface loss is evident, either by erosion from acidic foods and drinks, or by attrition due to tooth grinding, so that the progression of the tooth wear can be monitored and treatment determined

Photographs

These can be taken to record various aspects of the dentition or soft tissues, for future reference. They can be produced using conventional cameras (especially 'Instamatic' types), digital cameras with 'macro' lenses for close-up shots, or by using specialist intra-oral digital cameras. Specialised computers and equipment are required for this last technique.

Photographs are useful to record:

- Soft tissue lesions to aid diagnosis
- Extent of injury following trauma
- Before and after views of dental treatment

Provision of support during oral health assessment

The regularity of attendance for dental examinations puts the dentist in a unique position to monitor normality and detect abnormality at an early stage. Patients tend to seek medical advice only when they detect a problem, and this is often when a medical condition has existed for some time and is therefore quite likely to be more advanced and serious in nature. Thorough and accurate recording of findings at these dental examinations is therefore of great importance.

The dental nurse's role during dental clinical assessment is to:

- Support and reassure the patient throughout the assessment
- Have all the necessary instruments and equipment ready for use
- Be able to make accurate clinical records as required
- Be proficient in the use of soft tissue record sheets, if used

- Be proficient in the charting of teeth
- Be proficient in the recording of periodontal conditions
- Be able to complete a full medical history form, with the patient
- Assist the dentist as necessary throughout the assessment

Clinical notes are taken either in writing or entered into a computer system. Many dentists write their own notes, for medico-legal reasons, to ensure that everything said and done is recorded accurately, but others rely on the dental nurse to 'take notes'. It is imperative that these are full, concise and accurate, and include details of verbal discussions too. When legal problems arise, the production of full and contemporaneous notes ensure that any investigations and complaints can be dealt with correctly.

Full clinical notes should include all of the following, as necessary:

- Name, address, telephone numbers, and date of birth
- Doctor's details
- Medical history
- Dental history
- Contemporaneous clinical notes of each attendance
- Tooth and periodontal chartings
- Soft tissue assessments
- Details of all appointments with others, such as hygienist
- Consent forms, and all legally required NHS or private paperwork
- Copies of all referral letters
- Radiographs, correctly mounted as necessary
- Copies of any laboratory slips
- Records of all payment transactions
- Copies of any letters sent to patient, especially account letters

Medical history forms should be completed at every oral assessment session, and it should be verified at each attendance whether changes have occurred or not. The patient should sign and date the form when each update is recorded. Various styles of medical history form are available, or a practice can issue their own. An example is shown in Figure 7.29.

The pertinent questions that need to be asked of the patient are:

- Are they attending a general practice or hospital for or receiving any medical treatment currently?
- Are they taking, or have taken steroids in the past two years?
- Are they taking any other medications, including those bought over the counter?
- Do they have any known allergies?
- Are they currently a pregnant woman or a nursing mother?
- Do they have an human immunodeficiency virus (HIV)-positive status?
- Have they ever had rheumatic fever?
- Have they ever had liver, jaundice, hepatitis, or kidney disease?

■ Do they have any history of heart murmur, angina, or high blood pressure?
■ Is there any history of other heart problems?
■ Do they have a history of a bad reaction to local or general anaesthetic?
■ Do they have a history of arthritis, if so where?
■ Is there any history of diabetes, of themselves or a family member?
■ Is there any history of respiratory disease, including asthma?
■ Is there any history of epilepsy or fainting?
■ Do they carry any medical warning cards?
■ Do they have any other medical conditions or concerns to be disclosed?
■ Are they a smoker or non-smoker, and how many per day?
■ What is their average daily alcohol consumption?

Details can then be given for any positive responses to any of the questions. Using the information provided, the dental surgeon can determine the necessity for taking any special precautions during dental treatment, or even whether the patient should be referred for specialist care. This may be necessary for patients such as those taking warfarin as an anti-coagulant and who require multiple tooth extractions. In particular, prescribed medication can be checked to determine if one type of dental local anaesthetic should be used over another, especially in patients with heart disease.

First aid and medical emergencies

The basic requirements for all dental practices are:

■ All staff must be trained in basic first aid on an annual basis, in accordance with clinical governance guidelines, and have a nominated first aider
■ All practices must have a first aid kit available, besides the emergency drugs box and oxygen cylinder which must be kept too
■ All practices must have an accident book, which is used to record all events occurring on the premises, to both staff and patients alike
■ The medical emergencies described below can occur in dental practice, and the dental nurse may well be the first on the scene, so correct knowledge and procedures are imperative
■ The aim of the dental nurse is to reassure and help the casualty until help arrives, including maintaining life if necessary

Basic life support (BLS) is covered in detail in Unit 3 (Chapter 4). Medical emergencies relevant to the dental workplace are covered here, with a summary of each condition and the first aid treatment that must be applied. The emergencies discussed below are:

■ Severe bleeding
■ Burns and scalds

CONFIDENTIAL MEDICAL HISTORY

To provide the best and safest treatment, your dentist needs to know of any problems that may affect your treatment.

NAME _____

SEX: MALE/FEMALE _____

ADDRESS _____

_____

TEL NO: HOME _____ WORK _____

DATE OF BIRTH _____ OCCUPATION _____

WHEN DID YOU LAST RECEIVE DENTAL TREATMENT? _____

DOCTOR'S NAME AND ADDRESS _____

_____

	YES	NO	IF YES, PLEASE GIVE DETAILS
Are you attending or receiving treatment from a doctor, clinic, hospital or specialist?			
Are you taking any medicines, tablets, drugs or injections or using any creams or ointments?			
Are you taking or have taken any steroids in the last 2 years?			
Are you allergic to Penicillin?			
Are you allergic to any medicines, foods or materials?			
Are you pregnant or a nursing mother?			
Are you HIV positive?			
Have you had Rheumatic Fever or chorea?			
Have you had jaundice, liver, kidney disease or hepatitis?			
Have you been hospitalised for any reason?			
Have you ever had your blood refused by the blood transfusion service?			

Figure 7.29 Example of a medical history form.

	YES	NO	IF YES, PLEASE GIVE DETAILS
Have you ever been told you have a heart murmur, heart problem, angina or high blood pressure?			
Have you ever had a bad reaction to a local or general anaesthetic?			
Have you had a joint replacement or other implant?			
Do you have arthritis?			
Do you have a pacemaker or have you had heart surgery?			
Do you suffer from hay fever, eczema or any other allergy?			
Do you suffer from bronchitis, asthma or other chest condition?			
Do you have fainting attacks, giddiness, blackouts or epilepsy?			
Do you or anyone in your family have diabetes?			
Do you bruise or bleed easily following a tooth extraction or injury?			
Do you carry a warning card?			
Do you think there are any other aspects concerning your health that your dentist should know about?			
Are your a smoker/drinker? If so, how many of the following do you consume per day?	Cigarettes		Alcoholic units

SIGNED   DATE

Figure 7.29 (*Continued*)

- Poisoning
- Electrocution
- Bone fractures
- Faint
- Epileptic fit
- Anaphylactic shock
- Myocardial infarction

Severe bleeding

- The first aid principle is to restrict blood flow to the wound and so encourage clotting and reduce blood loss
- Arterial bleeding will spurt rhythmically from a wound and be cherry red in colour
- Venous bleeding will gush quickly from a wound and be dark red/purple in colour
- Capillary bleeding will ooze slowly from a wound and be dark red in colour

Treatment

- Raise the injured body part above heart level if possible
- Apply direct pressure onto the wound with a clean dressing for 5–15 minutes
- Do not remove any foreign bodies, such as broken glass, from the wound
- As a last resort, apply indirect pressure for arterial bleeding by compressing the artery against underlying bone, for just 5–15 minutes at a time

Burns and scalds

- Burns are injuries to body tissues caused by heat, chemicals or radiation
- Scalds are wet heat burns, caused by steam or hot liquids
- The first aid principle is to prevent infection of the underlying tissues, which are no longer protected by the skin, and to prevent clinical shock developing due to blood serum loss

Treatment

- Remove the casualty from all sources of danger if safe to do so
- Reassure the casualty, if they are conscious
- Place the injured part under cold water for a minimum of 10 minutes
- Remove any jewellery likely to cause constrictions, before swelling occurs
- Do not remove clothing, as this may be stuck to the skin and cause further tissue damage
- Seek medical help
- Carry out BLS if necessary

Poisoning

The first aid principle is to limit the exposure of the casualty to the poison, and maintain life until medical help arrives.

Treatment

■ Consult any relevant COSHH documents for first aid advice
■ Remove the casualty from the source of the poison, if safe to do so
■ Do not induce vomiting, under any circumstances
■ Maintain the airway and carry out BLS if necessary
■ Seek urgent medical help, giving details of the poison if known

Electrocution

■ This is caused by the passage of an electrical current through the body, which causes burns and can interfere with the heart beat, such that it beats erratically (fibrillation) or actually stops (asystole)
■ The first aid principle is to stop the electrical current and maintain life until medical help arrives

Treatment

■ Isolate the electricity source with great care, if safe to do so
■ Treat any surface burns as above, and minimise the effects of shock
■ Give BLS if necessary
■ Seek urgent medical help

Fractures

■ These usually occur due to external trauma or falls, especially with older patients
■ The first aid principle is to prevent further damage by restricting movement while medical help arrives

Treatment

■ Do not move the injured part, and restrict any movement by the casualty
■ Cover any open skin wounds with clean dressings to prevent infection
■ Control bleeding, as above
■ Seek urgent medical help

Faint

■ This is a brief loss of consciousness due to a temporary reduction in oxygenated blood flow to the brain and is the likeliest medical emergency to be

encountered in dental practice. The casualty will appear pale and clammy, and have a weak and thready pulse
- The first aid principle is to restore the cranial blood flow immediately

Treatment

- If conscious, sit with the head down, loosen tight clothing and provide fresh air flow. If unconscious, lay down and raise the casualty's legs above their head
- Maintain the airway and loosen tight clothing
- Provide fresh air flow
- Give a glucose drink when consciousness returns, as the casualty often faints due to lack of nutrients

Epileptic fit

- This occurs due to a brief disruption of the normal electrical activity of the brain. They can be slight fits (petit mal) where the casualty may just appear to be daydreaming, or major fits (grand mal) where muscle spasms and convulsions occur
- The latter occur in two stages and are known as 'tonic-clonic' seizures, where initially the casualty loses consciousness and become rigid, before a period of convulsion occurs
- The fit can last up to 5 minutes, and the casualty may be dazed afterwards
- In some instances, the casualty may become incontinent during the fit
- The first aid principle is merely to allow the fit to progress, and ensure the casualty's safety throughout

Treatment

- Do not attempt to move the casualty
- Remove all possible sources of injury from the immediate area
- Keep onlookers away and preserve the casualty's dignity
- Allow recovery to occur, then arrange an escort home
- If recovery does not occur, seek urgent medical help

Anaphylactic shock

- This is an over-reaction by the casualty's immune system to combat exposure to an allergen, such as in allergy to penicillin. It produces sudden onset rash formation and facial swelling, with restricted breathing followed by loss of consciousness
- The first aid principle is to maintain life until medical help arrives

Treatment

■ Prevent further exposure to the allergen, if safe to do so
■ Maintain the airway
■ Give BLS if necessary
■ Seek urgent medical help

Myocardial infarction

■ This occurs when the blood flow to the heart is obstructed
■ The casualty will experience a sudden crushing pain in the upper body, they will become giddy, breathless and lose consciousness rapidly, and they will appear grey
■ The first aid principle is to maintain life until medical help arrives

Treatment

■ If still conscious, give an aspirin tablet and oxygen
■ Do not lay flat back, and restrict all movement by the casualty
■ Seek urgent medical help
■ If unconscious, maintain the airway and give oxygen
■ If cardiac arrest occurs, begin BLS
■ Seek urgent medical help

Materials used in oral assessment

Materials that may be required to carry out oral assessments are:

■ **Ethyl chloride** – a liquid which vaporises easily and produces a cold sensation on doing so, can be applied to teeth as an aid to detecting dental problems (Figure 7.30)

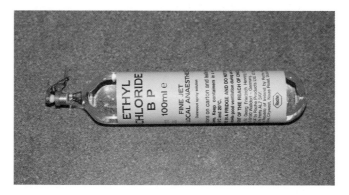

Figure 7.30 Ethyl chloride container.

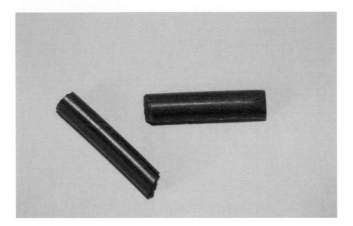

Figure 7.31 Greenstick composition.

- **Gutta percha** – a stick of green composition which can be heated and applied to a tooth to aid detection of dental problems (Figure 7.31)
- **Alginate** – an impression material consisting of calcium and alginate salts which are mixed with water at room temperature and loaded into trays for insertion into the mouth, so that accurate impressions can be taken
- **Dental stone** – a hardened calcium sulphate plaster mixed with water and used to produce a study model cast
- **Dental plaster** – a calcium sulphate plaster mixed with water and used to make a base for the dental stone cast

8 Unit 7: Contribute to the Production of Dental Images (OH4)

Knowledge specifications

Ionising radiation

K1 – A factual knowledge of ionising radiations – their nature and uses

K2 – A factual knowledge of the hazards associated with ionising radiations, including the effects which they may have on general health, and the likely effect of different doses of radiation on people

K3 – A factual knowledge of the risks associated with ionising radiations in general and the relative risks associated with dental radiographs

Health, safety and infection control

K4 – A working knowledge of the purpose, method of use, and function of protective wear and the reason for their use during assessment

K5 – A working knowledge of standard precautions and quality standards of infection control and your role in maintaining them

Radiation protection

K6 – A working knowledge of the practical protective measures which can be used to minimise risks to patients, self, the oral health care team, and the public

K7 – A working knowledge of why the radiation dose should be as low as possible

K8 – A working knowledge of methods for monitoring the ionising radiations which staff receive (eg Personal Radiation Monitors) and the purpose of these

K9 – A working knowledge of your role in relation to current legislation to protect persons undergoing medical examination and treatment (such as the Ionising Radiations Act, the Ionising (Medical Exposures) Regulations – including Local Rules, Control of Substances Hazardous to Health, Health and Safety at Work Act)

K10 – A working knowledge of the organisation's practices and policies relating to ionising radiations and the taking of radiographs

K11 – A working knowledge of the purpose of quality assuring dental radiographs and the relationship of this to radiation protection

K12 – A working knowledge of the organisation's quality assurance policy for processing dental radiographs, and your role in relation to this

K13 – A factual knowledge of the role of the Radiation Protection Supervisor and Radiation Protection Advisor in the organisation, their responsibilities and contribution to radiation protection

Principles of dental imaging

K14 – A factual knowledge of the dental imaging process (including digital and film)

K15 – A factual knowledge of the nature of dental imaging and their uses

Dental imaging – equipment and materials

K16 – A factual knowledge of the different sizes and types of radiographic film, how they are used and how to select the right one

K17 – A working knowledge of methods for cleaning the different equipment used, the reasons for doing this and the potential risks of not doing so

K18 – A working knowledge of methods of confirming the correct functioning of the equipment

K19 – A working knowledge of action to take in case of equipment failure

K20 – A working knowledge of the purpose and use of intensifying screens in dental radiography

K21 – A factual knowledge of the purpose of the different chemicals used in processing

K22 – A working knowledge of correct, safe methods of storage and disposal of the different chemicals

K23 – A factual knowledge of the reasons for storing films away from ionising radiations, the reasons for rotating film stock, and why film stock which has deteriorated should not be used

Patient management

K24 – A working knowledge of the concerns which patients may have regarding dental imaging, and methods of supporting patients during the taking of dental images

Dental radiography – processing films

K25 – A working knowledge of the reasons for protecting the processing environment from accidental intrusion, including the use of safe lights

K26 – A working knowledge of methods of handling the different films so as to maintain their quality

K27 – A working knowledge of correct methods of processing both extra- and intra-oral films, and the reasons for these

Dental radiography – mounting radiographs

K28 – A working knowledge of methods of mounting dental radiographs and the consequences of not doing so

K29 – A working knowledge of the organisation's policy for the filing of dental radiographs, and the records which should be attached to them

Dental radiography – assuring the quality of images and fault finding

K30 – A working knowledge of process defects (including fogging, density, contrast and handling marks), and criteria for determining whether a radiographic image is of an acceptable quality

Communication

K31 – A working knowledge of methods of communicating information clearly and effectively

K32 – A working knowledge of methods of modifying information and communication methods for different individuals, including patients from different social and ethnic backgrounds, children (including those with special needs), and the elderly

---

Dental radiography is an important aspect of dentistry with regard to diagnosing the cause of dental problems. Radiographs are used for the following reasons:

- To detect **dental caries**
- To detect levels of bone loss in **periodontal disease**
- To detect periodontal and periapical **abscesses**
- To detect cysts affecting the dental tissues
- To detect **iatrogenic problems** (that is, those caused by the dentist), such as overhanging restorations, perforations
- To aid in **endodontic treatment**
- To determine the number and position of tooth roots before **extraction**
- To detect **supernumerary** teeth and **unerupted** teeth
- To diagnose **hard tissue lesions**, such as bone cysts and tumours, salivary calculi, jaw fractures

Nature of ionising radiation

Ionising radiation is commonly referred to as 'x-rays'. X-rays are a type of electro-magnetic radiation that possess energy, like ultraviolet light and visible light. The radiation types differ from each other in the amount of energy they possess. X-rays having more energy so that they are capable of passing through matter such as human tissue. When they do so, one of three events will occur:

■ X-rays pass cleanly between the atoms of the matter and are **unaltered**
■ X-rays hit the atoms of the matter and are **scattered**, releasing their energy as they do so
■ X-rays hit the atoms of the matter and are **absorbed**, releasing their energy as they do so

With larger atoms of matter, such as some metals (including calcium), most of the x-rays are absorbed or scattered, and these are known as **radiopaque** substances. Those substances that allow the majority of the x-rays to pass through unaffected are called **radiolucent** substances.

As enamel contains a high calcium content, it is radiopaque to x-rays, and so are dentine and cementum to a lesser extent.

Effect of ionising radiation on the body

The energy released when the x-rays interact with human tissue is capable of causing tissue damage. This effect requires that x-rays are used only as necessary and at the lowest dose possible, to reduce the amount of energy released and therefore reduce the amount of tissue damage which occurs.

The effects occur when the x-rays hit the atoms of the cells in the tissues and are either scattered or absorbed, because of the energy that is released during these events. The energy released can **damage** the cells in the human tissues. The cells contain chromosomes, which are made up of DNA – the building blocks of life that determine exactly the organism that we are. If the energy hits the chromosomes it can damage them so that they undergo change (**mutation**) or even die.

This ability of x-rays to cause cell death is used in medicine to treat some types of cancer, during radiotherapy. The cancer cells can be accurately targeted to be hit by the ionising radiation beam so that they are killed outright, or so that the cancerous tumour is reduced to a size that can undergo surgical removal. High doses of x-rays are used for this treatment, and tissue cells that divide and grow rapidly, such as skin cells and the cells of children, are also easily affected.

However, cell death is an undesirable effect during the production of dental images. As there can be no 'safe' level of exposure to ionising radiation, strict legislation and guidelines have been introduced to ensure that the following occur when x-rays are used in dentistry.

- All use of dental imaging has to be **clinically justified**
- The dose of x-rays used must be kept **as low as reasonably achievable**
- Only the patient should be exposed to the x-ray beam
- Machines must be well maintained and serviced regularly
- No untrained personnel can be involved in radiation exposure procedures
- **Quality assurance systems** must be operated to ensure that dental images are produced to a consistently high standard

Principles of dental radiography

As stated previously, there are many sound reasons for dental radiographs to be taken. However, to avoid their indiscriminate use, guidelines have been drawn up for the safe prescription of dental radiographs in dental practice, and must be followed by all. These are as follows:

- A history and a clinical examination must be performed before any radiograph is taken
- Only new patients with clear evidence of some dental disease should have full mouth radiographs taken
- Regularly attending child patients in the mixed dentition stage who have orthodontic problems developing can have radiographs taken as necessary
- Recall patients with a low caries risk should have radiographs no more frequently than every 18 months
- Those with a moderate caries risk should have radiographs every 12 months
- Those with a high caries risk should have radiographs at six-monthly intervals, with a gradual reduction in this rate as the caries is brought under control
- Patients exhibiting evidence of periodontal disease can have selective radiographs taken of problem areas, as necessary
- Edentulous patients should only have selective radiographs taken if there are any clinically suspicious areas (such as retained roots, or hard tissue lesions)

Types of views used in dental radiography

Various types of film are used, depending on the reason for taking the dental image. However, all are either used within the oral cavity – **intra-oral films** – or outside the oral cavity – **extra-oral films**.

Intra-oral films are supplied in child and adult size packets that contain the following (Figure 8.1):

- Plastic envelope to protect the contents from fluid contamination
- Wraparound black paper to prevent exposure of the film to light
- Film, which is exposed to the ionising radiation and produces the dental image once processed or loaded onto the computer (digital imaging)

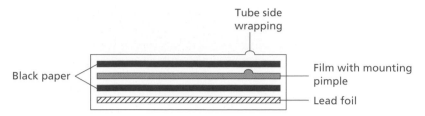

Figure 8.1 Contents of intra-oral film packet. Source: *Levison's Textbook for Dental Nurses,* 10th edn, C. Hollins, 2008, Wiley-Blackwell.

- Lead foil to prevent scatter of the ionising radiation past the film packet
- Raised pimple marker to correctly determine the left and right side of the image produced

The views that can be produced using these films are:

- **Horizontal bitewing** (Figure 8.2) – to view interproximal areas of the posterior teeth
- **Vertical bitewing** – to view periodontal bone levels of posterior teeth
- **Periapical** (Figure 8.3) – to view full length of any tooth
- **Anterior occlusal** (Figure 8.4) – to view either the upper or the lower anterior teeth and the surrounding bone

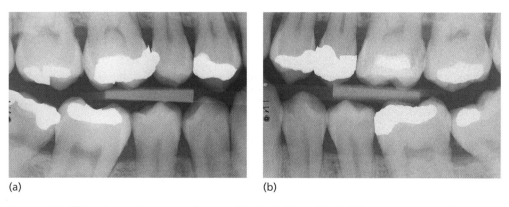

(a)   (b)

Figure 8.2 Bite-wing radiographs. Source: *Basic Guide to Dental Procedures,* C. Hollins, 2008, Wiley-Blackwell, Oxford.

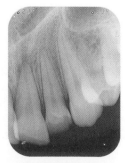

Figure 8.3 Periapical radiograph.

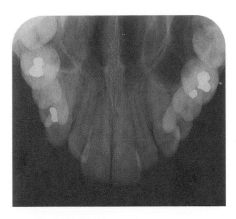

Figure 8.4 Anterior occlusal radiograph.

Extra-oral films are supplied in cassettes that contain the following (Figure 8.5):

■ Cassette case that is loaded into special imaging machines for use
■ Intensifying screens in both sides of the cassette, to reduce the dose of radiation exposure required to produce a dental image
■ Film, of a compatible type with the intensifying screens, to produce the dental image once exposed and processed
■ Marker to correctly determine the left and right side of the image produced

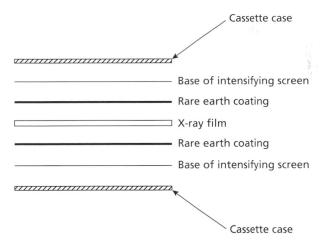

Figure 8.5 Contents of extra-oral cassette.

The views that can be produced using these films are:

■ **Dental panoramic tomograph (DPT)** (Figure 8.6) – to view both jaws in full and their surrounding bony anatomy
■ **Lateral oblique** to view the position of unerupted third molar teeth (these are used infrequently now)

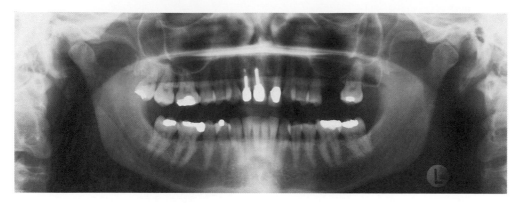

Figure 8.6 Dental panoramic tomograph.

Radiographic techniques

Any dental image is produced by the correct placing of the film on the far side of the area to be exposed from the x-ray machine. In other words, the radiation beam passes from the machine through the area to be exposed and then hits the film inside either the plastic envelope or the cassette.

Intra-oral films are held in the correct position by the use of film holder devices where possible, as described below, loaded with the film packet and placed inside the oral cavity for the patient to bite upon. If a digital imaging technique is used, the film is replaced by a special sensor that is positioned in exactly the same way, but instead of an exposed film being produced which is then chemically processed, the digital image is transmitted directly to a computer, where it can be viewed immediately.

Intra-oral films can be exposed in two ways, depending upon which is the best method for the given clinical situation: the **paralleling technique** and the **bisecting angle technique**.

In the paralleling technique, the film is held exactly parallel to the long axis of the tooth being exposed, so that the image produced is exactly the same size as the actual tooth. This is especially important during endodontic procedures, when the correct diagnostic length of the tooth has to be determined to ensure accurate root filling of the canal (Figure 8.7).

Sometimes the film cannot be placed parallel to the tooth, because of the size restriction of the patient's mouth. In these situations the bisecting angle technique is used. The film is placed intra-orally and the angulation of the long axis of the tooth against the film is determined by the operator. This angle is then halved (bisected) and the tube head is angled to be at right angles to it (Figure 8.8), before the film is exposed.

Lateral oblique cassettes are held in position by the patient's hand, on the far side of the head from the radiation machine. The tube head is angled so that the

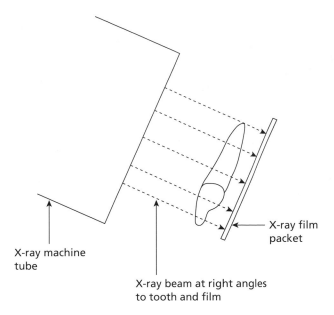

X-ray machine
tube

X-ray beam at right angles
to tooth and film

X-ray film
packet

Figure 8.7 Paralleling technique.

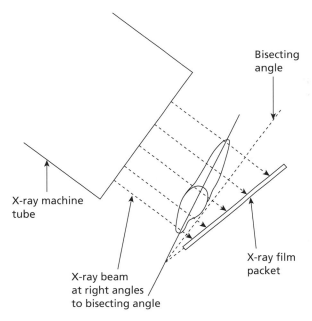

Bisecting
angle

X-ray machine
tube

X-ray beam
at right angles
to bisecting angle

X-ray film
packet

Figure 8.8 Bisecting angle technique.

x-ray beam passes through the angle of the jaw, exposing the third molar teeth on that side of the mouth.

Extra-oral DPT film cassettes are loaded into their special radiation machine, and then the patient is accurately placed within the machine and the cassette is revolved around their head during the exposure process.

Within the cassettes, the intensifying screens glow when they are hit by the x-ray beam. It is this glowing that exposes the film itself and produces the image. If intensifying screens were not used, a far higher dose of radiation would have to be used to create the same image – as discussed earlier, this is likely to produce significant tissue damage.

Formation of the image

An intraoral x-ray film packet contains a celluloid film coated with light-sensitive silver bromide salts in an emulsion, surrounded by black paper to protect it from unwanted light. This is all enclosed in a waterproof plastic packet. On one side of the film is a lead foil which prevents the emulsion coat being exposed twice, by absorbing scattered radiation during the exposure.

The passage of the x-rays through the tissue causes the energy release discussed earlier, and an exact pattern of the tissue is produced within the chemicals on the film itself, as a **latent** (hidden) image – with radiopaque tissues causing the most energy release and therefore a clearer image. Unless a digital imaging technique is used, the latent image can only be seen on the film by the use of special chemicals to make it visible during the processing procedure, in much the same way that photographs from a camera are developed before being able to be viewed.

Role of the dental nurse during imaging

Although legally only dental nurses holding a registerable qualification in dental imaging may act as the operator during the procedure, all dental nurses have a valuable role and contribution in the preparation for and taking of dental images. A dental nurse will:

- Have the correct patient records available beforehand
- Switch on the x-ray machine and ensure no warning lights or alarms sound, so that the equipment is known to be functioning correctly
- Ensure the correct patient is identified for the procedure by checking their name, address and date of birth
- Confirm the view to be taken and have ready the correct film and holder or loaded cassette, as required
- Ensure the film used is in date and has been stored correctly, that is, away from all sources of ionising radiation and heat
- Communicate effectively with the patient beforehand, allaying any fears that they may have with regard to dental imaging

- Refer any concerns or questions beyond your role to the dentist or other operator
- Ensure that all facial items of jewellery and any removable prostheses have been removed by the patient, so that they do not become superimposed over the dental image and limit its quality
- Handle these items while wearing gloves, to avoid cross-infection and to maintain a good standard of infection control
- Reassure the patient while they are being positioned for the exposure, and ensure that all escorts remain outside the imaging area – this must be at least 2 m away, but ideally they should not enter the actual room. The only exception to this is when small children are to have a radiograph taken – a parent may have to remain with them to ensure co-operation. In such cases, the parent must be given a lead apron to wear and stay behind the head of the x-ray machine to avoid exposure to themselves
- Assist the operator in placing the film, patient and machine, as necessary
- Assist the patient from the area once the exposure is complete
- Will handle any intra-oral films wearing gloves, and wipe the film with a disinfectant to remove saliva contamination from the packet
- Wear clean gloves to process the film
- Switch off the x-ray machine when the imaging procedure is complete
- Record the type of view and number of images taken on the patient's record card, or computer notes, or within the surgery's own record system

Film processing

As mentioned earlier, intra-oral digital images are transmitted directly to the computer and can be viewed immediately. All other films require chemical processing to convert the latent image to a visible image for viewing, and this can be done using an **automatic processing machine**, or **manually** with the film being passed through the chemical tanks by hand, and in the correct sequence.

Automatic processing

The machine used consists of a base containing the chemical and water tanks, with a conveyor belt style of rollers that carry the film through the machine during processing (Figure 8.9). These are all beneath a removable, light-tight lid which has hand entry ports so that the film packet or cassette can be put into the light-tight environment before being opened. If the film is exposed to visible light before being processed, the image will be lost.

The procedure of automatic processing is as follows:

- Remove the lid and check that the chemical and water levels are adequate
- Replace the lid and switch on the machine, so that the water is flowing and the tanks are heated to the correct temperature (range of 18–22°C)
- Once the correct temperature is reached, warning lights go out and the machine is ready for use

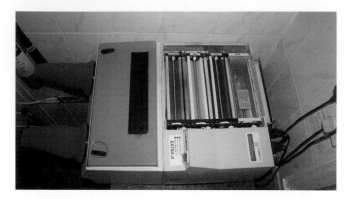

Figure 8.9 Velopex® machine.

- Intra-oral film packets are taken into the machine through the hand ports, while wearing clean gloves
- Extra-oral cassettes are placed into this section by lifting and replacing the lid, and then can be opened and handled via the hand ports
- The rollers become operational once their start button is pressed
- The film packet is carefully opened and the plastic envelope, black paper and lead foil are all dropped to the base of the tank
- The film is then held by its sides only, as finger marks on the surface will damage the image
- The film is carefully inserted into the entrance to the rollers, and it will be gently tugged into the machine to be processed
- Once the film has passed through the machine, processed and dried, it will reappear at the delivery port and can be safely handled and viewed

Manual processing

This is carried out in a 'dark room', a light-tight lockable room containing the processing chemicals and water tanks, sitting in a main water tank that is heated and maintained in the correct temperature range of 18–22°C.

The four tanks will be present as follows (Figure 8.10):

- **Developing tank**, with lid, where the chemicals will cause the image to initially develop on the film so that it can be seen. The image is still unstable in visible light at this point
- **Water tank**, to wash off the developer solution after a suitable time has elapsed
- **Fixing tank**, where the image will be permanently fixed onto the film so that it can be viewed in visible light
- **Water tank**, to wash off the fixer solution after a suitable time has elapsed

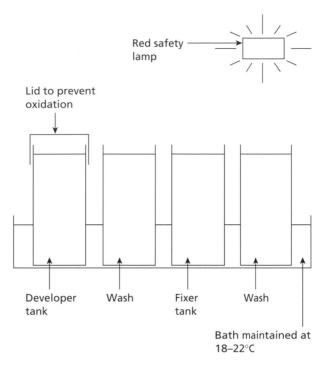

Figure 8.10 Darkroom layout.

Some vision is required within the room, so an orange or red **safe light** will be present under which the processing can be carried out without exposing the film to actual visible light. The room must be lockable from within, so that the door cannot be opened by anyone else. If the door is opened it will result in the accidental exposure of the film to light and the destruction of the image.

The procedure of manual processing is as follows:

(1) Check that the chemical and water levels are adequate
(2) Check the temperature of the solutions, and determine the developing and fixing times required from the chemical manufacturers guidelines provided
(3) Check that a timing clock and suitable film hangers are available in the room
(4) Wipe surfaces dry of any previously spilt chemicals or water, if necessary
(5) Lock the door and switch off all lights except the safe light
(6) Open the film packet or cassette, locate the film and clip it to one of the hangers available, carefully handling the film by its edges only, to avoid spoiling it with fingerprints
(7) Remove the developer lid, immerse the hanger into the solution so that the film is completely covered, and start the timer
(8) When the timer sounds, remove the hanger and film and immerse in the first water tank, agitating the hanger to ensure thorough washing occurs

(9)   Shake off excess water, then fully immerse the hanger and film into the fixer solution, and start the timer

(10) Replace the developer lid to prevent the solution being weakened by exposure to air

(11) When the timer sounds, remove the hanger and film and immerse in the second water tank, agitating the hanger to ensure thorough washing occurs

(12) Switch on the ordinary light

(13) Shake off excess water and dry the film, a small hairdryer is suitable for this

Once dry, the films can be correctly mounted as necessary, and returned to the dentist for viewing.

Role of the dental nurse during processing

All dental nurses are able to process films, once suitable training has been received from the surgery or organisation producing the films. The processing must be carried out correctly though to ensure that the films produced are readable, and so that no repeat exposures are required due to a faulty processing technique. For these reasons, the dental nurse must also be aware of the correct procedures to follow when cleaning and using the equipment, as well as what to do if the equipment is faulty.

The role of the dental nurse is as follows:

- Follow the training given in image processing techniques accurately
- Always carry out the pre-processing checks correctly
- Always wear suitable personal protective equipment when handling any of the chemicals used, to avoid personal injury – this should include gloves, mask, safety glasses, and a plastic apron over the uniform
- Be aware that the chemicals are toxic, and must be handled with great care at all times
- Follow the policies with regard to topping up or changing spent solutions – they should usually be fully replaced every month
- Clear away all spillages as soon as they occur, for health and safety reasons and also to avoid spoiling any films processed afterwards
- Be aware of the COSHH emergency advice for all of the chemicals used
- Dispose of the solutions as special waste in accordance with health and safety policy, using the storage containers provided by the waste collector (see Unit 1 (Chapter 2))
- Follow the training given in, and the manufacturer's guidelines on, cleaning the automatic processor or the manual processing area, so that processing faults due to dirty equipment do not occur. This is especially important in the cleaning of the automatic processor rollers, as films can become stained or stuck in the machine, making them unreadable so that the patient has to be re-exposed

■ Have knowledge of the correct functioning of the processing equipment, so that if equipment failure occurs, it can be recognised, the equipment switched off safely, and the correct person notified of the failure

Mounting and viewing films

Once the films have been successfully processed, they will be viewed by the dentist so that diagnoses can be made and treatment plans formulated. Ideally, a light box and magnifier will be available for viewing the films (Figure 8.11), but it is imperative that they are mounted and positioned correctly, otherwise the right teeth may present as the left, and *vice versa*.

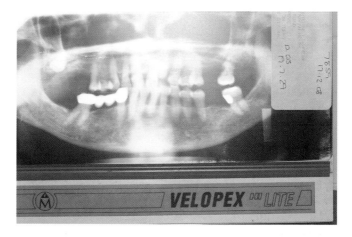

Figure 8.11 Viewing screen.

Extra-oral cassettes are marked with an 'L' to indicate the patient's left side, and unless the cassette has been placed upside down in the machine, the film is easily orientated on the viewer so that it is viewed as if looking at the patient from the front (see Figure 8.6).

Various plastic envelope designs are available to mount all types of intra-oral films nowadays, but they must be loaded correctly by the dental nurse first. All intra-oral films have a raised pimple in one corner which must be facing out to view the film correctly, and not back to front. It is irrelevant which corner of the film the pimple appears in, but it must face out. Also, the dental nurse should use their knowledge of oral anatomy to check themselves. Molar teeth are posterior to all other teeth, so correct mounting of bitewing films for instance should result in the molar teeth appearing on the outer side of both films, with their pimples palpable in one corner (see Figure 8.2).

Surgeries and organisations may use different methods of patient identification and storage of the films, and the dental nurse has to be aware of the methods in use and use them appropriately. These may include any of the following:

- Digital images stored on computer or downloaded onto discs
- Intra-oral films mounted in plastic envelopes, with patient identification details written on in indelible ink. These may be stored within each patient's record card and filed. If clinical notes are computerised, there may be a separate filing system used exclusively for films
- Extra-oral films may be too large to store within the record cards, so may also have their own exclusive filing system

Whichever system is used, all films must be marked with the patient's identification details (such as name, computer number, etc.), the date the image was taken, and a note of the view used, before being stored or filed.

Processing faults

Faults occur for two reasons; poor handling technique of the exposed film during processing, or poor preparation of the processing equipment. Obviously, both can be avoided by proper training and by carrying out procedures correctly. Some of the more common handling faults are shown below.

Fault	Reason
Scratches (Figure 8.12)	Catching film on tank side during immersion
Fingerprints	Not holding film at edges only
Blank spots	Film splashed with fixer before being placed in developer solution
Black line across film (Figure 8.13)	Film bent or folded during processing
Brown or green stains (Figure 8.14)	Not kept in fixer solution for adequate time
Crazed pattern on film (Figure 8.15)	Dried too quickly over a strong heat source
Presence of crystals on film (Figure 8.16)	Insufficient washing after removal from fixer solution

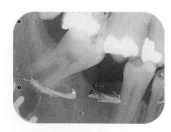

Figure 8.12 Scratches.

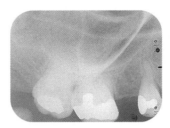

Figure 8.13 Bent film.

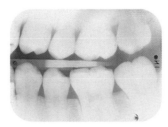

Figure 8.14 Inadequate fixing.

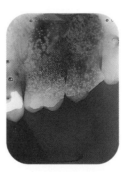

Figure 8.15 Dried too quickly.

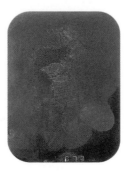

Figure 8.16 Insufficient washing after fixing.

Some of the more common equipment preparation faults are shown below.

Fault	Reason
Dark film (Figure 8.17)	Developer solution too concentrated Developer solution temperature too high Film kept in developer solution for too long
Blank film (Figure 8.18)	Film placed in fixer solution before developer solution, so image is destroyed
Partly blank film (Figure 8.19)	Film only partially immersed in developer solution
Fogged film (Figure 8.20)	Inadequate control of light source in processing room, film exposed to visible light
Faint image on film (Figure 8.21)	Developer solution too weak Developer solution temperature too low Film removed from developer solution too soon
Fading image	Inadequate fixing time, so image not held permanently on film
Loss of film	Stuck in automatic processor rollers, due to inadequate roller cleaning
Visible artefacts (Figure 8.22)	Film contaminated by solution spillages, either on work surfaces or in cassette cases

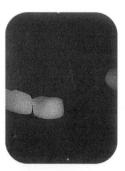

Figure 8.17 Over developed.

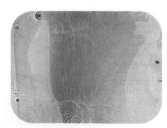

Figure 8.18 Blank film.

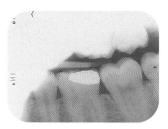

Figure 8.19 Partial immersion in developer.

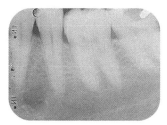

Figure 8.20 Fogged film.

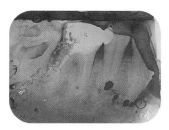

Figure 8.21 Under developed.

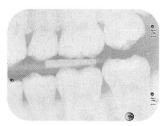

Figure 8.22 Solution splash contamination.

Quality assurance

To protect both patients and the dental team from unnecessary ionising radiation exposure, it is everyone's duty to ensure that the occurrence of these faults is kept to a minimum, or eliminated completely. To do this involves assessing the **quality** of the films processed to determine the following:

- How readable is the film?
- Is a fault present?
- What is the fault?
- How has it occurred?
- How can it be prevented from recurring?
- Is re-exposure of the patient necessary?

By going through this list of points for each film processed, a simple quality assurance system is developed that aims to achieve the following:

- Have a simple-to-use scoring system for the films
- Identify any areas of concern
- Develop solutions to the problems identified
- Limit the number of ionising radiation exposures to the minimum required for clinical necessity (**As Low As Reasonably Achievable – ALARA**)

The scoring system places each film into its level of quality:

- **Score 1** – **excellent** quality, no errors present
- **Score 2** – diagnostically **acceptable** quality, some errors present, but the film is still useful for diagnosis
- **Score 3** – **unacceptable** quality, errors present which make diagnosis too difficult to achieve

The aim is to have a minimum of 70% films scoring 1, and a maximum of 10% scoring 3.

Formal written records will need to be kept to show that the quality assurance (QA) system is in use and is being operated correctly – this is a legal requirement for all surgeries. Following adequate training, the dental nurse can play a valuable role in running the system for the surgery or organisation.

Similarly, a QA system can be developed to monitor and improve the quality of all of the following:

- Ionising radiation equipment
- Dark room and films
- Working procedures
- Staff training

To ensure that ALARA is achieved and patient exposure to x-rays is kept to an absolute minimum, all dental organisations should follow 'best practice' guidelines by carrying out the following:

- All radiographs taken must be **clinically justified**
- Only **qualified personnel** must take radiographs
- A **QA system** should be in place to ensure consistently good quality radiographs are produced, so that repeat exposures are avoided
- The **fastest speed** of film is used, to reduce the exposure time
- All staff processing radiographs are **correctly trained** to do so
- **Regular analysis** of rejected films is undertaken, to discover where errors lie so that procedures can be modified
- A system of **reporting machine breakages** should be in place, so that unknown or inadvertent exposure is avoided
- A **clinical audit** should be carried out, so that radiographs and techniques are constantly monitored and improved on as necessary
- Ideally, all clinical staff should wear **monitoring badges** so that inadvertent exposure or faulty machines are detected early
- The use of lead aprons is not normally necessary for dental radiography unless the pelvic area is in the main beam of the x-rays (this usually only occurs during a specialised view called a 'vertex occlusal' radiograph)

Staff safety

As the developer and fixer solutions are toxic and classed as **special waste**, the dental nurse should take the necessary precautions when handling them.

- Wear gloves when handling either solution, including during the processing of exposed films, to avoid skin contact
- Ensure there is adequate ventilation in the developing room, to avoid the unnecessary inhalation of fumes
- Wear a plastic apron to avoid chemical splashes onto the uniform
- Take adequate care when replenishing or changing the developer and fixer tanks
- Follow the practice policy for the storage and disposal of both solutions, normally they are stored in drums provided by a special waste contractor and collected accordingly when spent
- They can only be disposed of into the sewage supply with the written permission of the water supplier to the area, and this is unlikely to be given nowadays
- All spillages must be cleaned away immediately
- Any suspected medical problems related to either solution, such as skin irritation or breathing difficulties, must be reported to the dentist or other senior person immediately
- If an accident does occur, the information and advice provided on the relevant COSHH risk assessment sheet must be followed

Ionising radiation legislation

Despite its valuable uses in dentistry, ionising radiation presents a hazard to the whole dental team, their patients, and the general public. There is no 'safe' level of use – every exposure can cause some amount of tissue damage in the patient, or in anyone else in the imaging area.

The aim at all times should be to keep the numbers of exposures required to a minimum, and the practical methods that are followed to achieve this are:

- The principle of **ALARA**
- Formal **staff training** in all the necessary areas
- **Training updates** as required, in accordance with continuing professional development (CPD) requirements
- Exposures to be carried out by qualified personnel only
- **QA system** in place, and operated correctly
- Use of **personal monitoring badges** for all clinical staff, to identify the dose levels received and any inadvertent exposures (say, due to faulty equipment). However, this is not a legal requirement unless more than 50 DPTs or 150 intra-oral exposures are carried out per week
- Adequate **equipment failure mechanism** in place, to avoid inadvertent exposure
- **Non-use** of lead aprons for routine dental imaging

In addition to these 'best practice' pointers, legislation is in place to ensure full compliance with the health and safety aspects of ionising radiation by all surgeries and organisations. The specific regulations and legislation in force with regard to the use of ionising radiation in the dental workplace are covered by the following:

- **Ionising Radiation Regulations 1999 (IRR99)**
- **Ionising Radiation (Medical Exposure) Regulations 2000 (IRR(ME)2000)**

The role of the dental nurse in relation to this legislation can be summarised as follows:

- Assist in the identification of the correct patient before exposure
- Comply with all of the policies and rules in relation to ionising radiation as per the training received
- Assist in running the QA systems
- Comply with all health and safety legislation to protect themselves, all other personnel and patients, at all times
- Wear monitoring badges correctly, where provided
- Never carry out duties beyond their training or legal responsibility

The other points of relevance for the dental nurse to be aware of in relation to the ionising radiation legislation are the **formal appointments** required, and knowledge of the written **local rules**.

Formal appointments

These are a legal requirement in all surgeries and organisations using ionising radiation:

- **Legal person** – a designated person who is to ensure the organisation's full compliance with both sets of regulations (this is usually a senior dentist)
- **Radiation protection adviser (RPA)** – a medical physicist who is appointed in writing by the dental organisation, and is available to give advice on staff and public safety in relation to IRR99
- **Radiation protection supervisor (RPS)** – a designated person who can assess risks and ensure precautions are taken to minimise them, in accordance with IRR99 (this is usually a senior dentist or a radiographically qualified dental nurse)

Local rules

These should be written and displayed at each imaging area, so that they can be referred to by all personnel. They must include all of the following:

- Name of the designated **RPS**
- Identification of each imaging area as a **controlled area**, in relation to access by personnel and patients
- Standard **warning signs** at these areas to notify the use of ionising radiation (Figure 8.23)
- Summary of **working instructions** for the controlled areas, to include the designated 2 m safety zone from the machine head
- Summary of **contingency plans** in the event of machine failure
- Details of the **dose investigation levels**
- Use of **visible** and **audible** signs to indicate the actual exposure (usually a red light and a buzzer)

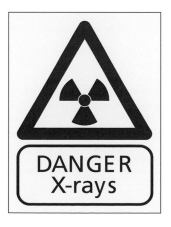

Figure 8.23 Radiation warning sign. Source: *Levison's Textbook for Dental Nurses*, 10th edn, C. Hollins, 2008, Wiley-Blackwell.

9 Unit 8: Provide Chairside Support During the Prevention and Control of Periodontal Disease and Caries and the Restoration of Cavities (OH5)

Knowledge specifications

Anatomy and physiology

K1 – A factual knowledge of primary and secondary dentition and the dates of eruption

K2 – A factual knowledge of the structure and functions of teeth and gingivae

Oral diseases and caries

K3 – A factual knowledge of the development of dental plaque and methods for controlling it

K4 – A factual knowledge of the main causes and treatment of periodontal disease and caries

K5 – A factual knowledge of the nature and progression of dental and oral disease

Retracting tissues and aspirating

K6 – A working knowledge of methods of protecting and retracting the soft tissues

K7 – A working knowledge of methods of aspirating during treatment

Preventing dental and oral disease

K8 – A factual knowledge of the ways in which periodontal disease can be prevented and/or minimised including effective oral hygiene techniques

K9 – A factual knowledge of the different forms of fluoride (systemic and topical) and its optimum levels

Equipment, instruments, materials and medicaments used in periodontal therapy and the preparation and restoration of cavities

K10 – A working knowledge of the function of the different kinds of equipment, instruments and materials/medicaments used in:

a)   periodontal therapy
b)   the preparation and restoration of cavities
K11 – A working knowledge of the equipment used in the administration of local and regional anaesthesia

Cavity preparation

K12 – A working knowledge of the different stages in cavity preparation for both deciduous and permanent teeth

Restorations

K13 – A working knowledge of the different types and purposes of linings, and their relationship to the type of restoration which is being used
K14 – A working knowledge of the advantages and disadvantages of the different types of:
a)   amalgam
b)   temporary restorations
c)   composite restorations
d)   glass ionomer restorations
K15 – A working knowledge of safe handling and disposal of amalgam and mercury spillage
K16 – A working knowledge of the purpose and different types of etchants, when and where they are used
K17 – A working knowledge of the purpose and different types of bonding agents, when and where they are used
K18 – A factual knowledge of the importance of finishing restorations, and the equipment, instruments and materials that may be used
K19 – A factual knowledge of the importance of matrix systems and the equipment and instruments that may be used

Health and safety and control of infection

K20 – A working knowledge of the potential hazards of curing lights
K21 – A working knowledge of standard precautions and quality standards of infection control, and your role in maintaining them
K22 – A working knowledge of the purpose, method of use and function of protective wear and the reason for their use during dental treatment
K23 – A factual knowledge of the hazards associated with amalgam, including:
a)   the reasons for, and importance of, preparing amalgam in ventilated areas
b)   the appropriate precautions that should be taken to prevent mercury spillage
c)   the correct action to take in the event of mercury spillage

Communication

Communication

K24 – A working knowledge of methods of communicating information clearly and effectively

K25 – A working knowledge of methods of modifying information and communication methods for different individuals, including patients from social and ethnic backgrounds, children (including those with special needs), and the elderly

Charts and records

K26 – A working knowledge of the different types of records used in the organisation (including medical history, personal details, dental charts, radiographs, photographs and study models for assessment and treatment planning), and their purpose

K27 – An in-depth understanding of confidentiality in relation to patient records

Team working

K28 – A working knowledge of methods of effective team working in oral health care

The causes and prevention of both periodontal disease and dental caries are covered in detail in Unit 5 (Chapter 6). For ease of reference, they will be summarised here along with the relevant background knowledge of dental anatomy necessary to have an understanding of their treatments.

Periodontal disease

This term covers a group of diseases that affect the supporting structures of the teeth (**the periodontium**):

- The gingivae
- The periodontal ligament
- The alveolar bone

Periodontal disease is an infection of these supporting structures by various species of oral bacteria that colonise plaque accumulations at the gingival margins of the teeth. The severity of the disease increases as the deeper supporting structures become involved. So it progresses as follows:

(1)   Initial inflammation of the gingivae due to the build up of marginal plaque – this is called **gingivitis**

(2)   Lack of oral health measures to remove the plaque allows increased inflammation – this forms **false pockets**

(3)   Continued failure to remove the plaque allows its progression under the gingivae, and it becomes mineralised and hardened – this is called **calculus**

(4)   Calculus scratches the gingivae, allowing bacterial toxins to enter the supporting tissues

(5)   Non-removal of the calculus allows further plaque development and toxin production to occur

(6)   Underlying periodontal ligament is gradually attacked and destroyed – this allows the formation of **true pockets**

(7)   Continued non-treatment allows the tissue damage to continue so that the alveolar bone is also destroyed – the condition is now called **chronic periodontitis**

(8)   When sufficient bone has been destroyed the tooth will become loose in its socket – **tooth mobility**

In summary then, the main causative factor for periodontal disease is poor oral hygiene allowing plaque accumulation at the gingival margin of the tooth. Other factors that increase the severity of the damage include:

■   Smoking
■   Some medical conditions, such as diabetes, leukaemia, vitamin C deficiency
■   Stress
■   Some prescribed drugs, including some for epilepsy and hypertension
■   Hormonal imbalance, especially during pregnancy or puberty

Periodontal disease can occur in both children and adults, although it often takes several years for chronic periodontitis to develop. As the disease is also painless, it can remain undetected by the patient for some considerable time.

Treatment of periodontal disease involves:

■   Reinforcement of good oral hygiene techniques
■   Removal of all calculus and plaque
■   Modification of other factors if possible, such as smoking cessation

When extensive pocketing has occurred and calculus is deeply placed, periodontal surgery may be required.

Dental caries

Dental caries is a bacterial infection which affects the mineralised tissues of the teeth. Again, it involves the accumulation of plaque, but with caries the plaque must be in contact with the tooth itself. This allows the bacteria involved to release their acidic by-products of digestion directly onto the tooth enamel, where the acid attacks the tooth structure in a process called **demineralisation**, and forms a cavity. Its progression is as follows:

(1) Attachment of the plaque to the enamel surface of the tooth
(2) Lack of oral health measures to remove the plaque allows the amount present to increase
(3) **Weak acids** are produced by the bacteria involved as they digest food particles stuck in the plaque. Dietary intake of **carbohydrates** massively increases the amount of acid produced by the bacteria
(4) Acids **demineralise** the enamel tooth surface – this shows as an **early white spot lesion**
(5) Removal of the plaque and a reduction in the frequency and amount of carbohydrates in the diet will allow enamel to repair itself at this point – a process called **remineralisation**. Otherwise, the acid attack continues through the enamel and into dentine – this allows **cavity formation**
(6) As the cavity extends deeper into the tooth, it causes inflammation of the pulp – **pulpitis**
(7) If the caries progression is stopped at this point and the tooth restored with a filling, all the symptoms will settle – this is called **reversible pulpitis**. Otherwise the pulp will become too badly inflamed and the tooth will die – this is called **irreversible pulpitis**
(8) An infection will occur and the tooth will require endodontic treatment to save it (see Unit 10 (Chapter 11)), or it will require extraction (see Unit 11 (Chapter 12))

In summary then, the two main causative factors for dental caries are:

■ Poor oral hygiene allowing plaque to develop on the tooth enamel (especially in stagnation areas)
■ A diet high in carbohydrates which provides the bacteria involved with the necessary food to produce acid

Dental caries affects all age groups, from the moment that the teeth are erupting into the oral cavity and for the rest of the patient's life. Unlike periodontal disease, it causes sensitivity or pain in the affected tooth once dentine is under an acid attack, so treatment is usually received in time to save the tooth.

Treatment of dental caries involves:

■ Reinforcement of good oral hygiene techniques
■ Modification of the diet to reduce the carbohydrate and acid content
■ Strengthening of the tooth enamel using fluoride
■ Restorative treatment of cavities

Dental anatomy

Full details of the primary and secondary dentition and their relevant eruption dates are covered in Unit 6 (Chapter 7). They are summarily covered here in the following tables.

■ **Deciduous dentition**

Tooth	Letter	Eruption date (months)	
		Upper teeth	Lower teeth
Central incisor	A	10	8
Lateral incisor	B	11	13
Canine	C	19	20
First molar	D	16	16
Second molar	E	29	27

■ **Permanent dentition**

Tooth	Number	Eruption date (years)	
		Upper teeth	Lower teeth
Central incisor	1	7–8	6–7
Lateral incisor	2	8–9	7–8
Canine	3	10–12	9–10
First premolar	4	9–11	9–11
Second premolar	5	10–11	9–11
First molar	6	6–7	6–7
Second molar	7	12–13	11–12
Third molar	8	18–25	18–25

Similarly, full details of the structure and function of teeth and gingivae are covered in Unit 6 (Chapter 7) and are summarised below.

Tooth structure, from the outer surface inwards, is as follows:

(1) **Enamel** – non-living tissue forming the outer part of the tooth crown, made up of mineral crystals lying in prisms, arranged at right angles to the tooth surface and the amelo-dentinal junction (ADJ)

(2) **Dentine** – living tissue forming the bulk of the crown and root, made up of hollow tubules containing nerve endings

(3) **Pulp** – soft tissue within the root chamber and canal, composed of nerves and blood vessels that keep the tooth alive and allow it to feel sensations

(4) **Cementum** – outer covering of the tooth root, lying beneath the gingiva and forming part of the tooth attachment to its supporting structures

The function of teeth is to cut into and chew food (**masticate**), so that it can be swallowed in small pieces and digested in the body to provide the chemicals required for the body to live and function.

The supporting structures are:

- **Gingivae** – commonly known as the gums, this is the pink soft tissue covering the jaw bones and forming a tight collar around the necks of all the teeth
- **Periodontal ligament** – a specialised fibrous tissue which attaches the teeth to the gingivae and the underlying alveolar bone
- **Alveolar bone** – the bony ridges of the maxilla and mandible that support the teeth in the jaws

The function of the supporting structures is to hold the teeth in the jaw bones, so that they can be used for mastication.

Treatment of periodontal disease

Once it has been determined that a patient has periodontal disease, a treatment plan will be made, depending on the severity of the disease present, and the patient's wishes. As mentioned previously, there are several factors that can worsen the extent of the disease–some of which are out of the patient's control (such as medical conditions, medication, hormone imbalances) – and others that they may not wish to change, such as smoking. Any treatment plan must accept these points and have realistic expectations with regard to the level of success that can be achieved following treatment. Good communication skills are very important in helping to explain treatment options to the patient (or their parent, guardian or interpreter) and these are discussed more fully in Unit 5 (Chapter 6).

The treatment options available depend on the severity of the disease present, and can be categorised as non-surgical or surgical. The treatment options are as follows:

- **Gingivitis** – removal of all plaque and calculus present above the gingival margin (**supragingival calculus**), using a variety of scaling instruments
- **Periodontitis** – with calculus present beneath the gingival margin (**subgingival calculus**) in true pockets but with no bone involvement, plaque and calculus removal using a variety of scaling and debridement instruments
- **Chronic periodontitis** – with alveolar bone loss and deep pocketing, plaque and calculus removal, and possible use of other techniques such as localised medicaments or surgical flap therapy

In the worst cases where teeth are mobile and other exacerbating factors are involved, it may be decided that periodontal treatment is unlikely to succeed and that a tooth or teeth may require extraction instead.

Non-surgical treatment of periodontal disease

Prevention is always better than cure, so sound oral health instruction to prevent plaque accumulation in the first instance is by far the best course of action. Plaque suppressants are available in various oral health products, the commonest being chlorhexidine, but its use is only advised on a short-term basis, due to the staining capabilities that some of the products possess.

The oral health message needs to be reinforced regularly if problems persist, and the advice given will be different for different age groups. In patients with chronic gingivitis, the removal of all plaque and the reinforcement of oral hygiene instructions should bring about a complete resolution of the problem. See Unit 5 (Chapter 6) for details.

Supragingival calculus

However, if matters have deteriorated and calculus is present, it needs to be professionally removed by either the dentist or the hygienist to allow healing of the periodontium. This is achieved for supragingival calculus by **scaling and polishing**. A variety of hand scaling instruments are in use to remove supragingival calculus (Figure 9.1):

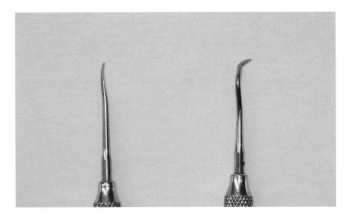

Figure 9.1 Supragingival scalers. Source: *Levison's Textbook for Dental Nurses,* 10th edn, C. Hollins, 2008, Wiley-Blackwell.

- Sickle scaler
- Cushing's push scaler
- Jaquette scaler

Ultrasonic scalers are also available with differing tips. All these instruments are used to dislodge calculus from the tooth surface.

Scaling by hand is tiring for the operator but gives superb tactile sensation, so specks of residual calculus are detectable. The use of an ultrasonic scaler is less tiring and faster, but the cold water spray required for its action can be uncomfortable for patients with sensitive teeth. Once all the calculus has been removed, the teeth are polished with prophylactic paste and a bristle brush or rubber polishing cup in the slow handpiece. This gives a smooth tooth surface and therefore slows down further plaque accumulation.

Subgingival calculus

With chronic periodontitis, any bone loss is permanent. However, if subgingival calculus is removed thoroughly and good oral hygiene is then maintained, there is every chance that the periodontal ligament will reattach and periodontal pockets will heal. Several instruments are available for subgingival calculus removal (Figure 9.2):

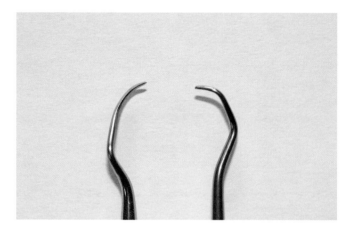

Figure 9.2 Subgingival scalers.

- Subgingival curette
- Periodontal hoe
- Ultrasonic scaler

The shanks of the curettes and hoes are longer so that they can pass deep into periodontal pockets and reach the subgingival calculus. This and the contaminated layer of cementum beneath are then scraped off and removed from the pockets by both aspiration and irrigation. This is called **subgingival debridement**. Healing of the periodontium can then occur, with reattachment of the junctional epithelium and the elimination of periodontal pockets. Subgingival scaling sometimes has to be carried out under local anaesthesia, as the procedure can be quite uncomfortable for some patients.

Continued periodontal health is dependent to a very large degree on the co-operation and motivation of the patient to maintain a good standard of oral hygiene.

Surgical treatment of periodontal disease

Gingivectomy

Sometimes, successful treatment of periodontal disease is hindered by the failure of established false pockets to be eliminated. These can be surgically eliminated by cutting off the hyperplastic gingivae level with the point of epithelial reattachment, a procedure called **gingivectomy** (Figure 9.3). This allows thorough cleaning of the teeth surfaces once exposed, and thus prevents further plaque accumulation and calculus formation. The point of reattachment is marked on the gingivae, and then all hyperplastic tissue is removed with a Blake's knife. This leaves a raw wound, which is covered with a zinc oxide and eugenol dressing (such as Coepak), to aid healing. The procedure is often carried out to remove drug-induced hyperplastic tissue too.

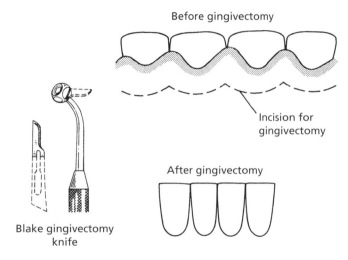

Figure 9.3 Gingivectomy. Source: *Levison's Textbook for Dental Nurses*, 10th edn, C. Hollins, 2008, Wiley-Blackwell.

Surgical recontouring of the gingivae can also be carried out once periodontal health has been achieved, to aid thorough cleansing of the area. This is called **gingivoplasty** and is often carried out using an electrosurgery unit, which coagulates cut blood vessels at the same time.

Flap surgery

Often, only certain teeth are affected by periodontal disease, rather than the whole dentition. These localised areas of disease can be individually investigated by raising a partial or full thickness **surgical flap** of mucoperiosteal tissue, to expose the persistent periodontal pockets to direct vision and cleaning. Any granulation tissue present, due to the body's attempts to heal the area itself, is also removed. Contaminated cementum, subgingival calculus and toxin impregnated soft tissue are all removed before the flap is sutured back into place to allow full healing (Figure 9.4).

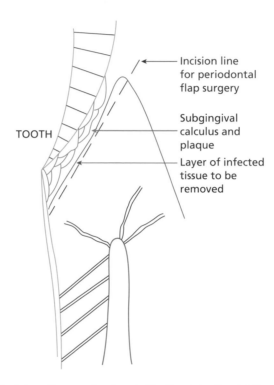

Figure 9.4 Flap incision. Source: *Levison's Textbook for Dental Nurses,* 10th edn, C. Hollins, 2008, Wiley-Blackwell.

Some operators make use of local delivery antibiotics in these areas to destroy bacteria and aid healing. These are available as gels (such as minocycline) which are squirted into the pocket bases, or more long term products with cellulose chips impregnated with slow-release antibiotics (such as Periochip).

In summary then, the instruments required are designed to be used either above or below the gingival margin, to scrape and dislodge the plaque and calculus off the tooth and root surfaces. Good aspiration is required if the scaling instruments are electrically driven, as they produce copious amounts of water during use. A list of instruments that are likely to be used and their function is given below.

Item	Function
Sickle scaler	Hand instrument used for supragingival calculus removal, especially on the lingual and buccal/labial tooth surfaces
Push scaler	Hand instrument used to remove interproximal calculus from the anterior teeth
Curette	Various designs, used for subgingival calculus removal and debridement in true pockets. Have long shanks to allow access to deep pockets
Ultrasonic scaler	Electrically driven multi-use scaler, water jet assists in dislodging calculus as well as cooling the operative tip
	Some patients may require treatment under local analgesia
Periodontal hoe	Hand instrument used to debride root surfaces in deep pockets
Medicaments	Various gels or coated chips impregnated with antibiotics or anti-inflammatories, placed within the pockets to release their chemicals exactly where required
Polishing items	Rubber cups or brushes used in the slow handpiece with prophylactic polishing paste, to produce a smooth tooth surface after scaling and prevent plaque adherence for a time. Gritty composition also helps to remove enamel surface staining

As mentioned, some patients and some periodontal procedures will require the use of local analgesia so that the treatment can be fully carried out while the patient remains comfortable. The local analgesic equipment routinely required is as follows:

Item	Function
Topical analgesic gel	To numb the oral soft tissues at the site of the injection, for patient comfort
Syringe – single use or autoclavable	To hold the needle and cartridge together for use – may be aspirating type to avoid injecting into the surrounding blood vessels
Needle – single use	Long – 27 gauge for nerve block injections
	Short – 30 gauge for infiltration injections
Cartridge – single use	Glass or plastic tube containing the local anaesthetic, buffering agents, vasoconstrictor to prolong anaesthesia in some makes, sterile water

Role of the dental nurse during periodontal treatment

There are some duties that are specific to periodontal treatment, and others that are very similar in other areas of dentistry, but the good dental nurse must be competent and proficient in all. The role of the dental nurse is summarised below:

- Have a good understanding of the procedure to be carried out
- Be aware of their position in the dental team for the procedure – this will be as the chairside nurse and directly assisting the dentist
- Have all the patient records, charts, radiographs, and consent forms completed and available for the appointment

- Have all the required instruments, equipment, materials and medicaments in good order and available for the procedure
- Communicate effectively with the patient throughout the procedure, inspiring confidence and trust
- Monitor the patient throughout the procedure, ensuring their comfort and well-being and giving reassurance where necessary
- Assist during the administration of local analgesia – this will be necessary for patients with sensitive teeth, and when deep scaling and debridement is carried out
- Provide careful but efficient moisture control to remove all irrigants and any specks of dislodged calculus from the oral cavity
- Careful soft tissue retraction to provide a clear operative field, without being so forceful as to cause trauma to the tissues
- Anticipate and pass instruments, etc. to the dentist in the correct order during the procedure
- Have ready any localised medicaments to be placed, and assist with their placement as necessary
- Follow the infection control policy to fully decontaminate the surgery after use – see Unit 4 (Chapter 5)
- All sharp items are carefully disposed of in the sharps box – this includes local anaesthetic needles
- All autoclavable items are debrided then sterilised in the autoclave
- Follow the health and safety policy with regard to hazardous waste disposal – see Unit 1 (Chapter 2)
- All contaminated waste and single-use items are placed in hazardous waste sacks
- All surgery surfaces are disinfected using the correct solution
- Ensure that all records, charts, etc. are correctly and securely stored for future use after being completed by the dentist, maintaining patient confidentiality at all times – see Unit 6 (Chapter 7)

Treatment of dental caries

Once it has been determined that a cavity is present in a tooth, a treatment plan will be decided, based on the following information:

- **Cavity size** – is restoration of the tooth feasible with a filling alone, or should a fixed restoration (such as a crown) be considered?
- **Cavity position** – which tooth surface or surfaces are involved, do aesthetics need to be considered?
- **Tooth involved** – is a posterior chewing tooth involved, which will require a strong and long lasting restoration, or is an anterior tooth involved where chewing forces are less, but aesthetics have to be considered?
- **Extent of caries** – is it possible that full caries removal will cause pulp exposure, so that endodontic treatment will be required?

- **Patient wishes** – is the patient amenable to restorative treatment, especially younger children and some patients with special needs?

Taking into consideration all of the points above, the restoration provided may be on a temporary or permanent basis.

- **Temporary restoration** – in less co-operative patients, and if a fixed restoration is being considered in the short term
- **Amalgam restoration** – in posterior teeth, where restoration strength and longevity are more of an issue than aesthetics
- **Composite restoration** – in anterior teeth for aesthetics, although more modern composites materials are suitable for use in restorations in posterior teeth too
- **Glass ionomer restoration** – in deciduous teeth (because of their fluoride release) and in certain cavity sites where retention of the restoration is difficult

The aims of cavity preparation are the same, whatever restorative material is to be used:

- To remove all caries from the cavity
- To remove the minimum amount of healthy tooth tissue while doing so
- To avoid accidental pulp exposure, by poor technique
- To protect the pulp after treatment by using linings or bases as necessary
- To produce a retentive cavity for restoration, if necessary
- To restore the tooth to an adequate appearance and full function

Cavities are prepared using a combination of high- and low-speed dental drills, with a variety of cutting dental burs. As the majority of the teeth involved are vital, a suitable method of pain control is required before the tooth is cut, the commonest being the use of local anaesthesia.

Local anaesthesia

The term 'anaesthesia' is defined as 'the loss of all sensation', but in dentistry when local anaesthetics are given, they produce the loss of the sensation of pain only. They would be more correctly termed 'local analgesics' then.

Teeth and their surrounding periodontium are highly innervated with a sensory nerve supply which responds to temperature, pressure and pain. If dental treatments were carried out without administering local analgesics by injection first, many procedures would be extremely painful for the patient.

Local analgesics act by **blocking the nervous impulses** from the source of the stimulation (the tooth or surrounding periodontium) so that the information that a painful procedure is being carried out does not reach the brain. The patient is fully aware of the treatment, as they are conscious, but can feel no unpleasant or painful stimuli.

Dental local anaesthetics

These are supplied in 2.2 ml or 1.8 ml cartridges with the following constituents in most:

- **Sterile water** – as a carrying solution
- **Buffering agents** – to maintain neutral pH
- **Preservative** – to give adequate shelf life
- **Anaesthetic** solution
- Possibly a **vasoconstrictor** – to give adequate duration of analgesia

The constituents which vary between different makes of cartridge are the anaesthetic agent and the vasoconstrictor. Vasoconstrictors act by narrowing the blood vessels in the immediate vicinity of injection so that the solution is not carried away so quickly. This then acts to prolong the duration of the anaesthetic and allow adequate time for the dentist to carry out the procedure, without the patient feeling any pain.

Commonly used local anaesthetics are:

- Lidocaine – 2% lidocaine hydrochloride with 1:80 000 adrenaline (**Lignospan** and **Xylocaine**)
- Prilocaine – 3% prilocaine hydrochloride with 0.03 IU felypressin (**Citanest**)
- Mepivacaine – 3% mepivacaine hydrochloride (**Scandonest**)
- Carticaine – carticaine with 1:100 000 adrenaline (**Articaine**)

Adrenaline is the commonest vasoconstrictor used. However, it is a potent **cardiac stimulant**, which acts to increase the rate and depth of the patient's heart beat generally. Therefore, caution is necessary with the following medical conditions to avoid adverse cardiac effects:

- **Hypertension** (high blood pressure)
- **Cardiac disease**
- **Hyperthyroidism** (over-active thyroid gland)
- **Older** patients with complicated medical histories
- Patients receiving **hormone replacement therapy**, as hypertension may be present

The following drugs were thought to be affected by adrenaline previously (nowadays this is considered to be a theoretical problem only):

- Tricyclic antidepressants
- Monoamine oxidase inhibitors

However, older patients taking several drugs should still be treated with caution, as interactions are difficult to predict.

Similarly, felypressin-containing local anaesthetics should be avoided in **pregnant women**, as theoretically it may induce womb contraction and cause the onset of premature labour.

Local anaesthetic equipment

Various designs of syringe are available, some side-loading and some breech-loading. The majority are metallic and autoclavable, although it is possible to purchase disposable syringes today. The plungers of some are adapted to be used with an aspirating technique, for safety reasons, by either screwing into the cartridge bung or being designed to press onto special bung diaphragms, without actually administering the contents (Figure 9.5).

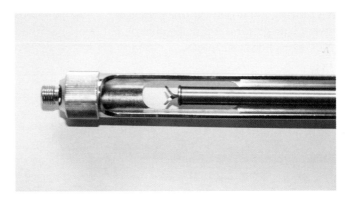

Figure 9.5 Aspirating syringe end.

All designs have a universal sized threaded end for the needle to be positioned, and various sizes, or gauges, of needle are available. Smaller sizes are less painful to use, but are too fine for some sites of injection in the mouth, especially when having to pass through muscle (Figure 9.6).

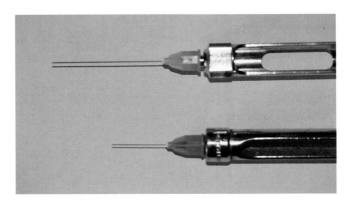

Figure 9.6 LA needles.

Administration techniques

There are four methods of administering local anaesthetics in dentistry:

- **Infiltration**
- **Nerve block**
- **Intra-ligamentary**
- **Intra-osseous**

Infiltration injections place the local anaesthetic solution just under the mucosal surface of the oral cavity, where it penetrates the pores of the alveolar bone so that the nerve endings in the immediate vicinity are affected. It is a technique used to anaesthetise all the gingivae, all the upper teeth and the lower incisor teeth.

Nerve block injections act by anaesthetising the main nerve trunk either before it enters bone or after it leaves it, producing regional anaesthesia. The commonest nerve block injections used are:

- **Inferior dental nerve block** – to anaesthetise the whole of the inferior dental nerve trunk, before it enters the mandible through the mandibular foramen (Figure 9.7)
- **Mental nerve block** – to anaesthetise the end portion of the inferior dental nerve, as it leaves the mandible through the mental foramen (Figure 9.8)
- **Posterior superior dental nerve block** – to anaesthetise this nerve before it enters the maxillary antrum

Thus, the inferior dental nerve block anaesthetises all lower teeth and their lingual gingivae, and the buccal or labial gingivae of all these teeth except the molars. The mental nerve block anaesthetises the premolar, canine, and incisor teeth and their buccal or labial gingivae. The posterior superior dental nerve block anaesthetises

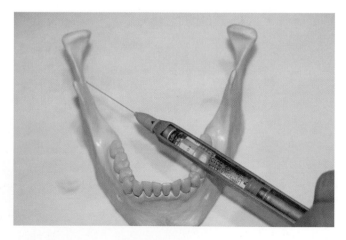

Figure 9.7 Inferior dental nerve block technique.

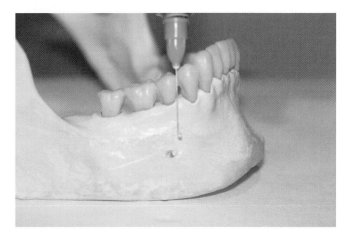

Figure 9.8 Mental nerve block technique.

the upper second and third molar teeth and their buccal gingivae, and part of the first molar tooth.

The nerve block technique is useful when an infection is present around a tooth which requires treatment. It produces anaesthesia without risking the spread of the infection by being able to place the injection at a distance from the tooth involved. However, all nerve trunks run in close proximity to blood vessels, and great care is required in avoiding an intra-vascular injection when nerve blocks are administered. An **aspirating type** of local anaesthetic syringe and cartridge are used, whereby once the needle point is positioned the dentist can aspirate and detect if a blood vessel has been pierced, as blood will flow back into the cartridge. If so, the needle point can be repositioned before the local anaesthetic is administered.

Intra-ligamentary injections tend to be used in conjunction with either infiltration or nerve block techniques, to produce deeper anaesthesia around hypersensitive teeth. Various specialised syringes are available, and one called the Ligmaject is shown in Figure 9.9. The local anaesthetic is administered into the periodontal ligament around the tooth, and requires relatively high force to be given, so the cartridge tends to be enclosed in a plastic sheath for patient protection, in case it shatters during use. The gingivae around the tooth can be seen to blanch as the anaesthetic is given, but the force required to administer it often produces some degree of post-operative soreness.

Intra-osseous injections are given through the outer cortical plate of the alveolar bone, directly into the cancellous bone where the nerves run. It produces profound anaesthesia of the immediate tooth, with no generalised soft tissue effects, and is therefore better for the patient. However, specialised burs to gain access through the bony plate, and then needles of the same size are required but can be used with normal syringes and cartridges. The technique can be used for all teeth, but the area of the mental foramen is best avoided, to prevent nerve damage to the mental nerve as it exits the mandible at this point (Figure 9.10).

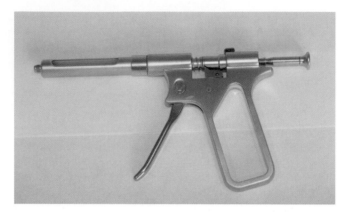

Figure 9.9 Ligmaject syringe. Source: *Levison's Textbook for Dental Nurses,* 10th edn, C. Hollins, 2008, Wiley-Blackwell.

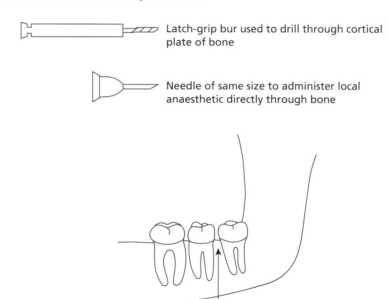

Latch-grip bur used to drill through cortical plate of bone

Needle of same size to administer local anaesthetic directly through bone

Injection site needs to be carefully chosen, between teeth and without damaging roots

Figure 9.10 Intra-osseous system. Source: *Levison's Textbook for Dental Nurses*, 10th edn, C. Hollins, 2008, Wiley-Blackwell.

Dental nurse safety after injections

Once the local anaesthetic has been administered, the needle is a very real source of cross-infection, as it has pierced the patient's tissues and will be contaminated with blood, no matter how small the amount.

Re-sheathing of the needle is the commonest cause of needle stick injuries to dental staff, and various needle guard devices have been developed to lower the incidence. Ultimately, the needle sheath should be placed in any container that will hold it firmly upright, so that the syringe can be held by its back end while the needle is re-sheathed. In this way, fingers are kept well away from the dirty needle and injury is unlikely. Ideally, the needles should be re-sheathed by the dentist after use, rather than passed to the nurse, as then the potential number of injured persons is reduced.

Dirty needle stick injury

The real causes for concern are from those patients infected with blood-borne viruses for which there is no protection, such as human immunodeficiency virus (HIV). In the event of a dirty needle stick injury, the following actions should be carried out immediately:

(1) Stop work immediately
(2) Wounded area should be squeezed immediately, to encourage bleeding
(3) Under no circumstances should the wound be sucked
(4) Area should be flushed with alcohol, dried and covered with a waterproof dressing
(5) Dentist should be informed immediately
(6) Patient's medical history form should be checked for known cross-infection risks
(7) Matter should be reported to the local occupational health adviser (OHA) if necessary, based at the local hospital. Any advice given by the OHA should be followed immediately
(8) Incident should be recorded in the accident book

Advice to patients after receiving local anaesthetic

Patients need to be informed of the effects of local anaesthesia, especially if receiving it for the first time, so that they are not unduly concerned nor do they injure themselves. It is often the dental nurse who gives this information. The advice should include:

- Sensation will be lost in the area for several hours
- No eating nor drinking must occur until sensation has returned, as the patient may bite or burn themselves
- Chewing should be avoided directly on teeth restored that day, to prevent damaging new restorations (not necessary for light cured restorations)
- A 'pins and needles' sensation indicates that the anaesthetic is wearing off (**paraesthesia**)
- Nerve blocks may produce tenderness locally for the day
- Intra-ligamentary injections may cause soreness in the surrounding gingivae

Classification of cavities

Cavities are classified into five different types, depending on the site of the original caries attack. This is called **Black's classification**, after the American dentist who devised it. In general usage his classification of cavities also applies to the fillings inserted in each class of cavity.

- **Class I** cavities are those involving a **single** surface in a pit or fissure. Thus a class I filling could be an occlusal filling or a buccal or lingual filling
- **Class II** cavities involve at least **two** surfaces, the mesial or distal, and the occlusal surface of a **molar** or **premolar**. Thus a class II filling could be a mesial-occlusal (MO) filling in a premolar, for example, or a mesial-occlusal-distal (MOD) filling in a molar
- **Class III** cavities involve the mesial or distal surface of an **incisor** or **canine**
- **Class IV** cavities are the same as class III but extend to involve the **incisal edge** on the affected side
- **Class V** cavities involve the **cervical margin** of any tooth. Thus a class V filling could be a labial cervical filling in an upper incisor, or a lingual cervical filling in a lower molar, for instance

The classification of cavities enables their accurate recording on the dental chart, so that a restoration can be placed.

Cavity preparation

Every dentist has their own personal preferences for the instruments used during restorative procedures, and the table below shows the more usual items and an explanation of their function. They are usually set out on a tray for use, which is often referred to as a **conservation tray** (Figure 9.11).

Item	Function
Mouth mirror	To aid the dentist's vision; to reflect light onto the tooth; to retract and protect the soft tissues
Right-angle probe	To feel the cavity margins; to feel softened dentine within the cavity; to detect overhanging restorations
Excavators	Small and large spoon shaped, used to scoop out softened dentine
Amalgam plugger	To push filling materials into the cavity, leaving no air spaces and forcing excess mercury to the surface
Burnisher	Ball shaped or pear shaped, to press the restoration margins fully against the cavity edges so that no leakage occurs under the restoration
Flat plastic	To remove excess filling material from the restoration and create a shaped surface
College tweezers	To pick up, hold and carry various items such as cotton wool pledgets
Gingival margin trimmer	To trim the margin of the cavity to ensure no unsupported enamel nor soft dentine remains
Enamel chisel	To remove any unsupported enamel from the cavity edges

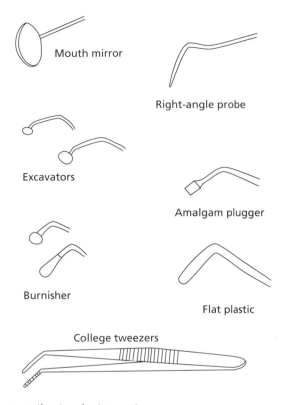

Figure 9.11 Conservation tray instruments.

Once local analgesia has been administered and has taken effect, the dentist will gain access to the caries within the tooth using diamond burs in the high-speed turbine, then change to a variety of stainless steel and other burs in the slow-speed handpiece when the carious dentine is encountered (Figure 9.12).

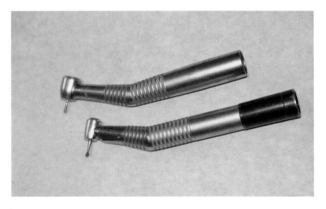

Figure 9.12 Handpieces.

As the cavity becomes deeper towards the pulp, the dentist will use the hand instruments, as detailed above, until the cavity is caries-free. Particular care is taken with deciduous teeth and the permanent teeth of younger patients because the pulp chambers are bigger and more easily breached.

Once the cavity is correctly shaped for retention (if necessary), the restoration can be placed.

Moisture control during tooth restoration

Adequate moisture control during restorative procedures is one of the most important duties of the dental nurse. It is vitally important for the following reasons:

- To protect the patient's airway from the inhalation of fluids
- It is uncomfortable for the patient to lie supine, with fluids in their mouth
- The dentist's visibility will be reduced, and injury to the patient may occur
- The setting of dental materials is adversely affected by moisture contamination
- Cements and linings do not adhere to moist tooth tissue
- Materials applied to the tooth are washed off, and this is especially undesirable with acid etchants as they can cause soft tissue burns

Many methods of moisture control are available:

- **High-speed aspiration** – suction with a wide bore tube
- **Low-speed aspiration** – saliva ejector placed in the floor of the mouth (Figure 9.13)
- **Rubber dam** – an isolating sheet of rubber with just the tooth being restored projecting through (see Unit 10 (Chapter 11))

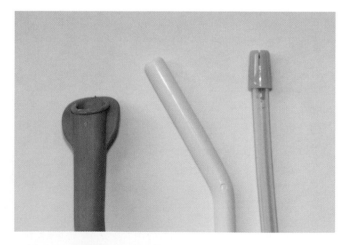

Figure 9.13 Aspirator and ejector tips. Source: *Levison's Textbook for Dental Nurses*, 10th edn, C. Hollins, 2008, Wiley-Blackwell.

- **Cotton wool rolls** – placed anywhere in the mouth to absorb pools of moisture
- **Cotton wool pledgets** – small balls used to dab cavities dry
- **Dryguards** – special discs containing absorbent material and placed over the parotid salivary gland duct
- **Compressed air** – from the triple syringe of dental unit, used to blow dry cavities and teeth

Role of the dental nurse during tooth restoration

There are some duties that are specific to the preparation and placement of restorations, and others that are very similar in other areas of dentistry, but the good dental nurse must be competent and proficient in all. The role of the dental nurse is summarised below:

- Have a good understanding of the procedure to be carried out
- Be aware of their position in the dental team for the procedure – this may be as the chairside nurse assisting directly with the procedure, or as a second nurse available to mix materials as they are required
- Have all the patient records, charts, radiographs, consent forms completed and available for the appointment
- Communicate effectively with the patient throughout the procedure, inspiring confidence and trust
- Monitor the patient throughout the procedure, ensuring their comfort and well-being and giving reassurance where necessary
- Assist during the administration of local analgesia; having the correct syringe and needle loaded with the correct cartridge as directed, passing them safely to the dentist for use, then retrieving them after use and safely re-sheathing the needle using a hands-free device to avoid needle-stick injury
- Provide careful but efficient moisture control and soft tissue retraction throughout the procedure, ensuring that no soft tissue trauma is caused
- Anticipate and pass instruments, etc. to the dentist in the correct order during the procedure
- Be aware of the required lining, base and restorative material to be used for the procedure, and mix each accordingly when directed
- Be proficient in the four-handed technique of passing instruments, etc. to the dentist as required, ensuring all items are passed safely
- Follow the infection control policy to fully decontaminate the surgery after use – see Unit 4 (Chapter 5)
- Follow the health and safety policy with regard to hazardous waste disposal, especially in relation to waste amalgam – see Unit 1 (Chapter 2)
- Ensure that all records, charts, etc. are correctly and securely stored for future use after being completed by the dentist, maintaining patient confidentiality at all times – see Unit 5 (Chapter 6)

Tooth restorations

Plastic restorations, which are those inserted at the chairside rather than being constructed in a laboratory include the following:

■ Temporary restorations
■ Linings and bases
■ Permanent restorations

Temporary restorations

These are those placed as a temporary measure, before the tooth is restored permanently, and are used for a variety of reasons:

■ As an emergency measure to seal a cavity and prevent carious ingress
■ During endodontic treatment, as repeated access may be required to the pulp chamber over several appointments
■ During inlay construction to seal the preparation while the permanent inlay is constructed
■ To allow a symptomatic tooth to settle and become symptom-free, before being permanently sealed

There are several materials available for use as a temporary restoration, some of which have other uses in dentistry – they are multipurpose materials. Their key features are:

■ Quick mixing and placement
■ Cheap compared with permanent restorative materials
■ Easily removed from the cavity when required
■ Not strong enough to be chewed on routinely
■ Have varying degrees of adhesiveness to the tooth
■ Some contain sedative ingredients to help settle inflamed pulps

A variety of materials are available, under many trade names, but temporary restorations can generally be categorised into one of the following groups:

■ Zinc oxide and eugenol
■ Zinc phosphate
■ Zinc polycarboxylate
■ Gutta percha

Zinc oxide and eugenol

■ Preparation as zinc oxide powder and eugenol liquid
■ Mixed by spatulation on a glass slab with a metal spatula

■ Used as a temporary filling, as a lining in deep cavities, during root filling and as a sedative dressing

Zinc phosphate

■ Preparation as zinc oxide powder and phosphoric acid liquid
■ Mixed by spatulation on a cool glass slab with a metal spatula
■ Used as a temporary filling, as a lining, as a luting cement and for endodontics

Zinc polycarboxylate

■ Preparation as zinc oxide and polyacrylic acid as powder, and sterile water as liquid
■ Mixed by spatulation on a glass slab with a metal spatula
■ Used as a temporary filling, as a luting cement, as a lining, and for endodontics

Gutta percha

■ Preparation as pre-formed cones or sticks of rubber
■ Only requires heat to become plastic
■ Used as a temporary filling with zinc oxide, and in endodontics and vitality testing

The main categories of temporary restorative materials, with their advantages and disadvantages are outlined below:

Material	Advantages	Disadvantages
Zinc oxide and eugenol	Cheap; sedative to inflamed pulp	Reacts with composites; eugenol can burn soft tissues
Zinc phosphate	Sets quickly; sets hard; adhesive to dentine	Irritant to pulp in deep cavity; moisture sensitive
Zinc polycarboxylate	Most adhesive cement	Sticks easily to instruments so difficult to place
Gutta percha	None over other cements listed	Messy to use; poor margin adaptation in cavity

Linings and bases

These are materials placed in the deepest part of the cavity, over the pulp chamber, before a restoration is placed. Their aim is to protect the pulp from thermal and chemical shock, by providing a barrier between the permanent restoration and the living pulp tissue, so that temperature fluctuations in the mouth are not transmitted, nor is any adverse chemical stimulation from restorations.

Zinc oxide and eugenol can be used as a sedative base beneath permanent restorations if allowed to set fully before the restoration is placed, and if an adequate thickness of the base can be placed. Zinc polycarboxylate and zinc phosphate can be used as bases too, but the acidic nature of the latter requires that a lining of calcium hydroxide is placed beneath it to further protect the pulp. Again, space is required for an adequate thickness of the base to be placed.

Calcium hydroxide

■ Preparation as calcium hydroxide and resin in a solvent
■ Usually supplied in ready-mixed paste form
■ Used as a lining under other materials, in pulp capping procedures, and in endodontics
■ Advantages – alkaline, so it counteracts acidic zinc phosphate, and kills the bacteria causing caries
■ Disadvantages – it is soluble in water, and not strong enough to use alone except as a thin liner in shallow cavities
■ Modern calcium hydroxide cements are available as light-cured liners, which are quick and easy to apply and can be set with a curing light in seconds

Permanent restorations

These are the restorations used to restore the tooth to full function and appearance (where necessary). They must have the following general properties:

■ Set hard enough to chew on without fracture
■ Easy to use and place, using the usual conservation instruments
■ Have a reasonable working lifespan (years rather than months)
■ Be safe in the oral cavity
■ Do not deteriorate in saliva

The three materials commonly used as permanent restorations are:

■ Amalgam
■ Composite
■ Glass ionomer

Amalgam restorations

This is the commonest permanent restorative material and has been used for over 150 years. It is supplied as a powdered alloy containing:

■ Silver up to 74%
■ Variable quantities of tin
■ Variable quantities of copper up to 30%
■ Small quantities of zinc

Modern amalgams are provided in sealed capsules containing the alloy powder and liquid mercury, separated from each other within the capsule by a plastic or rubber diaphragm (Figure 9.14). When the capsule contents are mixed within an amalgamator machine, the amalgam is produced (Figure 9.15).

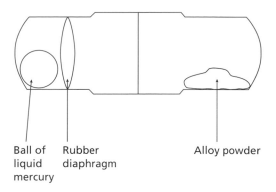

Ball of   Rubber   Alloy powder
liquid   diaphragm
mercury

Figure 9.14 Amalgam capsule. Source: *Levison's Textbook for Dental Nurses,* 10th edn, C. Hollins, 2008, Wiley-Blackwell.

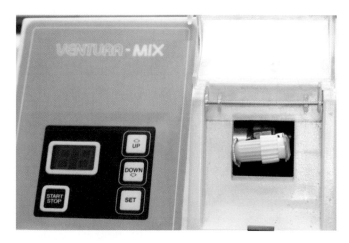

Figure 9.15 Amalgamator. Source: *Levison's Textbook for Dental Nurses,* 10th edn, C. Hollins, 2008, Wiley-Blackwell.

When used to restore class II cavities, a metallic matrix band and retainer are required to prevent the amalgam mix being squashed out of the cavity inter-proximally, as it is packed occlusally (Figure 9.16). Better adaptation to the tooth shape is achieved using wooden wedges inserted against the deeper edge of the matrix band.

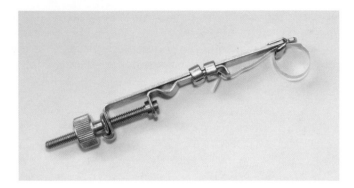

Figure 9.16 Siqveland matrix system. Source: *Levison's Textbook for Dental Nurses*, 10th edn, C. Hollins, 2008, Wiley-Blackwell.

Advantages	Disadvantages
Easy to use	Mercury is toxic
Relatively cheap	Not retentive to tooth, so cavities have to be undercut
Good set strength	Can transmit thermal shocks, so liners and bases are required in deeper cavities
Able to withstand normal occlusal forces	Has to be mixed very accurately to be dimensionally stable
Lasts for many years	Aesthetics are poor

Safe handling and usage of amalgam

Mercury is a toxic liquid metal that can enter the body in the following ways:

- **Inhaled** as a vapour
- **Absorbed** through the skin
- **Ingested** if swallowed

Special precautions have to be taken during its use to eliminate the risks to all concerned, and for the safety of the patient and the dental team, as follows:

- **Well-ventilated surgery** – so that mercury vapour does not build up
- **Personal protective equipment** – to avoid absorption and inhalation, but use of this equipment should be routine during all dental treatment
- **Use of amalgam capsules** – to avoid spillage that could occur when topping up the amalgamator
- **Health and safety policy** – developed in each dental workplace to assess and reduce the risks involved when using amalgam (see Units 1 and 4 (Chapters 2 and 5, respectively))

- **Mercury spillage kit** – system in place to deal with a mercury spillage safely, if one does occur
- **Thorough aspiration** – to remove all waste amalgam and mercury from the oral cavity, and prevent ingestion by the patient

Any waste amalgam and mercury produced have to be stored safely until they can be collected and removed from the premises, by a contracted waste removal company. Amalgam and mercury are categorised as **special waste**, and have to be stored in lidded containers containing chemicals to absorb any mercury vapour present (Figure 9.17). As the vapour production increases with temperature, these containers should be stored away from all heat sources, including sunlight.

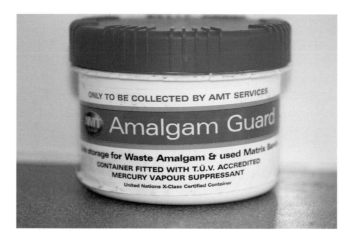

Figure 9.17 Waste amalgam tub.

If a small mercury spillage does occur, the following actions must be taken:

(1) Report the incident to a senior colleague immediately
(2) Wear full personal protective equipment
(3) Collect small mercury droplets into a syringe or bulb aspirator, and place in the waste amalgam container
(4) Collect waste amalgam with damp paper towels
(5) Use the mercury absorption paste from the mercury spillage kit to cover larger mercury spillages
(6) Gather the paste and spillage when dry with damp paper towels
(7) Risk assess the incident to determine if protocols require amendment and change

If a larger spillage occurs, the premises require evacuation while the incident is dealt with and the spillage cleared by Environmental Health. The Health and Safety Executive must be notified, so that a full investigation can be carried out.

Mercury poisoning

- Early stage symptoms:

  - Fatigue
  - Headache
  - Nausea
  - Irritability
  - Diarrhoea

- Later stage symptoms:

  - Hand tremors
  - Visual disturbance

End stage will be kidney failure and death if exposure continues or the patient is left untreated.

Monitoring devices are available nowadays, and blood and urine tests can be carried out on staff to detect abnormal levels of mercury in the body. If sound Health and Safety policies are followed at all times, there should be no cause for concern unless a large spillage occurs.

The procedure for the placement of an amalgam restoration is described below, along with the additional instruments, equipment and materials that may be required for the procedure besides the standard conservation tray.

Amalgam restoration procedure

(1)   All dental personnel and the patient wear the correct personal protective equipment throughout the procedure
(2)   All caries is removed from the cavity as described previously, without breaching the pulp chamber
(3)   The cavity is **undercut** so that the amalgam restoration does not fall out (Figure 9.18). **Moisture control** techniques are used so that the cavity remains dry
(4)   Adequate **soft tissue retraction** is applied, without causing trauma
(5)   **A lining or base** is placed on the floor of the cavity to protect the pulp, if required
(6)   A **metal matrix band** in its holder will be adapted to the tooth to prevent amalgam spillage during placement, if required
(7)   The amalgam is mixed and inserted into the cavity in increments, each one being fully pushed and **condensed** into the cavity
(8)   Once filled, any excess amalgam is carved off the tooth and the surface of the restoration is shaped
(9)   All excess amalgam and mercury are removed through the **high-speed suction**
(10)   The matrix band is removed and the restoration is checked for **overhangs**
(11)   The **occlusion** is checked and adjusted as necessary

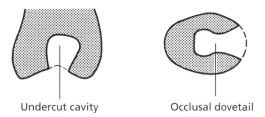

Undercut cavity   Occlusal dovetail

Figure 9.18 Cavity preparation for plastic fillings. Source: *Levison's Textbook for Dental Nurses,* 10th edn, C. Hollins, 2008, Wiley-Blackwell.

Item	Function
Liner or base material	To protect the pulp from thermal shock
	Various available including calcium hydroxide and some of the temporary cements, all suitable under amalgam restorations
Matrix system	To prevent overspill in cavities of two or more surfaces
	Usual systems are Siqveland or Tofflemire, the bands are single use
Wedges	Placed interdentally with matrix system, to tightly adapt the band to the tooth
	Both wooden wedges and plastic wedges available
Amalgam carrier (Figure 9.19)	Autoclavable 'gun' used to pick up and carry the amalgam to the cavity, where it is squeezed out
Amalgam plugger	Instrument to pack and condense the amalgam into the cavity so that no air spaces remain
Finishing instruments	To ensure the restoration is adapted to the tooth and is not high in occlusion
	Various items used – Ward's carver, burnisher, greenstone drills

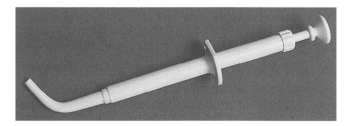

Figure 9.19 Plastic amalgam carrier. Source: *Levison's Textbook for Dental Nurses*, 10th edn, C. Hollins, 2008, Wiley-Blackwell.

Throughout the procedure (and that of all other restorative procedures), the dental team will be positioned for maximum comfort and visibility, with each team member aware of their own role in the treatment. When instruments and materials are transferred from one person to another, it is done so carefully and safely (and especially not over the patient's face), and in a manner that avoids cross-infection between items and team members.

At the end of the treatment, the area and all its contents need to be disposed of or disinfected and sterilised according to the infection control policy in place, and abiding by current legislation. This is an important duty of the dental nurse, and the routine is as follows:

(1) All sharps are carefully disposed of in the sharps box – this includes all metal matrix bands, which are classed as single use
(2) All autoclavable items are placed in an ultrasonic bath or a washer-disinfector unit and treated, before being placed in the autoclave for sterilisation
(3) All contaminated waste is placed in hazardous waste sacks
(4) All waste amalgam and mercury is carefully placed into the special waste container, and sealed
(5) All empty amalgam capsules are carefully placed in their own special waste container, and sealed
(6) All surfaces are disinfected using the correct solution
(7) All static equipment is wiped down using the correct solution

In addition, the clinical records should be fully completed before being filed away, whether this involves a paper or computer system, and any radiographs taken should be stored accordingly too. As always, the records system must ensure the full confidentiality of the patient's details and notes, by being securely stored.

Composite restorations

Composites are tooth-coloured restorative materials that are presented in a wide range of shades, to match the darkest or lightest tooth. They consist of the coloured particles suspended in a resin binder, and although usually used in anterior teeth, some systems are available for posterior teeth too.

Modern systems are set quickly by exposure to a blue curing light, rather than the older systems that relied on a chemical reaction to occur.

Advantages	Disadvantages
Excellent aesthetics	Technique-sensitive
Adhesive to tooth, using acid etch and bond	Longer procedure than for amalgam restoration
Little marginal leakage occurs	More expensive material than amalgam
Sufficient strength in smaller posterior restorations	Not as strong and hard wearing as amalgam
Usually only require lining	
Indirect inlay technique possible for larger restorations	Possible safety issue with resin bond
	Can only use glass ionomer as a base, as composites react with other bases
Fast set with curing light	Acid etchant can burn soft tissues
Available in pre-mixed compoules for easy insertion into cavity (Figure 9.20)	Safety issue with curing light causing eye damage

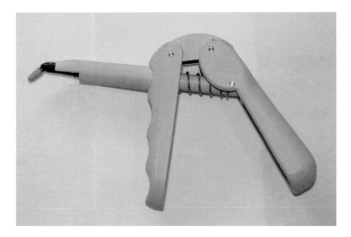

Figure 9.20 Compoule in gun.

Safe handling and usage of composite

Great care is required when using the acid etch liquid or gel during the place-ment of a composite restoration, to prevent soft tissue damage to the patient or the dental team. It consists of a **33% concentration of phosphoric acid**, and this is more than sufficient to cause acid burns and permanent scarring of the patient's soft tissues, including their facial skin.

Also, the **blue curing light** used to fast-set the restoration can cause damage to the retina of the eyes if looked at directly, so the patient must wear correctly tinted safety glasses during treatment (orange tinted are best). An orange-tinted protec-tive shield should also be held over the fibreoptic end of the light during use, to prevent the dental team from having to look at the light without eye protection too.

The procedure for the placement of a composite restoration is described below, along with the additional instruments, equipment and materials that may be required for the procedure.

Procedure for composite restorations

- All dental personnel and the patient wear the correct personal protective equipment throughout the procedure, especially tinted safety glasses
- All caries is removed from the cavity, without breaching the pulp chamber. Moisture control techniques are used so that the cavity remains dry, this may involve the placement of rubber dam (see Unit 10 (Chapter 11)). Adequate soft tissue retraction is applied, without causing trauma
- Calcium hydroxide lining, or glass ionomer base, is placed to protect the pulp if required
- **Transparent cellulose acetate matrix strip** is placed interdentally if required, to separate the tooth from its neighbours (Figure 9.21)

- Cavity edges are chemically roughened by being coated with **acid etchant** for about 15 seconds. This is thoroughly and carefully washed off and collected by the high-speed suction, and the cavity is wiped dry
- **Dentine primer** may be placed at this point
- **Resin bond** is wiped over the etched enamel and cured for about ten seconds
- Shade is determined using the shade guide and the composite material is pumped into the cavity in increments of 2 mm, and cured with the curing light (Figure 9.22)
- Cavity is gradually fully filled and cured, while the matrix strip is adapted tightly to avoid any overhangs
- Occlusion is checked and adjusted as necessary

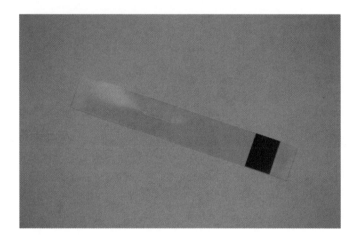

Figure 9.21 Cellulose matrix strip.

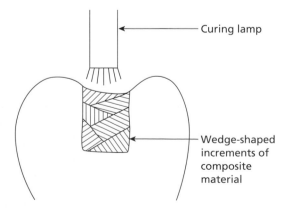

Curing lamp

Wedge-shaped increments of composite material

Figure 9.22 Composite curing technique.

Item	Function
Liner or base material	To protect the pulp from chemical shock
	Calcium hydroxide lining, and glass ionomer base in deep cavities
Matrix system	Transparent cellulose acetate strips, to allow curing of the composite through it
	Various holder systems available
Plastic instruments	To place the composite and remove excess before curing
	Various designs available, the commonest one being a flat plastic instrument
	Can acquire ceramic tipped instruments to avoid sticking
Finishing instruments	To ensure no overhangs are left and that the surface of the restoration is smooth
	Various items used – specially shaped plastic instruments, abrasive strips, polishing discs, polishing burs of various designs

The procedure is carried out and completed as for other restorative treatments (see earlier), and the surgery made ready for the next patient as usual.

Glass ionomer restorations

Glass ionomers are tooth-coloured restorative materials that are adhesive to all of the hard tissues of the teeth, so they tend to be used in situations when little natural retention of the restoration is available. They are composed of powdered glass particles and polyacrylic acid mixed with water, and although they have a range of shades available, their aesthetics are inferior to composites.

Various other forms are available, such as mixed with silver to produce a harder wearing posterior restoration, mixed with composite (as a compomer) to achieve a restoration with the advantages of both materials, or mixed with other metals (as cermets) for use in tooth core build-ups. Some glass ionomer products set chemically, others by exposure to the blue curing light as for composites.

Advantages	Disadvantages
Adhesive to enamel, dentine and cementum	Low strength compared with amalgam or composite
Ideal for use with abrasion cavities	Very technique sensitive
Good marginal seal, preventing leakage	Requires calcium hydroxide lining
Release fluoride over time, so very useful when restoring deciduous teeth	Moisture contamination causes failure of restoration
Better aesthetics than amalgam	Requires protection from moisture during full setting

Safe handling and usage of glass ionomers

The acid content of the material can damage metal spatulas during mixing, so plastic spatulas are best. If the make of glass ionomer being used is to be light-cured, then all the usual precautions must be taken to avoid eye damage to both the patient and the dental team.

The procedure for the placement of a glass ionomer restoration is described below, along with the additional instruments, equipment and materials that may be required for the procedure.

Procedure for glass ionomer restorations

(1) All dental personnel and the patient wear the correct personal protective equipment throughout the procedure
(2) All caries is removed from the cavity, without breaching the pulp chamber
(3) Moisture control techniques are used so that the cavity remains dry, this may involve the placement of rubber dam (see Unit 10 (Chapter 11))
(4) Adequate soft tissue retraction is applied, without causing trauma
(5) **Calcium hydroxide lining** is placed in deep cavities
(6) A **conditioner** is applied to the cavity, which increases the adhesion of the material to the tooth and improves the marginal seal. This is washed off after about 20 seconds and collected by the high-speed suction, then the cavity is dried
(7) Shade is determined and the material is carefully apportioned and mixed
(8) Material is placed into the cavity and allowed to achieve its initial set, or it is light-cured
(9) **Foil matrix** is used when restoring abrasion cavities, to produce a smooth surface (Figure 9.23)

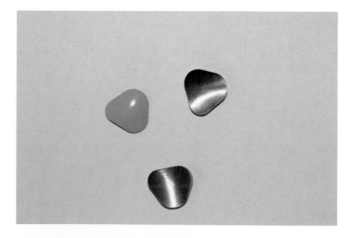

Figure 9.23 Glass ionomer class V matrix system.

(10) Excess material is carefully removed, without touching its surface as this will produce a chalky appearance

(11) Surface is coated with **varnish** while fully setting, to prevent moisture contamination

Item	Function
Liner	Calcium hydroxide, if any is required, to protect the pulp from the acrylic acid
Plastic instruments	To place the glass ionomer and remove any excess material
Matrix	Foil coated and pre-shaped for use when restoring abrasion cavities
	Cannot be used if the glass ionomer is a light-cured make
Finishing materials	Varnish, wiped over the restoration surface to prevent moisture contamination

10 Unit 9: Provide Chairside Support During the Provision of Fixed and Removable Prostheses (OH6)

Knowledge specifications

Anatomy and physiology

K1 – A factual knowledge of dental anatomy in relation to the mandible and maxilla

K2 – A factual knowledge of jaw movements of the temporo-mandibular joint

Replacement of teeth

K3 – A factual knowledge of the options available for replacing missing teeth and the relative benefits of each, including:
a)   fixed prostheses
b)   removable prostheses
c)   implants

Fixed prostheses

K4 – A factual knowledge of the purpose of crown, bridge, inlay and veneer techniques

K5 – A factual knowledge of the purpose of temporary crowns and bridges, and their construction

K6 – A working knowledge of the equipment and instruments used in preparing teeth for fixed prostheses

K7 – A working knowledge of the equipment, instruments and materials for retraction before impression taking

K8 – A working knowledge of selecting and preparing impression trays, and mixing and loading the appropriate impression material

K9 – A working knowledge of preparing and planning temporary crowns and bridges, cements, and hand instruments (such as flat plastics)

K10 – A working knowledge of shade taking (such as shade guides)

K11 – A working knowledge of methods of taking occlusal registrations, and why these are necessary

K12 – A working knowledge of the instruments and materials required for:
a) the removal of temporary prostheses
b) the checking and adjusting of fixed prostheses before final fitting
c) protecting and retracting the soft tissues (such as rubber dam)

K13 – A working knowledge of different types of cements, and correct methods of mixing and the methods of isolation during cementation

Prosthodontics

K14 – A factual knowledge of the use of impression materials in making study models or working casts for the construction of the appliance and of the opposing arch or tooth

K15 – A working knowledge of the different forms which impression materials take (alginates, reversible hydrocolloid, puttys), the relationship of these to the treatment being undertaken

K16 – A working knowledge of the preparation, application, storage and after-care of impressions to preserve the accuracy of the impression

K17 – A factual knowledge of why impression materials should be disinfected prior to the attachment of a laboratory ticket

Removable prostheses – types, functions and stages of treatment

K18 – A factual knowledge of the different stages in making complete and partial removable prostheses, relines, rebases and additions

K19 – A factual knowledge of the purpose of:
a) pre-prosthetic surgery
b) tooth preparation prior to partial denture constructions
c) using obturators
d) tissue conditioners
e) using spoon dentures

K20 – A factual knowledge of the options available for replacing missing teeth, and their relative benefits

K21 – A working knowledge of the equipment, instruments, and materials which are used in taking initial and second impressions

K22 – A working knowledge of the equipment, instruments, and materials which are used in taking occlusal registrations (such as wax occlusal rims, additional sheets of pink wax, heat source, markers, shade guides and mould guides)

K23 – A working knowledge of the equipment, instruments, and materials which are used in try-ins (such as the waxed-up removable prostheses, heat source, shade guides, wax knife, Le Cron carver, sheet wax, mirrors)

K24 – A working knowledge of the equipment, instruments, and materials which are used at the fitting of removable prostheses (such as individual mirror, handpiece, polymeric stone, polymeric trimming burs, pressure relief paste, articulating papers)

K25 – A working knowledge of the differences between constructing dentures for adults, children, and the elderly

Orthodontic treatment and appliances

K26 – A factual knowledge of the range of orthodontic treatments available and the different type of appliances used

K27 – A factual knowledge of the equipment, instruments and materials which are used in the fitting, monitoring and adjusting of orthodontic appliances

Liaison with manufacturers of custom-made prostheses

K28 – A factual knowledge of the role of the dental technician in the oral health care team, and purpose of close liaison with technical staff and the dental laboratory in relation to timing, materials, etc

K29 – A factual knowledge of the relevance and importance of laboratory work tickets and record cards

Supporting individuals in the care of removable prostheses and in their oral health care

K30 – A working knowledge of the type of support which patients may need when obtaining new removable prostheses, and the worries which they may have

K31 – A working knowledge of how to care for removable prostheses

K32 – A working knowledge of aftercare for immediate dentures

Retracting tissues and aspirating

K33 – A working knowledge of methods of protecting and retracting the soft tissues

K34 – A working knowledge of methods of aspirating during treatment

Communication

K35 – A working knowledge of the importance of communicating information clearly and effectively

K36 – A working knowledge of methods for modifying information and communication methods for different individuals, including patients from different social and ethnic backgrounds, children (including those with special needs), and the elderly

Health and safety and infection control

K37 – A working knowledge of the purpose, method of use, and function of protective wear, and the reason for their use
K38 – A working knowledge of standard precautions and quality standards of cross infection control, and your role in maintaining them
K39 – A factual knowledge of the reasons for monitoring continuously the patient and the operator

Charts and records

K40 – A working knowledge of the different types of charts and records used in the organisation (including medical history, personal details, dental charts, radiographs, photographs and study models for assessment and treatment planning), and their purpose
K41 – An in-depth knowledge of confidentiality in relation to patient records

Team working

K42 – A working knowledge of methods of effective team working in oral health care

Prosthetics is the branch of dentistry that is concerned with fixed prosthetics and removable prosthetics. Fixed prosthetics include:

- Crowns and temporary crowns
- Bridges and temporary bridges
- Veneers
- Inlays

Removable prosthetics include:

- Acrylic dentures
- Chrome dentures
- Immediate replacement dentures
- Orthodontic appliances

Summary of anatomy and tooth morphology

A background knowledge of anatomy and physiology is required to understand the reasons for replacing teeth with prostheses, and the requirement to ensure that the prostheses function correctly. These areas are covered in full in Unit 6 (Chapter 7), and are summarised below.

Maxilla – the upper jaw

- Made up of two bones that form the roof of the mouth – **hard palate**
- Also form the base of the nose
- Hollow air-filled space between these two areas is called the **maxillary sinus** or **antrum**
- Nerves and blood vessels supplying the upper teeth and surrounding soft tissues run through the maxilla
- Horseshoe-shaped ridge of bone running around the maxilla called the **alveolar process**
- Alveolar process holds the upper teeth in the dental arch

Mandible – the lower jaw

- Made up of two bones joined in the centre-line to form a horseshoe shape
- Connected to the skull at the temporo-mandibular joint (TMJ) as a hinge, so that the mouth can be opened and closed
- **Alveolar process** holds the lower teeth in the dental arch
- Nerves and blood vessels supplying the lower teeth and surrounding soft tissues run through the mandible
- Sheet of muscle running across the base of the horseshoe forms the **floor of the mouth**
- **Tongue** lies above this muscle, within the oral cavity and enclosed by the mandible

The remaining soft tissue structures that complete the oral cavity are the surrounding muscles of the face (**muscles of facial expression**) and the muscles involved in closing the mouth and carrying out jaw movements, including chewing (**muscles of mastication**).

Temporo-mandibular joint

This is the hinge joint between the base of the skull and the mandible, which allows the mouth to open and close. The head of the **mandibular condyle** sits in a depression of the temporal bone of the skull (**glenoid fossa**) and the articulation of the bones at this point forms the TMJ. The two bones are separated by a pad of cartilage (**meniscus**) so that the bones do not grate against each other as the jaw moves.

Any excessive jaw movements, including clenching and grinding the teeth, can disrupt the position of the meniscus, so that the TMJ 'clicks' and 'pops' on opening or closing. If the meniscus is pulled completely out of position, the jaw can lock open or closed.

Muscles of mastication

These are four sets of muscles that run between the mandible and the base of the skull, and they act to **close** the mouth and to **chew**.

Their **point of origin** is the base of the skull and their **point of insertion** is the mandible. When each pair of muscles contracts, they move the mandible in relation to the skull, as shown below.

Name	Point of origin	Point of insertion	Action
Temporalis	Temporal bone of skull	Coronoid process of mandible	Back and closed
Masseter	Outer zygomatic arch	Outer ramus and angle	Closed
Lateral pterygoid	Lateral pterygoid plate	Head of condyle and into meniscus	Forwards to bite tip to tip; or swings jaw to side
Medial pterygoid	Medial pterygoid plate	Inner ramus and angle	Closed

Significance of the TMJ and the muscles of mastication

Overuse of the lateral pterygoid in particular, as when clenching and grinding, disrupts the TMJ and the meniscus itself. When fixed or removable prostheses are provided that have not been correctly adjusted to the patient's bite, strain is put on the TMJ and the muscles of mastication, and the patient will experience facial as well as dental pain.

The accurate recording of the patient's occlusion during the provision of fixed and removable prostheses is imperative if the prostheses are to be successful.

Tooth and root morphology of permanent teeth

The details of each tooth's morphology are summarised below.

Tooth	Number	Number of roots	Number of cusps (where applicable)
Central incisor – upper	1	One	N/A
Lateral incisor – upper	2	One	N/A
Canine – upper	3	One	N/A
First premolar – upper	4	Two	Two
Second premolar – upper	5	One	Two
First molar – upper	6	Three	Five
Second molar – upper	7	Three	Four
Third molar – upper	8	Three	Four
Central incisor – lower	1	One	N/A
Lateral incisor – lower	2	One	N/A
Canine – lower	3	One	N/A
First premolar – lower	4	One	Two
Second premolar – lower	5	One	Two
First molar – lower	6	Two	Five
Second molar – lower	7	Two	Four
Third molar – lower	8	Two	Four

Significance of individual tooth anatomy

The teeth have evolved with their individual morphology to provide the best ability to bite into, and chew, food – this is their main function. When they are being replaced by artificial prostheses, such as crowns, bridges or dentures, their original shape has to be copied exactly so as not to disrupt the patient's **occlusion**. The only exceptions are when the teeth being replaced are in a poor position or have a poor shape already. This can occur when fixed prostheses are placed on tilted teeth for instance, to restore the occlusion, or when removable prostheses are used to replace poorly aligned teeth, such as severely proclined incisors.

Treatment options to replace missing teeth

When one or several teeth are missing, they may require replacement for any of the following reasons:

- **Prevent damage** to other teeth due to excessive chewing forces
- **Prevent movement** of other teeth into the space present, so that the occlusion is disrupted
- Allow **adequate chewing** to occur, so preventing digestive problems caused by under-chewed foods, especially in older people
- **Prevent soft tissue trauma** of the alveolar ridges during chewing
- **Prevent over-eruption** of the opposing teeth, so that the occlusion is disrupted
- Provide **good aesthetics**

The options available to the patient are:

- Removable prosthesis – denture
- Fixed prosthesis – bridge
- Titanium implant

Each of these options has their own advantages and disadvantages, but in relation to each other their relative benefits are as follows:

- Dentures:
  - Cheapest option
  - Can be added to without the need of remakes
  - Rarely involves any tooth preparation
  - Easily cleaned by the patient
- Bridges:
  - Second cheapest option
  - Little soft tissue coverage involved
  - Good alternative for patients with a strong gag reflex
  - Maintain good aesthetics for many years

■ Implants:

  – No other tooth preparation involved
  – No soft tissue coverage involved
  – Good aesthetics
  – Long lasting

Other fixed prostheses are used to cover the teeth fully or partially (crowns or veneers), or instead of conventional filling restorations (inlays).

Fixed prostheses

All fixed prostheses described here are provided for varying reasons but involve the use of similar materials and similar instruments. These are: temporary or permanent crowns, inlays, veneers, and temporary or permanent bridges. Each of these prostheses has their own reasons for use as shown below, and can be constructed from various materials, depending on the following considerations:

■ **Tooth involved** – are high chewing forces likely to occur?
■ **Aesthetics** – is an anterior tooth involved?
■ **Longevity** – is the prosthesis temporary or permanent?
■ **Occlusion** – is the patient's bite unusual in any way?

Prosthesis	Purpose	Materials
Temporary crown (Figure 10.1)	To cover the prepared tooth while awaiting a permanent crown; as an emergency restoration	Preformed acrylic or polycarbonate; cold cure acrylic
Permanent crown (Figure 10.2)	To protect a heavily filled or root filled tooth from fracture during chewing; aesthetics; tooth shape change	Porcelain ceramic; bonded porcelain to metal; precious metal alloy; non-precious metal alloy
Veneer (Figure 10.3)	Aesthetics, to cover the labial surface of an anterior tooth when it is discoloured or mis-shaped	Porcelain
Inlay (Figure 10.4)	To restore a cavity in a tooth with a material stronger than conventional filling materials	Porcelain; precious metal alloy; non-precious metal alloy
Temporary bridge	To cover prepared teeth and replace missing teeth while awaiting the permanent bridge; to replace missing teeth after extraction while resorption occurs	Acrylic resin-based materials
Permanent bridge (Figure 10.5)	To replace missing teeth; aesthetics	Ceramic; bonded porcelain to metal; precious metal alloy; non-precious metal alloy

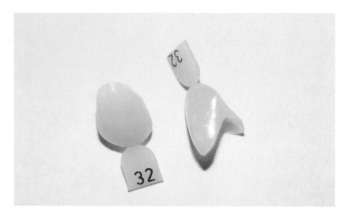

Figure 10.1 Temporary polycarbonate crown forms.

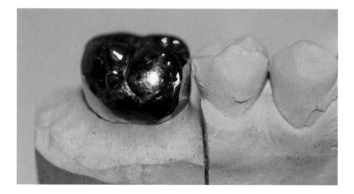

Figure 10.2 Full gold crown on model. Source: *Levison's Textbook for Dental Nurses*, 10th edn, C. Hollins, 2008, Wiley-Blackwell.

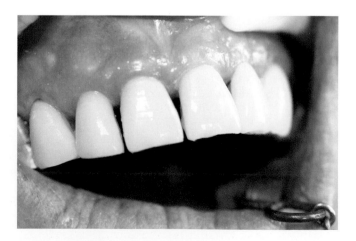

Figure 10.3 Porcelain veneers.

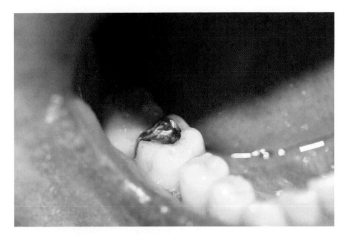

Figure 10.4 Cemented gold inlay. Source: *Levison's Textbook for Dental Nurses,* 10th edn, C. Hollins, 2008, Wiley-Blackwell.

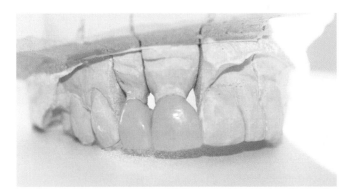

Figure 10.5 Permanent bridge on model.

Although temporary crowns and bridges can be constructed at the chairside, sometimes using stock crown-formers, all the other prostheses are sent to a laboratory for their construction. The chairside preparation procedure for all of them is as follows:

(1)   Suitable personal protective equipment for the patient and all staff
(2)   Administration of local analgesia, unless the tooth is non-vital
(3)   Preparation of the tooth (or teeth) using tapered diamond burs in the high speed turbine, ensuring that no undercuts are produced
(4)   Retraction of the gingival tissues away from the prepared tooth margins, using gingival retraction cord or electrosurgery
(5)   Taking of the working arch impression, using highly accurate elastomeric impression material in an impression tray

(6) Taking of the opposing arch impression, using alginate in an impression tray
(7) Recording of the occlusion, using wax wafers or an elastomer occlusal impression material
(8) Taking of the shade required, using the shade guide (Figure 10.6)
(9) Preparation of temporary tooth coverage, using crown-formers if necessary
(10) Cementation of a temporary crown or bridge, or placement of temporary coverage where a veneer or inlay are to be constructed

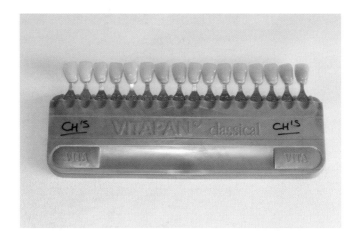

Figure 10.6 Shade guide.

Instruments

The majority of dentists have a normal 'conservation tray' set up as the basic requirements for instruments (see Unit 8 (Chapter 9)), but additional equipment and materials will also be required, as shown below.

Item	Function
Diamond burs (Figure 10.7)	Tapered so that no undercuts are produced on the prepared tooth or teeth, otherwise the fixed prosthesis will not seat onto the tooth
Retraction cord	Cord soaked in an astringent solution (adrenaline or alum) and packed into the gingival crevice to cause shrinkage of the gingiva away from the prepared tooth
Impression trays (Figure 10.8)	Variety of plastic or metal boxed trays, sized to fit fully over the dental arch – upper and lower styles
Crown-former	Pre-formed plastic or polycarbonate tooth-shaped formers, in a variety of sizes and available for each tooth shape
Beebee crown shears (Figure 10.9)	Short beaked shears for shaping the margins of temporary crowns
Shade guide	Shaded teeth in holder, to determine the required shade of the prosthesis by comparing each to the surrounding teeth

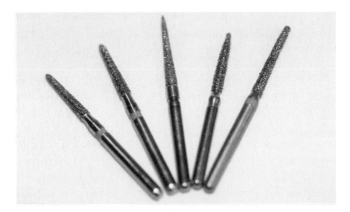

Figure 10.7 Tapered diamond crown preparation burs.

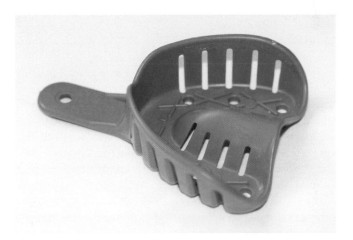

Figure 10.8 Impression tray. Source: *Levison's Textbook for Dental Nurses,* 10th edn, C. Hollins, 2008, Wiley-Blackwell.

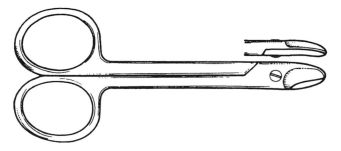

Figure 10.9 Beebee crown shears. Source: *Levison's Textbook for Dental Nurses*, 10th edn, C. Hollins, 2008, Wiley-Blackwell.

In addition, some dentists will carry out the preparation procedure using rubber dam, to provide complete moisture control and good gingival retraction (see Unit 10 (Chapter 11)).

Impression materials

The technique of crown construction is an indirect one, whereby the dentist prepares the tooth and then sends a copy of it to a technician (using impression materials) for the crown to be custom-made. This is then returned to the dentist for fitting to the patient's tooth. An impression of the opposing arch of the teeth is also sent so that the technician can ensure that the crown will not alter the patient's bite, once fitted.

The variety of impression materials available is vast, but all have to have the following properties:

- Should be easily mixed
- Should be cost effective
- Have an adequate working time before setting
- Have a relatively short setting time, for the patient's comfort
- Record the tooth details accurately
- Should be stable when set so that models cast from the impression are accurate and not distorted
- Should be elastic so that tearing on removal does not occur, and so that the impression maintains the details recorded accurately
- Should be able to be disinfected without affecting the accuracy of the details recorded, for cross-infection purposes

The more commonly used elastic types of impression material fall into one of the following categories:

- Irreversible hydrocolloids – alginate
- Addition silicones, from heavy bodied putty to light bodied paste
- Polyethers

A far less commonly used impression material is agar, which is a **reversible hydrocolloid**. Details of the more common materials available are shown below, but some of the more modern ones can be mixed automatically in special machines, rather than by hand.

Name	Type	Mixing
Alginate	Irreversible hydrocolloid	Powder and room temperature water in equal portions, mixed by spatulating in a bowl
Addition silicone	Elastomer	Base and catalyst, as putty and liquid or two pastes, mixed in equal portions by spatulation, or in pre-loaded tubes, or in a mixing machine
Polyether	Elastomer	Base and catalyst pastes, mixed in equal portions by spatulation, then loaded into a syringe for direct application
Agar	Reversible hydrocolloid	Gel in a sealed tube, becomes fluid by heating the tube and is mixed by manipulation within the tube before use Used in the laboratory to produce duplicate models

Alginate

This is the most commonly used impression material in the dental workplace, as it is easy to mix and relatively cheap. It is suitable for producing impressions for models for:

- Opposing arch models for crown, bridge, inlay, veneer construction
- Models for the construction of full and partial acrylic dentures
- Models for the construction of removable orthodontic appliances
- Study models
- Models for the construction of special trays, bleaching trays, orthodontic retainers

However, alginates are not accurate enough to be used to take the working model for crown, bridge, veneer, or inlay construction.

Alginates are presented as a dry powder of **calcium salt**, **alginate salt** and **filler**, with a measured scoop, which is mixed with **water at room temperature** using a similar measuring cup. Once the container has been shaken to ensure even distribution of the constituents, and then measured out, it is mixed in a plastic bowl with a large spatula, by folding the powder into the water initially, then vigorously spreading it against the bowl side (**spatulating**). The mix needs to be spatulated thoroughly to be free of air bubbles, to create a stiff and creamy consistency. The mix is then loaded into an impression tray (see below) before insertion into the patient's mouth.

The working time of alginate is affected by the temperature of the mixing water used, and the setting time is affected by the room temperature. In both cases, the higher the temperature, the lesser is the time required. There are also 'chromogenic' alginate materials available, which change colour during the mixing and setting stages, for ease of use and accuracy of set.

Addition silicones

These are highly accurate impression materials used specifically for fixed prosthetic work and some removable prosthetic work. They have a variety of presentations:

- Tubs of heavy bodied putty with liquid or paste activator (chemical which actually starts the reaction to produce the impression material)
- Tubes of light bodied paste with liquid or paste activator
- More recently, preloaded gun syringes which mix the constituents automatically (Figure 10.10)

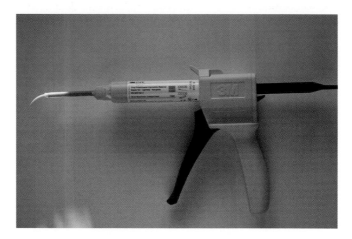

Figure 10.10 Silicone impression gun.

Again, measures are provided for accurate mixing, but it should be noted that it is possible for the mixing and setting times to be affected by some types of rubber PPE gloves used. If mixing is to occur by hand, it is advisable that vinyl gloves are worn as other types may affect the setting of the silicone impression. As each component is usually highly coloured, adequate mixing can be seen to have occurred when a non-streaky mix is produced. Silicones are not affected by temperature.

The silicones can be used either in a one-stage technique (using addition cured silicones) or a two-stage technique (using condensation cured silicones). With the former, both the heavy bodied putty and the light bodied paste are mixed at the same time. The putty is loaded into the impression tray while the paste is either syringed onto the prepared tooth, or placed onto it using a flat plastic instrument. Both materials then set and are removed together. With the latter, the putty is mixed, loaded into the tray, inserted into the mouth and allowed to set first. It is then carefully removed and spaced in the area of the preparation, while the mixed paste is syringed or wiped onto the tooth. The set putty and tray are reinserted and the whole is removed when the paste has set.

While the one-stage technique is obviously quicker, the two-stage ensures that adequate paste remains around the prepared tooth during tray insertion and gives a very accurate impression; whereas it can be displaced by the putty during tray insertion in the one-stage method. Adhesive is usually supplied by the manufacturer, but perforated trays can also be used.

Setting time is usually four minutes or more, so adequate moisture control to maintain patient comfort is of great importance during this period. Following removal from the mouth, the impression is again rinsed in cold water, then immersed in 10% sodium hypochlorite solution, but only for one minute. It is then rinsed again and, unlike alginate, the impression is blown dry (using a triple syringe) before being sealed in an airtight bag and despatched to the laboratory, ideally within 24 hours.

Polyethers

These are also highly accurate impression materials, used specifically for fixed prosthetic work and certain removable prosthetic work. They are presented as two pastes that are usually of different colours to ensure that uniform mixing occurs. The two pastes are mixed in equal proportions by spatulation on a waxed paper pad, and then collected into special syringes for administration to the prepared tooth (Figure 10.11). The remaining material is loaded into the impression tray. Again, adhesive is supplied by the manufacturer. The setting time is similar to that of silicones.

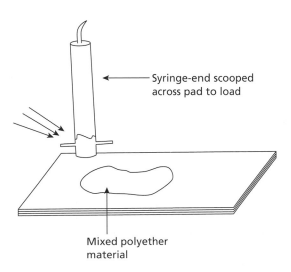

Syringe-end scooped
across pad to load

Mixed polyether
material

Figure 10.11 Polyether technique.

Polyethers set more stiffly than other elastomers, and therefore need to be removed with a sharp displacing action from the mouth, otherwise they can be difficult to remove. Disinfection is carried out in a similar manner to silicones, but polyethers are more dimensionally unstable if moist, so the impression must be thoroughly dried before sealing in an airtight bag and despatching to the laboratory, again preferably within 24 hours.

Impression trays

Impression trays are available as:

- Plastic **disposable** or plastic/metal **re-usable** (which need to be autoclavable)
- Upper or lower
- Variety of sizes from child to large adult
- **Stock trays**, which are mass produced, or **special trays**, which are made individually from the patient's first model
- **Boxed** for dentate patients, or ridge shaped for **edentulous** patients (those with no teeth)
- **Perforated** or requiring an adhesive, to prevent impression material pulling out of the tray while being removed from the mouth

For a single crown, inlay or veneer preparation, a type of **triple tray** can be used which records the prepared tooth, the opposing teeth and the patient's correct occlusion in one stage. These are single use, disposable trays made of a plastic frame and cloth infill, which save considerably on the more expensive types of impression material, as they do not require full arch impressions to be taken (Figure 10.12).

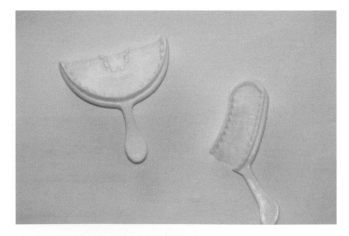

Figure 10.12 Triple Tray® impression system.

Impression handling

As the impressions have been inside the patient's mouth, they will obviously be contaminated by their saliva and perhaps even their blood. To avoid cross-infection from the patient to either staff or the technician, the impressions and bite records must be disinfected immediately after their removal from the mouth. This is done as follows:

(1) Rinse the impression under cold running water to remove any visible debris
(2) Fully immerse in a disinfectant bath of **10% sodium hypochlorite** (bleach)
(3) Immerse for up to ten minutes
(4) Rinse under cold running water again, to remove the disinfectant solution
(5) Alginate impressions – cover with wet gauze and seal in an air-tight bag; elastomer impressions – blown dry and seal in an air-tight bag
(6) Store at room temperature or below before transportation to the laboratory
(7) Enclose work ticket – detailing dentist, patient name and age, prosthesis to be constructed, material to be used, shade, additional features, date of delivery for fitting, disinfection details

The work ticket details should also be recorded onto the patient's record card or computer notes.

As indicated, the majority of impressions are sent away to a laboratory and this can take some considerable time, especially if they are posted. During this period, they must remain stable so that the cast models eventually produced are accurate, otherwise the fixed prostheses will not fit onto the patient's tooth. For this reason, they should not be exposed to any heat sources nor chemicals. Alginate impressions must be kept moist and not be allowed to dry out, otherwise they will distort and any models cast from them will be useless.

Role of the dental nurse during fixed prosthetics

There are some duties that are specific to the preparation and placement of fixed prostheses, and others that are very similar in other areas of dentistry, but the good dental nurse must be competent and proficient in all. The role of the dental nurse is summarised below:

- Have a good understanding of the procedure to be carried out
- Be aware of their position in the dental team for the procedure – this may be as the chairside nurse assisting directly with the procedure, or as a second nurse available to mix materials and load impression trays as they are required
- Have all the patient records, charts, radiographs, study models, completed prostheses, consent forms completed and available for the appointment
- Communicate effectively with the patient throughout the procedure, inspiring confidence and trust

- Monitor the patient throughout the procedure, ensuring their comfort and well-being and giving reassurance where necessary
- Assist during the administration of local analgesia; having the correct syringe and needle loaded with the correct cartridge as directed, passing them safely to the dentist for use, then retrieving them after use and safely re-sheathing the needle using a hands-free device to avoid needle-stick injury
- Assist with the placement of rubber dam, as necessary – see Unit 10 (Chapter 11)
- Provide careful but efficient moisture control and soft tissue retraction throughout the procedure
- Anticipate and pass instruments, etc. to the dentist in the correct order during the procedure
- Be aware of the correct trays and impression materials, or luting cements to be used for the procedure, and mix each accordingly when directed
- Load the impression trays efficiently and pass and retrieve them safely, avoiding the patient's facial area
- Be proficient in the four-handed technique of passing instruments, etc. to the dentist as required, ensuring all items are passed safely
- Assist during the construction and cementation of temporary prostheses, as necessary
- Record the accurate laboratory instructions for the prosthesis, and duplicate them exactly into the patient's records as necessary
- Follow the infection control policy in relation to the safe handling of all impressions and bite records taken
- Follow the infection control policy to fully decontaminate the surgery after use – see Unit 4 (Chapter 5)
- Follow the health and safety policy with regard to hazardous waste disposal – see Unit 1 (Chapter 2)
- Ensure that all records, charts, etc. are correctly and securely stored for future use after being completed by the dentist, maintaining patient confidentiality at all times – see Unit 6 (Chapter 7)

Surgery procedure for crown preparation

So, adapting the above procedure for a crown preparation, the actual surgery procedure can be summarised as follows:

(1) Unless the tooth is non-vital, **local anaesthetic** will be necessary
(2) An **alginate impression** of the opposing arch is taken, using the appropriate impression tray
(3) An **occlusal registration** is often taken, especially in complicated cases, using either softened wax which the patient bites into, or using face bows for articulation of the models at the laboratory
(4) The **tooth is prepared** by reducing its overall dimensions by 1 mm for metallic or ceramic crowns, or 1.5 mm for bonded crowns, using diamond burs which produce near parallel sides to provide optimum retention, but without producing undercuts (Figure 10.13)

(5) To ensure accurate recording of the crown preparation margins, **gingival retraction cord** can be pushed into the gingival crevice and removed immediately before the impression is inserted. This is cord soaked in either adrenaline or alum, both of which cause the gingivae to retract and pull away from the tooth, thus allowing impression material to flow in and accurately record the margins

(6) An **elastomer impression** is then taken of the working arch, as described above

(7) When satisfactory impressions have been produced, a **temporary crown** is made at the chairside and cemented temporarily to the prepared tooth

(8) A **shade** of the tooth is taken, to match accurately the adjacent teeth including any darkening towards the root, or hypomineralised areas

(9) All relevant details are **accurately recorded** on the laboratory slip, which is sent to the laboratory with the impressions and occlusal registration for construction of the permanent crown

(10) A correct return date should be given, to coincide with the patient's next appointment for fitting of the crown

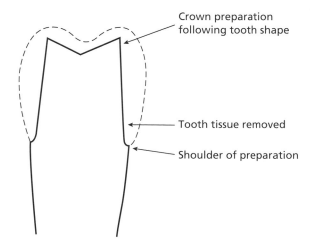

Crown preparation
following tooth shape

Tooth tissue removed

Shoulder of preparation

Figure 10.13 Crown preparation.

Temporary crowns

These are provided for aesthetic reasons, to prevent over-eruption of the prepared tooth and to avoid sensitivity problems in the prepared tooth while the permanent crown is being constructed. They can be hand-made at the chairside.

(1) An alginate impression of the tooth is taken before crown preparation begins

(2) A cold cure acrylic material is then mixed and placed in the impression after crown preparation, and reinserted into the mouth

(3) This takes just minutes to set, and produces a temporary crown of exactly the shape of the original tooth

Shades are rather restricted, so colour matching is as accurate as can be expected.

Temporary crowns can also be provided by mass production in various sizes, for each tooth shape. These can be cut and trimmed at the chairside to fit any prepared tooth, using either acrylic trimming burs, or 'Beebee' crown shears to ensure accurate marginal fit. They are then temporarily cemented to the tooth, using a zinc oxide and eugenol temporary cement, while awaiting the permanent crown construction.

Surgery procedure for crown fitting

Laboratories vary in the time required for the crown to be custom-made. Accurate and detailed information provided on the laboratory slip will ensure that unnecessary delays are avoided, and a professional and trusting relationship between the practice and the laboratory technician often allows for speedier completion on occasion. Again, the dental nurse's role is as detailed previously, and the fitting procedure can be summarised as follows:

(1) Provide suitable personal protective equipment for the patient and all staff
(2) Administration of local analgesia, unless the tooth is non-vital
(3) Application of rubber dam, if necessary
(4) Removal of the temporary prosthesis, using specific crown-removal instruments or a bur in the high speed turbine to cut the temporary prosthesis off the tooth
(5) Try in of the prosthesis onto the tooth (or teeth)
(6) Dentist will check the marginal fit, the correct occlusion, and the shade of the prosthesis
(7) Occlusion will be checked using articulating paper – high spots will leave a coloured mark to indicate the point that needs reducing
(8) Reduction is carried out using burs in the high-speed handpiece, and polishing burs or stones to smooth the area after
(9) When the dentist and patient are happy with the fit, the prosthesis can be cemented into place using one of a variety of luting cements. If the fit is poor or the occlusion is completely incorrect, the dentist will take new impressions and bite registration and request a remake of the prosthesis

Luting cements

A luting cement is one that is **adhesive to the dentine** of the tooth, and is mixed to a **creamy consistency** so that the prosthesis can be seated fully onto the tooth before the cement sets. There are many types available, some setting by a chemical reaction only, some requiring light curing, and others that set by both methods – **dual cure cements**. All require good moisture control during their use, otherwise their setting is affected and good adhesion will not be achieved. Types available are shown below:

Type	Action	Mixing
Zinc phosphate	Mechanically adhesive to rough inner surface of prosthesis, and surface of tooth	Glass slab and spatula
Zinc Polycarboxylate	Chemically adhesive to tooth and inner surface of prosthesis	Glass slab and spatula
Glass ionomer	Chemically adhesive to tooth and inner surface of prosthesis	Waxed pad and spatula
Polyester resin	Chemically adhesive, and inert in saliva	Waxed pad and spatula
Self-cure resin	Chemical bonding between tooth and prosthesis	Double syringe mix
Light-cure resin	Light-cure bonding between tooth and prosthesis	Double syringe mix
Dual-cure resin	Combination of self-cure and light-cure bonding between tooth and prosthesis	Double syringe mix

Modern types of cement tend to be provided in double syringe form with no mixing necessary, but older types (such as phosphate, polycarboxylate and glass ionomer cements) require correct proportioning and thorough mixing before use. All cements can be mixed on a cool glass slab with a small spatula, by incorporating increments of powder into the relevant liquid and spatulating thoroughly until a smooth, creamy mix is produced.

Working and setting times vary between products, and need to be followed closely for accuracy. If the mix is too stiff, the crown will be unable to be seated fully so that the occlusion will be incorrect. If the mix is too runny, the setting time will be prolonged and the cement will not set consistently throughout, so that loss of the crown is likely.

Post-crowns

These are crowns cemented onto a metallic post and core, which has been inserted into the empty root canal of a non-vital tooth (Figure 10.14).

Often, root-filled teeth become brittle with time and sometimes snap off at the gingival margin, leaving just the root of the tooth in the dental arch. Post-crowns provide a permanent method of restoring them.

(1) The remaining root face is shaped as for the margins of a crown preparation
(2) The root filling material is removed to a suitable depth from the root canal, using 'Gates-Glidden' drills (Figure 10.15)
(3) The empty canal is widened using a post preparation system, such as 'Parapost', which produce parallel sided post holes for maximum retention
(4) Either a prefabricated metal post or a carbon fibre post is then cemented in, or an impression of the preparation is taken, incorporating a wax post which will accurately record the post hole. If the former, then a core can be built onto

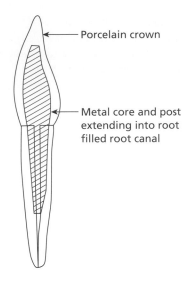

Figure 10.14 Post crown.

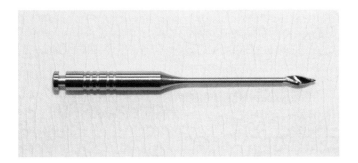

Figure 10.15 Gates-Glidden drill.

the protruding end of the post so that a conventional crown impression technique can be followed. If the latter, then the post and core will be custom-made by the laboratory. This can then be cemented permanently at the crown fit stage, using one of the luting cements described

Oral hygiene instruction for crowns

No matter how well fitting the crown is to the tooth, microscopically the junction between the two is a potential stagnation area for plaque to gather. Thorough brushing at the margins of the crown will ensure that plaque does not accumulate and cause recurrent caries or periodontal problems. The oral health messages to be relayed to the patient following crown cementation are:

- Regular and thorough toothbrushing daily
- Use of fluoride toothpaste and medium textured toothbrush
- Regular flossing to clean crown margins inter-proximally
- Careful use of floss so as not to dislodge crown
- Attend for dental examinations so that margins can be checked professionally
- Sensible diet, low in non-milk extrinsic sugars
- Regular use of good-quality mouthwash, to reinforce plaque control

Bridges

These are a type of fixed prosthesis that is used when a patient has one or more missing teeth in a dental arch and does not wish to have them replaced by a denture.

Missing teeth can also be replaced by titanium implants, which are surgically placed into the alveolar bone, but they are a specialist technique practised in few general dental practices, and are beyond the remit of this book.

Bridges have several advantages over removable prostheses:

- There is no embarrassment of a loose prosthesis falling out, as bridges are fixed to the teeth permanently
- On the whole, their aesthetics are superior to dentures
- They are more hygienic than dentures, because there is no involvement of any teeth except the retainers and therefore fewer stagnation areas
- Usually only two appointments are required for their provision
- The materials used in their construction are better able to resist occlusal forces than acrylic
- The shades available can be customised in any way by the laboratory technician to mimic the patient's other teeth, whereas those available for dentures are mass produced and unalterable
- They solve the problem of patients with a strong gag reflex who require tooth replacement, and who usually cannot cope with a denture
- They are also better tolerated because of the minimal amount of soft tissue coverage involved

However, the need for good oral hygiene control post-operatively is of paramount importance, as bridges produce stagnation areas unlike any others in the mouth (that is, **under the pontics**), and require special techniques for effective cleaning.

Several different types of bridge have been developed, but all designs rely on retaining teeth (**abutments**) to hold the bridge permanently in place, and they are joined to the missing teeth (**pontics**) in one structure. The different types are:

- **Fixed-fixed bridge** – the retaining teeth are involved to either side of the missing teeth, as one solid design (Figure 10.16)
- **Fixed-moveable bridge** – a joint is incorporated in the design to allow some degree of flexibility to the bridge (Figure 10.17)

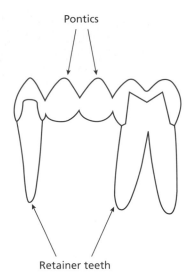

Figure 10.16 Fixed-fixed bridge.

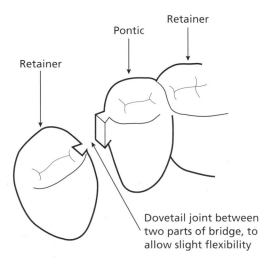

Figure 10.17 Fixed-moveable bridge.

- ■ **Cantilever bridge**:
  - – **Simple** design where retaining teeth are those immediately to one side of the pontic only (Figure 10.18)
  - – **Spring** design where the retaining teeth are to one side but several teeth away from the pontic (Figure 10.19)
- ■ **Adhesive bridge** – retaining teeth undergo minimal tooth preparation and retention is provided by metal wings only (Figure 10.20)

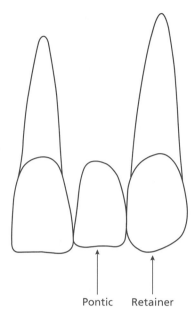

Pontic   Retainer

Figure 10.18 Simple cantilever bridge.

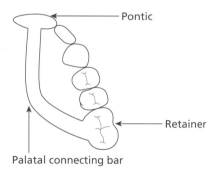

Pontic

Retainer

Palatal connecting bar

Figure 10.19 Spring cantilever bridge.

The choice of which type of bridge is used depends on several factors.

■ Whether an anterior or a posterior tooth is being replaced, as the latter usually undergo heavier occlusal forces so full crown retainers are generally required, rather than just the metal wings which may be used for anterior bridges
■ Like crowns, bridges can be constructed of all-metal or ceramic materials and obviously the former would not be provided anteriorly
■ Fixed-fixed bridges tend not to be used nowadays, as their inflexibility during use has been seen to be able to cause damage to retaining teeth
■ Wherever possible, adhesive bridges are used, as they involve minimal tooth preparation

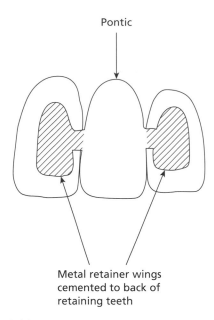

Pontic

Metal retainer wings
cemented to back of
retaining teeth

Figure 10.20 Adhesive bridge.

- If a patient has natural spaces between the teeth, only a spring cantilever design can be used so as to maintain the spaces and give good aesthetics
- The health of the retaining teeth is of paramount importance to the success of the bridge, and if there is any cause for concern, an adhesive type of bridge is advisable so that any problems would result in its dislodgement rather than causing damage to the retainers

All types of bridge except adhesive ones rely on the retaining teeth being of full crown coverage, indeed, the tooth preparation is exactly the same as for a single crown, as are the instruments and the impression materials used.

Temporary bridges

Temporary coverage of the prepared abutments is necessary as for crowns, the missing tooth or teeth being replaced temporarily either by a pre-existing denture or not at all.

Alternatively, the missing tooth and the retainers can be covered by a temporary bridge. Temporary bridges can be made in the laboratory, before tooth extraction, or at the chairside in a similar fashion to temporary crowns using an alginate impression taken before tooth extraction.

Their functions are:

- To provide reasonable aesthetics while the extraction site heals
- To provide reasonable aesthetics while the permanent bridge is constructed

- To hold the extraction space open, as teeth can drift naturally and close the space, or tip into it
- To maintain the occlusion
- To prevent sensitivity of the prepared abutment teeth

Once the permanent bridge has been constructed, any temporary bridge present can be removed in the same way as for a temporary crown. The same fitting checks are made before permanent cementation, using the same luting cement options as for crowns.

Adhesive bridges

Adhesive bridges, unlike the above, require special dual curing resin cements with primers, to provide a strong chemical bond between the retaining teeth and the metal wings of the bridge. There is little retention provided by tooth preparation with these bridges. Their use is generally restricted to areas of low occlusal force to prevent dislodgement, although new luting cements are being developed constantly to attempt to increase the use of adhesive bridges.

Oral hygiene instruction for bridges

Bridges provide a challenge to the patient with regard to adequate oral hygiene, as they are fixed prostheses producing stagnation areas beneath the pontics. As well as the oral hygiene instructions for crowns, patients with bridges need to be instructed in the use of **Superfloss** (Figure 10.21). This is a type of dental floss with a stiff end, which can be threaded under the pontic by the patient, and then drawn through to a sponge part which is used to clean beneath the pontic. When used

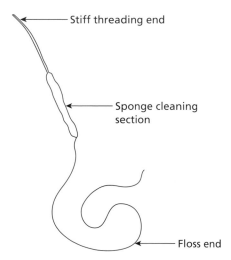

Stiff threading end

Sponge cleaning section

Floss end

Figure 10.21 Superfloss®.

regularly, it keeps this region of the bridge plaque-free and prevents caries under-mining the retainers, with catastrophic consequences.

More recently, the use of sonic toothbrushes has been shown to provide excellent cleaning in these areas, without dislodging the bridge, and these are being recommended more frequently in these cases.

Veneers

A veneer is either a composite or porcelain facing made to cover the labial surface of anterior teeth. They are used in the following situations:

- To mask a **discoloured tooth** (such as with tetracycline staining)
- To mask a darkened, root filled tooth
- To **close diastemas** between teeth
- To **change the shape** of rotated teeth so that they appear aligned
- To change the shape of malaligned teeth so that they appear aligned
- To **correct poorly shaped teeth**, such as peg laterals
- As a **cosmetic procedure**, to lighten the whole labial segment

Veneers are fragile once constructed, and can break if the patient is careless with them. Ideally, they are only fitted to patients with low incisal edge forces and they are often constructed so as not to cover the incisal edge of the tooth. This then gives the unlikeliest conditions for the veneer to fracture during normal use.

The instruments and impression materials used for veneer placement are the same as for crowns and bridges. However, often no opposing arch impression is required as veneers rarely encroach on the occlusion.

Surgery procedure for veneer preparation

The role of the dental nurse is as summarised for crown preparation.

(1) Unless the tooth is non-vital, local anaesthetic will be required
(2) On the rare occasion that an opposing arch impression is required, this is taken in a stock tray using alginate
(3) The labial surface of the tooth is prepared by removing enough enamel to allow the technician to construct the veneer, this is especially important if the veneer is to give the appearance of alignment to the tooth (Figure 10.22)
(4) An impression is taken of the labial segment using one of the highly accurate elastomer materials, as for crowns and bridges
(5) The prepared tooth is covered temporarily for appearance and sensitivity reduction, using composite material etched just to the centre of the tooth, so that it can be removed easily at the veneer fit appointment
(6) An accurate shade is taken, recording all tooth characteristics for the technician, as for crowns and bridges

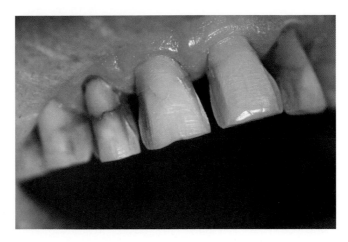

Figure 10.22 Veneer preparations.

Surgery procedure for veneer fitting

As with all fixed prostheses, veneers are custom-made in the laboratory, by a highly skilled technician. The shades selected in the surgery will be accurately replicated as the veneer is constructed from porcelain, before having the final firing in an oven to produce the surface glaze. The fitting surface of the veneer will be abraded in the laboratory, to produce a rough surface for cement adhesion. The finished product is then carefully returned to the surgery for fitting. The veneer fitting procedure is as follows:

(1) Local anaesthetic may be required
(2) The temporary veneer is removed, by flicking it off carefully with a hand instrument, such as a flat plastic or an excavator
(3) The veneer is carefully tried onto the tooth and the fit and shade are checked
(4) If satisfactory, the fitting surface of the veneer is coated with a **silane agent** which allows the dual cure resin cement to chemically bond to it for good adhesion
(5) The **tooth is isolated** with either rubber dam or celluloid matrix strips, and then etched, washed and dried
(6) The dual cure resin bond and cement are applied to the tooth and the veneer is carefully pushed onto it, in the correct position
(7) Excess cement is removed before light curing occurs
(8) Flecks of cement trapped inter-proximally can be removed using abrasive diamond strips, otherwise they will act as stagnation areas and accumulate plaque

Alternatively, composite veneers can be made at the chairside by the dentist. Good isolation of the adjacent teeth is of paramount importance, otherwise etch, resin and cement will adhere to these teeth and the patient will be unable to clean correctly in the interproximal areas.

The shades available for composite veneers are inferior to those for porcelain veneers, but the former are far cheaper to provide.

Inlays

Inlays are a fixed prosthesis constructed indirectly at a laboratory rather than placed directly into the tooth, as a filling would be (although a direct technique using wax patterns used to be carried out years ago, but is rarely seen nowadays). They are constructed of gold alloy, porcelain or a special type of composite which contains more filler than usual, and is therefore stronger than conventional composites.

The purpose of using an inlay is to produce a restoration of higher strength than the plastic materials, and of a more permanent nature, although with the continual improvement of filling materials, gold alloy inlays are being provided less frequently nowadays. As the inlay is inserted into the tooth rather than cemented onto it, less tooth preparation is also necessary than for a conventional crown. The equipment, materials and impression techniques are the same as for other fixed prostheses.

Inlay preparation is as for a conventional filling, with the full removal of all carious tooth tissue to sound dentine, but then the cavity preparation is adjusted to ensure that the sides are not undercut but **parallel** (Figure 10.23). This allows:

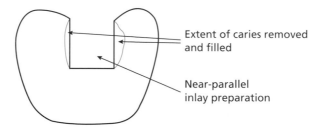

Figure 10.23 Inlay preparation.

■ The inlay to be inserted fully, without becoming stuck on an undercut
■ The maximum retention possible is produced, by ensuring that the inlay fits snugly against all the cavity walls
■ Only a fine cement layer will then be required, which reduces the risk of cement dissolution in saliva with time

Once the cavity has been prepared suitably and the necessary impressions and occlusal registrations have been taken, the tooth is restored with a temporary filling. At the time of fit of the inlay, the occlusion is checked as for crowns and when correct, the inlay is cemented using one of the luting cements available, as for crowns.

Gold alloy inlays have their margins well adapted to the tooth by **burnishing** at the fit stage, so that the wafer thin edge of the inlay is pressed firmly against the cavity wall. This prevents ingress of saliva and reduces the possibility of the cement being dissolved out (dissolution), with subsequent loss of the inlay.

Removable prostheses

Removable prostheses are all types of dentures – appliances that are made in the laboratory in various stages to replace missing teeth. They can be removed from the mouth by the patient, for example for cleaning, and reinserted again easily, without the use of cements. Generally, removable prostheses are made to replace several missing teeth rather than just one or two, as bridges do, or even to replace all the teeth in edentulous patients. When several teeth are missing, their replacement is necessary to:

■ Prevent **excess masticatory forces** on the remaining teeth, which may cause their eventual fracture
■ Prevent **over-eruption** of opposing teeth, which can cause occlusal problems
■ Prevent **tilting** of adjacent teeth into the edentulous spaces, which disrupts the occlusion and creates stagnation areas
■ Prevent **soft tissue trauma** to the alveolar ridges during mastication
■ Allow **adequate mastication** and avoid digestive problems, especially in the elderly
■ Provide **good aesthetics**, especially if anterior teeth are missing

Full and partial acrylic dentures

These are the commonest types of denture produced, full ones for edentulous patients and partial ones for any number of missing teeth. As dentures are removable prostheses, their retention in the mouth relies not on cements, as for fixed prostheses, but on the following:

■ A **suction film** of saliva developing between the denture and the patient's soft tissues
■ A **post-dam** along the back border of the denture, to help the suction film to develop
■ An **accurate design and fit** of denture, to allow the film to develop adequately
■ Use of any **natural undercuts** in the patient's mouth, such as the alveolar ridges or any natural teeth
■ Use of **stainless steel clasps** around standing teeth, to increase retention

Sometimes, the patient's own teeth are adjusted to provide undercuts, in the following ways:

■ Use of a crown to change the overall shape of the tooth
■ Use of composite build-ups to provide a retentive area for clasps to engage
■ Shape change of an existing restoration for similar reasons

With edentulous patients, the alveolar ridges can be changed surgically, to improve retention and comfort.

■ Gross undercuts which would prevent the denture being seated can be removed
■ Flat ridges can be built up by the addition of bone substitutes to increase natural retention
■ Sharp ridges can be smoothed to allow comfortable wearing of the denture (**alveolectomy**)

Not all patients are suitable for treatment involving the use of dentures, and the following points are considered for every case before treatment commences:

■ Is there any previous denture experience, and was it successful or not?
■ If not, is there a cause which can be remedied?
■ Is the shape of the patient's mouth naturally retentive for full dentures, with good ridges and a high palate, or might pre-prosthetic surgery be necessary?
■ Are there any potential retention problems for partial dentures? If so can they be remedied by tooth shape adjustment?
■ Might the patient's occlusion cause problems with the provision of a denture? Is there enough clearance without premature contact onto the denture?
■ Are there any medical contraindications to dentures, such as epilepsy or an adverse reaction to the acrylic material?
■ Are there other dental problems which need addressing first, such as caries or periodontal disease?
■ If the teeth have been lost within the previous six months, bone resorption is likely to occur and this will affect the fit of a denture adversely
■ Is the treatment affordable to the patient?
■ Good co-operation and perseverance by the patient are paramount to the success of dentures. If there is any doubt about these then treatment is likely to fail

Denture construction

As with fixed prostheses, dentures are constructed by the technician in the laboratory in several stages, as follows:

(1) **First impressions** – using stock trays and alginate impression material, tooth shade and shape (mould) are often decided at this stage too
(2) **Laboratory** – study models cast and special acrylic impression trays are custom made from them
(3) **Second impression** – using special trays and either alginate or elastomer impression material to produce a very accurate impression

(4)   **Laboratory** – working models cast and wax occlusal rims are constructed

(5)   **Bite registration** – occlusal face height of the patient is recorded, by warming the rims or using bite registration paste

(6)   **Laboratory** – models in their recorded face height positions are mounted onto an articulator, so the technician can construct the wax try-in dentures in these positions

(7)   **Try-in** – wax or wax and metal try-ins with the actual teeth mounted in them are inserted and checked for accuracy of fit and occlusion, as well as shade; any major inaccuracies will result in a retry being requested

(8)   **Laboratory** – stainless steel clasps are added as necessary, then the try-ins on their models are sealed into flasks and the wax is replaced by heat-cured acrylic, completed dentures are then cleaned and polished

(9)   **Fit** – acrylic or metal dentures are inserted and checked for comfort, fit and aesthetics, then specific denture care information is given

Each stage of the denture construction in the surgery involves the use of specific instruments, materials and equipment.

First impressions

Item	Function
Stock impression trays	To be sized and used to take the initial impressions, so that special trays can be constructed
Alginate impression material and room temperature water	To be mixed, loaded into the trays and inserted to produce the initial impressions
Shade and mould guides	To determine the colour and shape of the denture teeth, to be as close in appearance to any remaining teeth as possible
Work ticket	To record the patient and dentist details, the denture design and base material to be used, the tooth shade and mould, the type and position of any clasps, the return date

The work ticket information must be duplicated onto the patient record card or the computerised notes. The handling and after care of the impressions is as for fixed prostheses.

Second impressions

Item	Function
Study models and special trays	To take the more accurate second impressions, to produce the working models
Alginate or elastomer impression material	To take the more accurate second impressions
Work ticket	To record the next stage request and the return date

Bite registration

Item	Function
Wax bite rims	Adjusted in height so that correct face height of the patient can be recorded
Heat source	To warm the hand instruments and rims for adjustment
Wax knife (Figure 10.24)	To remove or add additional wax to the rims, as necessary
Bite registration paste	To be mixed and applied to the rims, so that they are held in the correct position once set
Pink sheet wax	For addition to the rims, as necessary
Willis bite gauge (Figure 10.25)	To record the desired occlusal face height in edentulous patients, where no natural teeth remain as a guide
Work ticket	To record the next stage request and return date

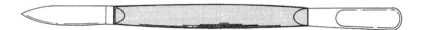

Figure 10.24 Wax knife. Source: *Levison's Textbook for Dental Nurses*, 10th edn, C. Hollins, 2008, Wiley-Blackwell.

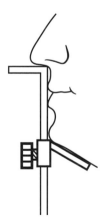

Figure 10.25 Willis bite gauge in position recording occlusal face height. Source: *Levison's Textbook for Dental Nurses*, 10th edn, C. Hollins, 2008, Wiley-Blackwell.

Try-in

Item	Function
Try-in prostheses	To determine if fit, occlusion and aesthetics are correct before finishing the dentures
Heat source	To warm the wax and make adjustments, as necessary
Le Cron carver (Figure 10.26)	To make fine adjustments to the try-in, as necessary
Wax knife	To warm and smooth the wax after adjustments, as necessary
Shade and mould guides	To check or alter the shade or mould, as necessary
Pink sheet wax	For addition to the try-in, as necessary
Patient mirror	To allow the patient to view the try-ins and decide if they are happy with the appearance, before completion
Work ticket	To record any changes required for a retry, or to record the fit return date

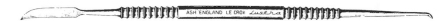

Figure 10.26 Le Cron carver. Source: *Levison's Textbook for Dental Nurses,* 10th edn, C. Hollins, 2008, Wiley-Blackwell.

If changes are required to the prostheses they must be requested at this point. Once the flasking process has been carried out, no further changes can be made, and the whole construction process would have to be started again. Any concerns that the patient may have must be identified and discussed at this point.

Fitting

Item	Function
Completed removable prostheses	To fit, to the patient and dentist's satisfaction
Straight handpiece and selection of trimming burs and polishing stones	To remove any acrylic pearls or occlusal high spots before polishing and smoothing the adjusted area for comfort
Patient mirror	To allow the patient to view the completed prostheses
Articulating paper	To identify occlusal high spots, for adjustment as necessary
Pressure relief paste	To identify high spots on the denture fitting surface, for removal as necessary

Once the removable prostheses have been successfully fitted, the patient will be given oral hygiene instruction and general advice, so that they can wear the dentures successfully. If the dentures have been provided for the first time, the patient may well have concerns with regard to:

- Whether they will get used to them
- Whether they will become loose and fall out

- Whether they will be able to chew successfully with them
- Whether friends or family will realise that they are wearing them

Good communication skills and a sound background knowledge of these concerns by the dental team will help allay the patient's worries. Care and oral hygiene advice should be given as follows:

- Demonstration of how to insert and remove the prostheses
- Avoid wearing the prostheses overnight if possible, to avoid the development of oral fungal infections (thrush)
- Clean after each meal if possible, using a toothbrush and toothpaste
- Clean over a bowl of water, to avoid damage to the denture if it is dropped
- Avoid soaking in bleach-based cleansers if any metal components are included in the design
- Eat soft foods initially, while the oral soft tissues acclimatise to the prostheses
- Take time to chew foods thoroughly, to avoid indigestion
- Harden oral soft tissues by carrying out hot salt water mouthwashes initially
- Return to the surgery if any ulceration occurs, for further adjustments

Older patients are more likely to require full dentures than other patients, and they will tend to have years of experience of wearing dentures too. However, as the alveolar ridges resorb away once teeth have been extracted, it may become more difficult to retain the dentures successfully especially as there will be no standing teeth to clasp. Special impression techniques may need to be used in these cases, to maximise the retention that can be achieved from the soft tissues alone.

On the other hand, younger patients and children will hopefully wear dentures on a temporary basis only, before bridges or implants can be considered. The use of dentures in these cases may be necessary when there has been traumatic loss of an anterior tooth, for instance.

Full and partial chrome cobalt dentures

Chrome-cobalt can be used as the base of the denture, rather than acrylic, but the teeth still need to be attached to this metal base by acrylic on the ridges. Metal-based dentures are more difficult to construct and cost more than acrylic ones, but the advantages are:

- A much **thinner palatal covering** is possible, which makes the denture more tolerable to patients with a strong gag reflex
- Overcomes any tissue reaction to acrylic monomer, as some patients are sensitive to it
- Denture base is **far stronger** and less likely to break
- Allows patients with deep overbites onto their palate to be able to wear denture

- Can design partial dentures as **'skeletons'**, giving minimal tissue coverage and making the denture more tolerable for the patients (Figure 10.27)
- As less tissue coverage is involved, chrome dentures tend to be more hygienic than acrylic ones

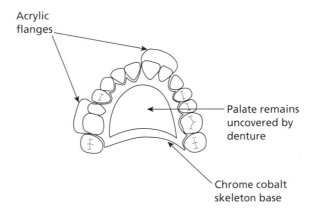

Acrylic flanges

Palate remains uncovered by denture

Chrome cobalt skeleton base

Figure 10.27 Skeleton denture design.

If the whole palate is covered by a chrome base, then retention is provided by the saliva suction film, as for acrylic dentures. However, if a skeleton design is used then clasps must be placed to retain the denture, so an adequate number of healthy and well-positioned teeth are required. The clasps will be part of the chrome base, and tooth adjustments can be carried out to provide undercuts, as for stainless clasps on acrylic dentures.

Chrome-cobalt denture construction

The surgery stages are as for acrylic dentures, the only differences being:

- Final impressions are often taken in a highly accurate **elastomer** material, rather than alginate
- The chrome-cobalt base is then made on the final model as a wax pattern by the technician, before being cast in a special furnace
- The casting of the metal base is sometimes carried out at specialised laboratories, so extra time between appointments may be necessary
- A try-in of the metal base only is often carried out, to ensure it is accurate
- A second try-in is then performed, with the teeth added and held by wax
- No adjustment of the metal base can be made in the surgery once it has been constructed, except minimal easing using a pink stone in the slow handpiece

- All instructions as for acrylic dentures except that bleach-based cleaners must **not** be used, as these will corrode the metal base of the denture
- Demonstration of how to insert and remove partial metal dentures may take some time, as some designs can be quite tricky

Immediate replacement dentures

These dentures are fitted on the day that a tooth or teeth are extracted, so that the patient has no unsightly gaps visible. There can be no try-in stage for this technique, but otherwise the procedure for construction is the same as for conventional dentures, until the final stage when the technician removes the teeth to be extracted from the model and replaces them with the new denture teeth.

The patient must be made aware that following the fitting of the immediate denture, alveolar bone resorption will occur and this could result in the prosthesis becoming loose quite quickly. Patients tend to accept this phenomenon readily, as the alternative is to have extraction spaces visible for months before a conventional denture is provided. However, as chrome cobalt cannot be adjusted once cast, immediate dentures are only constructed from acrylic.

If just one anterior tooth is to be replaced, the denture is usually designed in a 'spoon' shape, so that the gingival margins of other teeth are not covered by the denture, making it more hygienic (Figure 10.28).

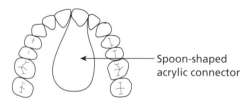

Spoon-shaped
acrylic connector

Figure 10.28 Spoon denture.

As the denture is fitted directly after extraction, the patient's soft tissues will be numb due to the local analgesia used, and some areas of discomfort will not be immediately obvious. The aftercare instructions that should be given are:

- Leave the denture in place overnight, to protect all the extraction sockets
- Return to the surgery the following day, for any adjustments to be carried out
- From then on, remove the denture after meals and carry out hot salt water mouthwashes to help heal the extraction sockets (see Unit 11 (Chapter 12))
- Return to the surgery when bone resorption has caused significant loss of retention, so that adjustments can be made or a permanent denture provided

Sometimes, tooth extraction results in prominent, sharp spicules of alveolar bone remaining around the sockets, and these can cause immense discomfort to the patient if the denture provided sat directly onto them. In these cases, a procedure known as **alveolectomy** is carried out to remove these spicules by surgically grinding them away. This can be done at the time of extraction, or before the denture is constructed in edentulous patients with sharp alveolar ridges.

As a surgical procedure is involved, a full flap would need to be raised, as for a surgical tooth extraction (see Unit 11 (Chapter 12)).

Other prosthetic procedures

Relines and rebases may be required as alveolar bone resorption occurs beneath the denture with time, and the retentive fit is lost so that the denture becomes loose. The bone lost can be replaced with an acrylic addition within the fitting surface of the denture.

(1) The denture is thoroughly cleaned at the surgery, ensuring that no food debris is present
(2) The patient is asked to carry out a vigorous mouthwash at the surgery, and toothbrushing if necessary, to remove any debris
(3) An accurate impression (**wash impression**) is taken within the denture itself, using an elastomer material
(4) The technician makes a cast within the denture so that the alveolar bone is recorded
(5) Wash impression is removed from the denture, and the space present between it and the model is filled with acrylic
(6) This creates a new base fitting surface to the denture, which will then sit against the oral soft tissues again

Additions of either teeth or clasps may be necessary, as teeth and retention are lost with the original prosthesis.

■ Alginate impression is taken over the denture while in the mouth
■ Technician casts the model with the denture in it
■ The denture is then exactly in place for the tooth or clasp addition to be added

Tissue conditioners are used when the soft tissues beneath the denture are continually sore, for whatever reason, so that the denture cannot be worn routinely. This is often a problem with older patients, and can cause medical problems due to their being unable to eat sufficiently well.

A special impression material is used that takes hours to set, so that it becomes well moulded to the oral soft tissues, and can be bitten on without causing pain to the denture wearer as it 'gives' under pressure. However, the conditioner requires regular replacement, as it deteriorates in time within the mouth.

Obturators are appliances used to seal off an abnormal cavity in the mouth, such as a cleft palate or the space left after significant oral surgery, such as for tumour removal. The area requires sealing to allow proper speech and to prevent food collecting here. The denture area of the obturator is constructed in the usual way, but an elastomeric impression material is used to record the cavity accurately, before being incorporated into the denture design.

Where large cavities are present, the extension area is hollow so that the obturator is not too heavy to wear.

Role of the dental nurse during removable prosthetics

There are some duties that are specific to the preparation and fitting of removable prostheses, and others that are very similar in other areas of dentistry. The good dental nurse must be competent and proficient in all. The role of the dental nurse is summarised below:

- Have a good understanding of the stages of the procedure to be carried out
- Be aware of their position in the dental team for the procedure – this may be as the chairside nurse assisting directly with the procedure, or as a second nurse available to comfort the patient, or mix materials and load impression trays as necessary
- Have all the patient records, charts, radiographs, study models, removable prostheses, consent forms available for the appointment
- Communicate effectively with the patient throughout the procedure, inspiring confidence and trust – this is especially important when impressions are being taken, as many patients find the procedure unpleasant
- Monitor the patient throughout the procedure, ensuring their comfort and well-being, giving assurance as necessary, and assisting them if they are unfortunate enough to vomit during impression taking
- Anticipate and pass instruments, etc. to the dentist in the correct order during the procedure
- Be aware of the correct trays and impression materials to be used, and mix and load each accordingly when directed
- Record the accurate laboratory instructions for the prosthesis, and duplicate them exactly into the patient's records as necessary
- Follow the infection control policy in relation to the safe handling of all impressions and bite records taken, as well as other construction stages
- Follow the infection control policy to fully decontaminate the surgery after use, especially in relation to clearing away vomit – see Unit 4 (Chapter 5)
- Follow the health and safety policy with regard to hazardous waste disposal – see Unit 1 (Chapter 2)
- Ensure that all records, charts, etc. are correctly and securely stored for future use after being completed by the dentist, maintaining patient confidentiality at all times – see Unit 6 (Chapter 7)

Orthodontic appliances

Orthodontic appliances are used to straighten (align) crooked teeth, so that effective oral hygiene is possible to prevent caries or periodontal disease developing (see Unit 8 (Chapter 9)). Two basic types of appliance are used:

- **Removable appliance** – similar to a denture in construction, and can be removed from the mouth for cleaning, eating and adjustment
- **Fixed appliance** – individual metal components bonded onto each tooth, and connected together by an archwire, they cannot be removed from the mouth by the patient

Greater and more complicated forces can be applied to the teeth using fixed appliances, and the range possible for both is as follows:

- Movement of teeth forwards or backwards in each arch – removable and fixed
- Movement of jaws in relation to each other – functional and fixed
- Alignment of slightly misplaced teeth in arch – removable and fixed
- Alignment of severely misplaced teeth in arch – fixed
- Derotation of teeth – fixed
- Guided eruption of unerupted teeth – fixed
- Guided reduction of deep overbite – removable and fixed

Removable appliances

These are similar to dentures in construction, in that alginate impressions of both arches and a wax bite registration are taken and sent to the laboratory, along with a work ticket detailing the exact design of appliance required. The technician casts the study models and then constructs an acrylic base for each appliance. The additional components that can be added are as follows:

- **Adam's cribs** to retain the appliance in the mouth, usually to fit onto molar or premolar teeth and made of stainless steel (Figure 10.29)

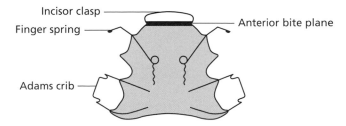

Figure 10.29 Removable upper orthodontic appliance. Source: *Levison's Textbook for Dental Nurses*, 10th edn, C. Hollins, 2008, Wiley-Blackwell.

- **Springs** in a variety of designs, to move the teeth along the arch as required (Figure 10.30)
- **Retractors** to push one or several teeth backwards (Figure 10.31)
- **Expansion screws** to move several teeth or each half of the upper arch outwards

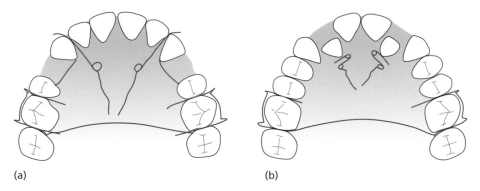

(a)   (b)

Figure 10.30 Types of springs. (a) Palatal finger spring; (b) 'Z' spring.

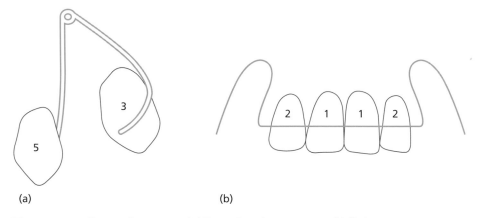

(a)   (b)

Figure 10.31 Types of retractor. (a) Buccal canine retractor; (b) Robert's retractor.

The equipment and instruments required for the monitoring and adjusting of the appliance are as follows.

Item	Function
Adam's crib pliers (Figure 10.32)	To adjust all metal springs and retractors, as necessary
Straight handpiece and acrylic trimming bur (Figure 10.33)	To adjust all acrylic areas of the appliance, as necessary
Measuring ruler	To record any measurable tooth movement, such as the overjet
Expansion screw key	To count the number of turns applied to the screw between visits, to ensure compliance

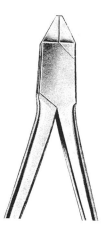

Figure 10.32 Adam's universal pliers. Source: *Levison's Textbook for Dental Nurses*, 10th edn, C. Hollins, 2008, Wiley-Blackwell.

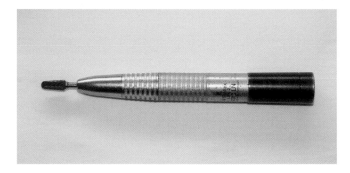

Figure 10.33 Acrylic trimming bur in straight handpiece.

Patient advice for removable appliances

As with removable prostheses, orthodontic appliances are capable of acting as stagnation areas and holding food debris and plaque against the teeth and gingivae, unless a good standard of oral hygiene is maintained. Although some dentists prefer patients to wear appliances during meals, it is possible that more acrylic breakages will occur if this is the case. The instructions necessary for patients wearing removable appliances are:

■ Wear as directed by the dentist
■ Clean the appliance and teeth after each meal, using a toothbrush and toothpaste
■ Avoid cariogenic foods and drinks, as advised
■ Attend all dental appointments for the necessary adjustments
■ Contact the surgery immediately if any breakages or loss of the appliance occur

- Expect the appliance to feel tight initially after each adjustment
- Contact the surgery if any prolonged or excessive symptoms occur
- If the appliance is to be removed for meals, ensure it is placed safely in a rigid container to avoid breakages

Functional appliances

These are a specialised type of removable appliance made of acrylic and stainless steel components, and worn in both arches at the same time, the commonest one currently being a **twin block** (Figure 10.34). They are used to correct skeletal Class II discrepancies, by holding the mandible forwards in the ideal Class I position and allowing mandibular growth to occur and correct the malocclusion. As their success depends on the growth of the mandible, they can only be used while the patient is still growing but after the premolars have erupted, so the ideal age is up to 14 years.

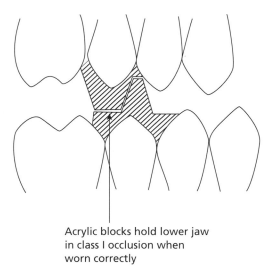

Acrylic blocks hold lower jaw
in class I occlusion when
worn correctly

Figure 10.34 Functional appliance. Source: *Levison's Textbook for Dental Nurses*, 10th edn, C. Hollins, 2008, Wiley-Blackwell.

The materials, instruments, and patient advice are as for removable orthodontic appliances.

Fixed appliances

These consist of separate components that are individually bonded onto each tooth, using either a light-cured composite or glass ionomer material (see Unit 8 (Chapter 9)).

The procedure is carried out in the surgery, with no laboratory input required except to cast up the before and after study models required. Bonding of the components causes no tooth damage, and they are 'snapped off' at the end of the treatment harmlessly.

The equipment and instruments required for the monitoring and adjusting of the fixed appliance are given below.

Item	Function
Archwire	Flexible nickel titanium or stainless steel wires, to fasten into the brackets or bands
End cutters	Right-angled cutters to trim the ends of the archwire after replacement
Elastic modules (Alastik)	Rubber bands to hold the archwire into each bracket
Alastik holders	Ratcheted holders (similar to artery forceps) to apply the Alastik modules
Brackets (Figure 10.35)	Metal components to attach to teeth, if any have been lost since last appointment
Bands	Metal rings to attach to molars especially if any have been lost
Bracket holders	To hold and position each bracket to the centre of the tooth, if any replacements are required
Bracket and band removers (Figure 10.36)	To remove brackets, bands and any residual bond material before replacing, if necessary
Band removers	To remove molar bands before replacement, if necessary
Bonding materials	Acid etch and orthodontic bond material, to hold brackets onto the tooth
Band cement	Any luting cement material, to hold bands onto the molar teeth

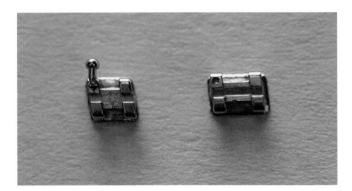

Figure 10.35 Orthodontic brackets.

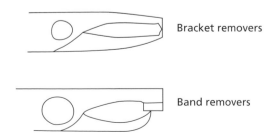

Figure 10.36 Bracket and band removers.

Patient advice for fixed appliances

Every tooth is incorporated into a fixed appliance, so the number of stagnation areas, and the potential for oral damage to occur, is far greater. Routine toothbrushing twice daily is insufficient to ensure good oral hygiene standards are maintained. So besides all other instructions as applicable to removable appliances, special oral hygiene instructions are recommended for patients undergoing fixed therapy.

- Careful manual toothbrushing should be carried out after each meal
- Use of fluoridated toothpaste
- Use of **interdental brushes** daily to clean around each bracket individually
- Avoidance of cariogenic food and drinks, for the full length of treatment
- Use of **fluoride mouthwash** daily, to minimise risk of decalcification
- Regular use of **disclosing tablets**, to highlight problematic areas

The wearing of any type of orthodontic appliance demands a high level of motivation and co-operation from the patient. Their diet has to be restricted to minimise the risk of caries developing, and in the teenage years this is often unacceptable, and motivation will wane. This is more likely for prolonged courses of treatment.

Co-operation and levels of motivation need to be assessed at each adjustment appointment, and reinforced as necessary by both the dental nurse and the dentist. Warning signs include:

- Failed appointments
- Recurrent breakages
- Reporting of problems wearing appliances, which have resulted in non-wear
- Falling standards of oral hygiene
- Obvious disinterest during adjustment appointments
- Requests for early removal of fixed appliances
- Failure to wear removable or functional appliances during daytime

Any combination of the above signs should alert the oral health team to reinforce co-operation, for the patient's benefit, or failure of treatment is likely to occur. A system of discontinuation of treatment must be in place, so that patients are aware that failure to comply will result in the early removal of the appliance and incomplete treatment. This may mean that malocclusions remain as they were for life, with all of the consequences that that will infer.

If a patient persistently fails to wear the appliance or to attend appointments for adjustment and review, treatment is best discontinued at an early stage before too much surgery time has been wasted. Patients who have discontinued treatment once and then re-present for continuation should be treated with great caution, as the likelihood of a second failed course is greater still.

11 Unit 10: Provide Chairside Support During Non-surgical Endodontic Treatment (OH7)

Knowledge specifications

Anatomy and physiology

K1 – A factual knowledge of primary and secondary dentition and dates of eruption

K2 – A factual knowledge of the structure and functions of teeth and gingivae

Non-surgical endodontic treatment

K3 – A factual knowledge of the purpose of non-surgical endodontic treatment, the different forms which it may take, and its relationship to other forms of dental treatment

K4 – A factual knowledge of the reasons why it may be necessary to undertake non-surgical endodontic treatment

K5 – A working knowledge of the potential risks, complications and traumas that may arise during and after non-surgical endodontic treatment

K6 – A working knowledge of methods of cleaning and preparing root canals

K7 – A working knowledge of the equipment, instruments, materials and medicaments which are used in identifying, locating, filing and measuring the roots of teeth

K8 – A working knowledge of the different materials used in the sealing, filling and restoration of the root canal

K9 – A working knowledge of equipment used in moisture control

K10 – A working knowledge of the equipment used in the administration of local and regional anaesthesia

Providing close support and assistance to the oral health team

K11 – A working knowledge of the ergonomics of dental practice; eg seating, positioning of the patient and team, instrument passing and protecting and retracting the soft tissues

K12 – A working knowledge of methods of aspirating during treatment and facilitating a clear view of the treatment area for the operator, and the consequences of doing this incorrectly (such as tissue damage)
K13 – A working knowledge of the importance of monitoring the patient
K14 – A working knowledge of why it is important that the worker's actions complement the work of other team members, and how this is achieved

Health and safety and control of infection

K15 – A working knowledge of standard precautions and quality standards of infection control, and the dental nurse's role in maintaining them
K16 – A working knowledge of the purpose of protective wear, and the reasons for the different kinds which might be necessary

Charts and record keeping

K17 – A working knowledge of the different types of charts and records used in the organisation (including medical history, personal details, dental charts, radiographs/photographs, and study models for assessment and treatment planning), and their purpose
K18 – An in-depth understanding of confidentiality in relation to patient records

Communication

K19 – A working knowledge of the importance of communicating information clearly and effectively
K20 – A working knowledge of methods of modifying information and communication methods for different individuals, including patients from different social and ethnic backgrounds, children (including those with special needs), and the elderly

Summary of dental anatomy and dentition

Non-surgical endodontics covers three techniques of attempting to dentally treat a dead or dying tooth, so that it is retained in the dentition and restored to function. The alternative is extraction of the tooth and the likely requirement for a permanent artificial replacement. The three techniques discussed in this chapter are:

- **Pulp capping**
- **Pulpotomy**
- **Pulpectomy** – root canal treatment (RCT)

The need for endodontics occurs following injury to or infection of the **pulp**. In soft tissues the injury/infection would resolve rapidly after a period of swelling and possibly bruising, but in the closed chamber of the root canal, any swelling cuts off the apical blood supply to the tooth, and pulp death occurs. This eventually leads to a non-vital tooth and periapical infection. The patient often presents initially with pain, swelling and sometimes a sinus tract with pus present at its opening.

Inflammation of the pulp – **pulpitis** – can occur due to:

■ **Deep caries** which lies close to, or actually exposes, the pulp
■ **Thermal injury**, by heat transmission through unlined restorations, or inadequate cooling of air turbine during treatment
■ **Chemical irritation** from restorative materials
■ **Fracture** following trauma, possibly causing pulp exposure
■ **Irritation** from very deep fillings, over time

Any of these events will result in inflammation of the pulp tissue, and as it is confined within the closed root canal chamber of the tooth any swelling that occurs will squeeze the pulp contents, cutting off the blood supply to the tooth and ultimately resulting in its death.

Full details of the structure of teeth and their anatomy is covered in Unit 6 (Chapter 7), but in summary they are composed of the following tissues, in order from the outside surface inwards:

■ **Enamel** – non-living tissue forming the outer part of the tooth crown, made up of mineral crystals lying in prisms, arranged at right angles to the tooth surface and the amelo-dentinal junction
■ **Dentine** – living tissue forming the bulk of the crown and root, made up of hollow tubules containing nerve endings
■ **Pulp** – soft tissue within the root chamber and canal, composed of nerves and blood vessels that keep the tooth alive and allow it to feel sensations
■ **Cementum** – outer covering of the tooth root, lying beneath the gingiva and forming part of the tooth attachment to its supporting structures

Any tooth can be affected by pulpitis at any age, and the tooth involved and when it erupted, as well as the severity of the pulpitis, will determine which one of the three techniques listed above is used to try to save it.

Pulpitis can occur as either of the following:

■ **Reversible** – not causing pulp death and treated by filling the tooth only
■ **Irreversible** – causing partial or full pulp death and requiring one of the non-surgical endodontic techniques to save it

Deciduous teeth will eventually be resorbed and exfoliate, as a natural progression to the eruption and development of the permanent dentition, so full RCT is not required to treat them. Either pulp capping or pulpotomy is adequate. When permanent teeth erupt, it can take up to three years for the root end to close. So if they are recently erupted, these teeth will have a good blood supply and can also be maintained by either a pulp capping or pulpotomy procedure. Once the root end has closed, and in the full adult dentition, RCT is required to treat the tooth in an attempt to save it from extraction.

Full details of the primary and secondary dentition and their eruption dates are covered in Unit 6 (Chapter 7), but a summary is given below:

Deciduous dentition

| Tooth | Eruption date (months) | | |
	Letter	Upper teeth	Lower teeth
Central incisor	A	10	8
Lateral incisor	B	11	13
Canine	C	19	20
First molar	D	16	16
Second molar	E	29	27

Permanent dentition

| Tooth | Eruption date (years) | | |
	Number	Upper teeth	Upper teeth
Central incisor	1	7–8	6–7
Lateral incisor	2	8–9	7–8
Canine	3	10–12	9–10
First premolar	4	9–11	9–11
Second premolar	5	10–11	9–11
First molar	6	6–7	6–7
Second molar	7	12–13	11–12
Third molar	8	18–25	18–25

Diagnosis of irreversible pulpitis

The vitality of the tooth (that is, whether it is alive, dying or dead), can be assessed by the dentist using the following techniques:

■ Stimulation of the tooth by heat/cold application:
  – Hot gutta percha (as greenstick compound) onto the tooth
  – Cold ethyl chloride sprayed onto a cotton pledget and placed onto the tooth

■ Stimulation of the tooth by an electric current, using an electric pulp tester:

– Pen type, with digital numerical scale which gradually increases as the current increases until the patient indicates a tingling sensation in the tooth (higher scores indicate a loss of vitality)
– Older types with a box and wand applicator, applied as above

To function properly, all electric pulp testers require a dry tooth surface, and for an electrical circuit to be made between the patient, the dentist and the machine. Their use is not advised for patients who have cardiac pacemakers fitted, as they could interfere with the function of these devices.

■ Use of radiographs:

– As an indicator that the tooth is not fully healthy
– Usually using a periapical view to show a widened periodontal ligament around the suspect tooth root, or an actual radiolucent periapical area

Often, a tooth will have been giving symptoms for some time before deteriorating into irreversible pulpitis, and this is especially true when caries is the cause as it is a progressive infection of the dental hard tissues, rather than a sudden event.

The patient usually has symptoms that gradually increase in severity until the tooth dies, as follows:

(1) Occasional sensitivity to cold, then to hot and sweet stimulation
(2) Develops into spontaneous intermittent spasms of pain
(3) Becomes continuous throbbing pain with time
(4) Eventually not affected by hot, cold or sweet stimulation
(5) Becomes hypersensitive to vitality testing
(6) Not tender to percussion

With the full patient history taken, and any necessary radiographs viewed, the dentist can make a diagnosis of irreversible pulpitis and discuss treatment options with the patient.

Treatment option considerations

There are many factors to be considered by both the dentist and the patient (or their guardian) when discussing treatment involving non-surgical endodontics.

■ **Usefulness of the tooth in occlusion** – if the tooth stands alone and is not routinely used for mastication, nor involved in the retention of a prosthesis then there is little point in trying to save it from extraction
■ **Tooth restoration possibilities** – if the tooth is badly broken down with little structure remaining for restoration, the feasibility of restoring it to full function is unlikely

■ **Dental health of the patient** – if this is poor generally, with a lack of good oral hygiene and poor diet control, the tooth is unlikely to survive for any reasonable length of time

■ **Patient co-operation** – both child and adult patients may refuse the treatment offered for whatever reason, and their right to do so has to be respected by the dental team

■ **Medical history of the patient** – some medical conditions contraindicate endodontic treatment, whereas others contraindicate extraction

■ **Cost of treatment** – successful endodontic treatment usually culminates in the tooth being crowned eventually to preserve it for as long as possible. Both treatments can be too expensive for some patients to consider

All of these considerations need to be fully and clearly discussed with the patient, or their guardian in the case of children, before the decision can be made whether to proceed or not. Dental terminology may have to be avoided with some patients, to modify the necessary explanations to their level of understanding or language. However, this must never result in full information not being given, nor the patient being patronised. It is possible to issue patient leaflets in various languages nowadays to help explain dental treatment, and their availability should be investigated in each local area.

Patient consent

The patient cannot give valid consent to endodontic treatment until they have been informed of any risks and complications that may be involved, and have been made aware of the full procedure details.

Complications

■ The procedure carries a 70–80% chance of success, so extraction may still be necessary in some cases

■ Endodontically treated teeth become brittle with time, so long term restoration is likely to be a crown

■ If the root apices are close to underlying nerves, there is a possibility of nerve damage from over-instrumentation or from medicaments used

■ If the root apices are close to the floor of the maxillary antrum, there is a risk of creating an oro-antral fistula

Procedure details

■ Often one or two long appointments, where full mouth opening will be necessary

■ Local anaesthesia will usually be required initially

- Rubber dam may be used, which may be a new experience
- Antibiotics may be required to control infection
- Temporary dressings may be used, and care will be required not to dislodge them
- Post-operatively, anti-inflammatory drugs may be recommended
- Patient may have some tenderness and may need to contact the surgery if this worsens

Use of rubber dam in non-surgical endodontics

The use of rubber dam during endodontic procedures is now routine. It is a sheet of rubber which is pierced and placed over the tooth to be treated, so that it is effectively separated from the rest of the mouth. The technique is used to:

- Isolate the tooth to avoid contamination from the oral cavity
- Protect the patient's airway from endodontic instruments
- Protect the oral cavity from endodontic medicaments
- Allow good vision for the dentist
- Allow good aspiration by the nurse

Special instruments are required to use rubber dam (Figure 11.1):

- **Rubber dam sheet**
- **Hole punch**, to create the hole through which the tooth will project during treatment
- **Rubber dam clamp** to hold the dam tightly around the neck of the tooth during treatment. They come in different shapes depending which tooth is undergoing treatment
- **Clamp forceps** to hold the clamp during its placement on the tooth
- **Rubber dam frame** which holds the dam sheet taut over the lower face, for ease of application

There are several different techniques for applying the rubber dam to the tooth. Each dentist will use the one with which they are most familiar and successful. As long as the dam is applied correctly and causes no trauma or discomfort to the patient, the technique is irrelevant.

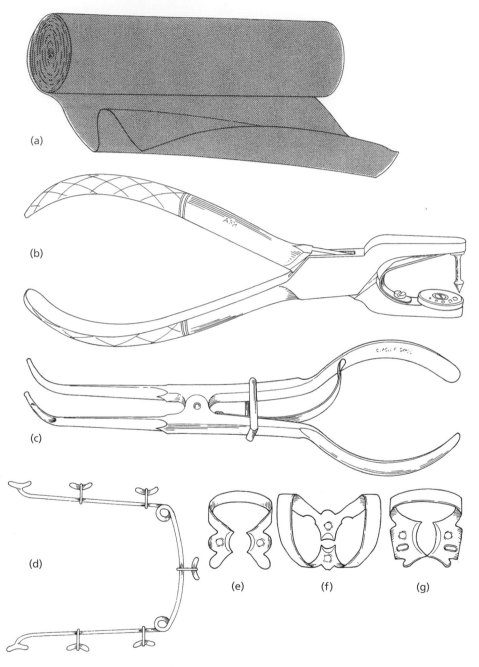

Figure 11.1 Rubber dam instruments. (a) Rubber dam. (b) Rubber dam punch. (c) Rubber dam clamp forceps. (d) Rubber dam frame. (e) Premolar clamp. (f) Incisor (butterfly) clamp. (g) Molar clamp. Source: *Levison's Textbook for Dental Nurses*, 10th edn, C. Hollins, 2008, Wiley-Blackwell.

Non-surgical endodontic techniques

Pulp capping

This can be carried out in either deciduous or permanent teeth, as a temporary measure before tooth exfoliation in the former, or before pulpotomy or RCT in the latter. It is carried out in the following instances:

- When routine restorative treatment produces a small, unexpected pulp exposure in an otherwise healthy tooth
- When a patient attends as an emergency with a small pulp exposure following trauma

The aim is to **seal the exposed pulp** from the oral cavity so that no oral microorganisms contaminate the tooth and cause an infection. This buys time for either the tooth to exfoliate naturally, or for the patient to be reappointed so that either pulpotomy or RCT can be carried out without the patient experiencing pain in the interim.

The technique is as follows (Figure 11.2):

(1) All dental personnel wear personal protective equipment (PPE) to protect their health and safety – safety glasses or visors, masks, non-latex gloves, uniform
(2) Patient wears PPE – safety glasses, protective bib
(3) Local analgesia is administered, if not already given
(4) The tooth is isolated from saliva contamination using moisture control techniques suitable for the situation
(5) The exposure is dried with sterile cotton wool, and carefully covered with **calcium hydroxide paste** to promote dentine repair
(6) A cap made from a cervical matrix is placed over the calcium hydroxide paste, to prevent excess pressure being applied to the exposure site while the tooth is dressed
(7) The cavity or fracture site is temporarily sealed with a sedative dressing

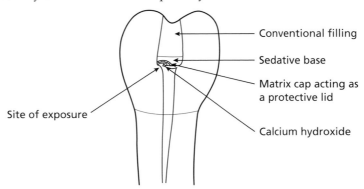

Figure 11.2 Pulp capping technique.

If a deciduous tooth is pulp capped, it can now be left to painlessly exfoliate naturally. If a permanent tooth is involved, it can be left for some time before any second procedure is carried out, or even just kept under observation by the dentist at three-monthly intervals.

Pulpotomy

This technique is used when **immature** permanent teeth are exposed. The apical foramen takes three years to close after tooth eruption. So when trauma occurs to teeth at this time, there is a good chance that the exposure can heal without loss of vitality of the tooth because the open apex ensures a good blood supply to the tooth.

As the main purpose of pulpotomy is to avoid contamination of the whole pulp tissue, it is vital that a high level of infection control is maintained throughout. However, it must be accepted that some surface contamination will have occurred if the exposure event happened outside the surgery environment. Nevertheless, all instruments and equipment used must be sterile, and good moisture control should be achieved to avoid further saliva contamination of the exposure site.

Moisture control techniques available are given below. These apply to all aspects of clinical dentistry.

Item	Function
Cotton wool, as rolls or pledgets	Rolls placed into sulcus against tooth being treated, to absorb any pooled saliva Pledgets used to dry cavity itself
High speed aspiration	Fast removal of saliva, debris, and coolant water from handpieces Can also be used to retract soft tissues of cheek, lip or tongue to provide good vision of operative field for the dentist
Low speed aspiration	Saliva ejector, placed under tongue to slowly remove any pooled saliva or water from the mouth
3 in 1 tip	Device to both wash and blow dry the operative field
'Dryguard'	Absorbent pad placed inside cheek, over the parotid salivary gland duct to absorb all saliva excretions from the gland
Rubber dam equipment	Kit of equipment designed specifically for endodontic use, provides full isolation of the tooth from the oral cavity, and full protection of the patient's airway from all dental instruments and materials used (see Figure 11.1)

Wherever possible, rubber dam is the moisture control technique of choice, but it may be unable to be used in younger or uncooperative patients, or it may not be physically possible to actually place it, especially if access is difficult to the tooth involved. Whichever technique is used, the dental nurse should be knowledgeable and competent in the handling of the equipment so that:

- Moisture is successfully controlled
- The operative field is kept visually clear

- The patient is comfortable
- Soft tissues are fully retracted without causing trauma to them

As with any clinical dental procedure, PPE should always be provided and worn by all dental personnel, and the patient. Failure to provide PPE by the employer, or for staff to fail to wear it, is a breach of health and safety legislation.

PPE usage is covered in full in Unit 4 (Chapter 5) and Unit 6 (Chapter 7), and is summarised below:

- **Safety glasses** – to avoid eye injury from flying debris, or infection from aerosol contamination, worn by staff. Tinted ones are worn by patients to also avoid retinal damage by the curing light
- **Mask or visor** – to prevent inhalation of debris, aerosols and micro-organisms, worn by staff
- **Gloves** – to prevent cross-infection by touch transfer of micro-organisms, worn by staff
- **Bib** – to prevent clothing contamination by aerosol spatter or fluids, worn by patient
- **Uniform** – to prevent clothing contamination, worn by staff in clinical areas
- **Plastic apron** – to prevent blood contamination of uniform, worn by staff during surgical procedures

The pulpotomy procedure is as follows:

(1)   All the necessary PPE is placed
(2)   Local anaesthetic is administered and allowed to take full effect
(3)   The tooth is isolated from saliva contamination
(4)   The pulp chamber is opened through the fracture site, using a dental bur and handpiece
(5)   Any potentially contaminated pulp tissue is removed from the pulp chamber only, using sharp sterile hand instruments to separate it from the pulp lying in the root canal
(6)   All bleeding of the pulp stump is stopped using sterile cotton wool pledgets
(7)   Once bleeding has stopped, the stump is covered with a calcium hydroxide material to encourage dentine repair
(8)   This is sealed beneath a base material and then the restorative material used to restore the tooth to function

If the permanent tooth loses vitality in a young patient, conventional orthograde root treatment is not an option until the apex has closed. This is because any attempt at inserting gutta percha will ensure its passage through the apex and into the peri-radicular tissues. Under these circumstances, a non-setting calcium hydroxide cement (such as Hypocal) can be used to fill the whole canal, and then left *in situ* while an apical calcific barrier forms and the apex closes. Progress can be monitored with periapical radiographs, and once the apex has closed conventional orthograde root canal therapy can be carried out.

Pulpectomy (RCT)

This is the non-surgical endodontic procedure carried out to try to save a tooth from extraction, once it has experienced irreversible pulpitis. The aim of the treatment is **to remove all of the pulpal tissue from the pulp chamber and root canal, and replace it with a sterile root filling material**. The material must be placed to fully seal the whole root canal system and prevent any contamination from causing a recurrent infection at the root apex. As discussed in Unit 6 (Chapter 7), permanent molar and upper first premolar teeth have multiple roots, and each one must be successfully debrided and sealed for the endodontic treatment to work.

Although the dentist will use many dental hand instruments during the endodontic procedure that are multi-functional and used in other dental disciplines, there are several instruments used exclusively for RCT. These are detailed below. Their functions are similar whether used as hand instruments or as rotary instruments in the dental handpiece.

Item	Function
Broach (Figure 11.3)	Plain broach to help locate the entrance to each root canal
	Barbed broach to remove (extirpate) the pulpal contents from the canal
Reamer	Hand or rotary – to enlarge the root canals laterally and to the root apex
File (Figure 11.4)	Hand or rotary – to smooth the root canal walls and remove any residual debris from them
Irrigation syringe (Figure 11.5)	Blunt ended with a side bevel, to irrigate and wash out debris from the root canal without injecting contents through the root apex
	Solutions used include chlorhexidine, sodium hypochlorite and local anaesthetic
Metal ruler	Used with a file in place, to work out the full length of each root canal by comparing with a periapical radiograph view of the tooth to the established working length
Apex locater	To determine the working length electronically
Spiral paste filler (Figure 11.6)	Used with the slow dental handpiece to spin sealant material into the root canal
Lateral condenser, or Finger spreader (Figure 11.7)	Used to condense the root filling points laterally into each root canal, so that no space remains for micro-organisms to return
	Not required if root filling material used is inserted while hot and flowable

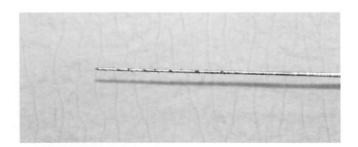

Figure 11.3 Barbed broach.

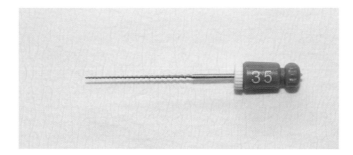

Figure 11.4 Hand file.

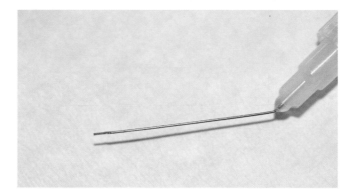

Figure 11.5 Monoject® syringe needle end.

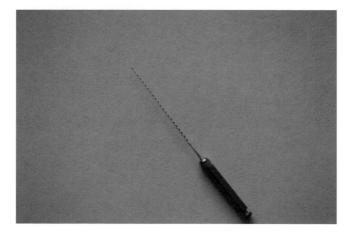

Figure 11.6 Spiral paste filler.

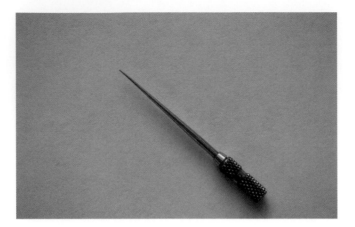

Figure 11.7 Finger spreader.

Similarly, there are materials and medicaments used exclusively in non-surgical endodontic treatment, all of which will have been risk assessed before their use in accordance with COSHH regulations (see Unit 4 (Chapter 5)). Their potential to cause both the patient and dental personnel harm if misused must be fully appreciated and understood by the whole dental team. Consequently, working safely as a member of the dental team throughout chairside procedures should be second nature to the dental nurse. This will ensure that there is no potential for accidents or mistakes during any treatment session.

The materials and medicaments used throughout RCT are:

- **Irrigation solution** – used during root canal preparation to lubricate the instruments and wash out any debris (individual choice between sodium hypochlorite (bleach), chlorhexidine, local anaesthetic solution)
- **Antiseptic paste** – non-setting and containing antiseptic anti-inflammatories; used to dress infected root canals for a time before root filling
- **Cresophene** – medical grade creosote used to dress infected root canals for a time, soaked onto paper points before insertion
- **Gutta percha points (GP points)** – various diameter tapered rubber points used to fill (obturate) the root canal system (Figure 11.8)
- **Sealing cement** – setting cement used to aid insertion of the GP points and to seal off any residual spaces in the root canal; some contain antiseptics and anti-inflammatories
- **Restorative materials** – used to restore the tooth to full function and appearance after root filling; see Unit 8 (Chapter 9) for full details

With knowledge of the specialised equipment, instruments, materials and medicaments used during the RCT procedure, the whole treatment session will now be run through. To limit the potential for recontamination of the root canal,

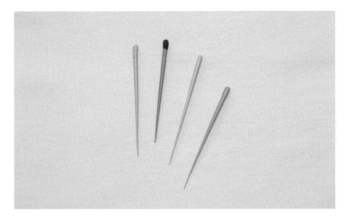

Figure 11.8 Gutta percha points.

the full procedure is ideally carried out in one session. However, when extensive infection is present the root canals are often dressed for a time with antiseptics, before the RCT procedure is completed at a later date.

The technique of pulpectomy is as follows:

(1)   All the necessary PPE is placed
(2)   Local anaesthetic is administered and allowed to take full effect
(3)   The tooth is isolated, by rubber dam preferably
(4)   Access is gained to the pulp chamber using a bur and dental handpiece
(5)   All root canals are located using a plain broach
(6)   The pulp contents are **extirpated** using a barbed broach
(7)   The root canal system is enlarged using reamers, and smoothed using files
(8)   Irrigation is provided as necessary
(9)   The diagnostic (working) length of each root canal is determined, using files and a radiograph or an apex locater
(10) The decision is made to continue or to dress the root canal system for a time
(11) If dressing, a paper point (Figure 11.9) soaked in antiseptic is placed in the root canals and sealed in with a temporary filling material (see Unit 8 (Chapter 9))
(12) If root filling, sealant cement is placed in the root canal using a spiral paste filler
(13) A correctly sized GP point is inserted to the working length
(14) A lateral condenser, or a finger spreader is used to allow the insertion of accessory points to fully seal the root canal – this is called **obturation**
(15) If an apex locater has not been used, a final periapical radiograph is taken to confirm that the working length has been reached, and that no apical perforation has occurred (Figure 11.10)
(16) The tooth is permanently restored using one of the permanent restorative materials available (see Unit 8 (Chapter 9))

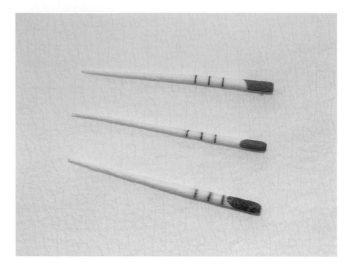

Figure 11.9 Paper points.

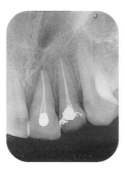

Figure 11.10 Radiograph of root filled tooth.

Throughout the procedure, the dental team will be positioned for maximum comfort and visibility, with each team member aware of their own role in the treatment. When instruments and materials are transferred from one person to another, it is done so carefully and safely (and especially not over the patient's face), and in a manner that avoids cross-infection between items and team members.

At the end of treatment, the area and all its contents need to be disposed of, or disinfected and sterilised according to the infection control policy in place, abiding by current relevant legislation. This is an important duty of the dental nurse, and the routine is as follows:

■ All sharps are carefully disposed of in the sharps box – this includes all endodontic hand instruments, which are classed as single use
■ All autoclavable items are placed in a washer – disinfector unit, or an ultrasonic bath, and treated before being placed in the autoclave for sterilisation

- All contaminated waste is placed in hazardous waste sacks
- All surfaces are disinfected using the correct solution
- All static equipment is wiped down using the correct solution

In addition, the clinical records should be fully completed before being filed away, whether this involves a paper or computer system. Any radiographs should be stored accordingly too. As always, the records system must ensure the full confidentiality of the patient's details and notes, by being securely stored.

Role of the dental nurse during endodontic procedures

There are some duties that are specific to non-surgical endodontic treatment; others are very similar in other areas of dentistry, but the good dental nurse must be competent and proficient in all. The role of the dental nurse is summarised below:

- Have a good understanding of the procedure to be carried out
- Be aware of their position in the dental team for the procedure – this may be as the chairside nurse, or as a secondary nurse available for material mixing, etc.
- Have all patient records, charts, radiographs, consent forms completed and available for the appointment
- Have all the required instruments, equipment, materials and medicaments in good order and available for the procedure
- Communicate effectively with the patient throughout the procedure, inspiring confidence and trust
- Monitor the patient throughout the procedure, ensuring their comfort and well-being, and giving reassurance where necessary
- Assist during the administration of local analgesia
- Assist during the application of rubber dam, if used
- Provide careful but efficient moisture control and soft tissue retraction throughout the procedure
- Anticipate and pass instruments, etc. to the dentist in the correct order during the procedure
- Correctly mix and pass any materials and medicaments as they are required
- Correctly process any dental radiographs after exposure – see Unit 7 (Chapter 8)
- Give accurate post-operative instructions to the patient after the procedure
- Follow the infection control policy to fully decontaminate the surgery after use – see Unit 4 (Chapter 5)
- Follow the health and safety policy with regard to hazardous waste disposal – see Unit 1 (Chapter 2)
- Ensure that all the records, charts, etc. are correctly and securely stored for future use after being completed by the dentist, maintaining patient confidentiality at all times – see Unit 6 (Chapter 7)

Use of antibiotics in endodontics

The aim of endodontic treatment is to attempt to save the tooth from extraction. When a patient presents with obvious signs of acute infection, a course of antibiotic therapy may be required before treatment of the tooth can commence.

Signs of infection are:

■ Presence of pus
■ Raised body temperature (pyrexia)
■ Obvious debilitation of the patient
■ Severe pain and loss of function of the affected tooth
■ Swelling, either intra-orally or extra-orally

The dentist will attempt to begin treatment and alleviate the symptoms if possible. They will either try lancing an intra-oral abscess or open the root canal and place the tooth on open drainage. At the same time they will prescribe the following antibiotics:

■ Amoxycillin or erythromycin (if the patient is allergic to penicillin) 250 mg four times daily
■ Metronidazole 200 mg three times daily for three days given concurrently, if a severe infection is present

12 Unit 11: Provide Chairside Support During the Extraction of Teeth and Minor Oral Surgery (OH8)

Knowledge specifications

Anatomy and physiology

K1 – A factual knowledge of the structures of the skull and oral cavity
K2 – A factual knowledge of nerve and blood supply to the teeth and gingiva
K3 – A factual knowledge of morphology of teeth and roots of teeth
K4 – A factual knowledge of primary and secondary dentition and the dates of eruption

Equipment, instruments, materials and medicaments

K5 – A working knowledge of the equipment, instruments, materials and medicaments which are used in the following procedures:
a) extraction of erupted teeth
b) extraction of unerupted teeth and roots including local and regional anaesthesia
K6 – A working knowledge of the purpose and correct methods of preparing and handling the range of equipment, instruments, materials and medicaments
K7 – A working knowledge of the relationship of the equipments, instruments, materials and medicaments to the different procedures, and the order in which they are likely to be used in each procedure

Extractions

K8 – A working knowledge of the different forms of pain and anxiety control that are available in dentistry (including conscious sedation)
K9 – A factual knowledge of the reasons why the extraction of teeth may be necessary
K10 – A factual knowledge of the purpose of removing roots and unerupted teeth, the different forms which this may take, and its relationship to other forms of dental treatment
K11 – A working knowledge of the purpose and reasons for raising muco-periosteal flaps and the dental nurse's role in providing chairside support for this procedure

K12 – A working knowledge of the purpose and reason for tooth sectioning or bone removal, and the dental nurse's role in providing chairside support for this procedure

K13 – A working knowledge of the potential risks and complications that may arise during and after extractions (including nerve damage, haemorrhage, oro-antral fistulas, equipment failure)

Health and safety and infection control

K14 – A working knowledge of standard precautions and quality standards of infection control, and the worker's role in maintaining them

K15 – A working knowledge of what is and is not a sterile field, and how the correct level of cleanliness may be maintained for the patient's condition, the treatment and the setting

K16 – A working knowledge of legislation and practice guidelines related to health and safety and control of infection, and how these affect the worker's actions (including COSHH and Health and Safety at Work Act)

Providing close support and assistance to the oral health care team

K17 – A working knowledge of the ergonomics of dental practice (eg seating, positioning of the patient and team, instrument passing, suction tip placement)

K18 – A working knowledge of methods of working which will complement the work of the operator, and the reasons for this

K19 – A working knowledge of the function, use and maintenance of suction equipment and aspirators

K20 – A working knowledge of methods of protecting and retracting the soft tissues

K21 – A working knowledge of methods of aspirating during treatment

K22 – A working knowledge of methods of facilitating a clear view of the treatment area for the operator, and the consequences of doing this incorrectly (such as tissue damage)

K23 – A working knowledge of your role in assisting haemostasis, including assisting the placement and cutting of sutures, and preparing packs

K24 – A working knowledge of methods of monitoring the patient

K25 – A working knowledge of how to recognise and respond to actual or potential emergencies

K26 – A factual knowledge of why the patient should be confirmed as fit prior to leaving the surgery

Communication

K27 – A working knowledge of methods of communicating information clearly and effectively

K28 – A working knowledge of methods of modifying information and communication methods for different individuals, including patients from different social and ethnic backgrounds, children (including those with special needs), and the elderly

Records

K29 – A working knowledge of the different types of records used in the organisation (including medical history, personal details, dental charts, radiographs and photographs, and study models for assessment and treatment planning), and their purpose

K30 – An in-depth understanding of confidentiality in relation to patient records

Many procedures carried out in daily dental practice can be collectively termed as 'minor oral surgery', and those discussed in this chapter are:

- **Simple extractions** – of roots or whole teeth, where no soft tissue or bone removal is required
- **Surgical extractions** – of roots or whole teeth, where soft tissue alone or with bone, has to be removed to gain access to the root or tooth
- **Operculectomy** – the surgical removal of the gingival flap overlying a partially erupted tooth, especially a lower third molar
- **Alveolectomy** – the surgical adjustment and removal of bone spicules from the alveolar ridge after tooth extraction, to produce a smooth base for denture seating
- **Gingivectomy and gingivoplasty** – periodontal soft tissue surgery to adjust the shape of the gingivae to aid oral hygiene measures
- **Periodontal flap surgery** – the surgical raising and replacing of surgical flaps, to enable subgingival debridement to be carried out
- **Soft tissue biopsies** – the partial or complete removal of soft tissue oral lesions, for pathological investigation and diagnosis

Arguably, these procedures constitute those most worrying to the patient, as bleeding and possible post-operative pain are quite likely to occur. The dental nurse has a very important role in the reassurance and monitoring of the patient during these procedures, so that the patient remains less anxious and co-operative throughout. As always, health and safety and infection control procedures must be strictly adhered to before, during and after the surgical procedure.

Reasons for tooth extraction

Both deciduous and permanent teeth may require extraction at some point. This is usually due to infection and pain being present following caries, periodontal disease or trauma. Tooth extraction may also be indicated for the following reasons:

- The tooth cannot be restored, whether or not pain and infection are present
- The position of the tooth prevents the placement of a fixed or removable prosthesis
- The tooth is poorly positioned to be aligned orthodontically
- The tooth may be selectively extracted to provide space in a crowded dental arch
- Attempts to save the tooth by root filling have failed
- The tooth may be partially erupted and impacted, and experience recurrent painful infections (pericoronitis) due to food trapping
- Deciduous teeth can be selectively extracted to encourage eruption of their permanent successors into more favourable positions
- The patient's choice, where attempting to save the tooth by root filling is not the preferred option

To ensure that any tooth is extracted painlessly and successfully, the dentist has an in-depth knowledge of the anatomy and physiology of the head and neck region, as well as the oral cavity. An efficient and supportive dental nurse must also have a background knowledge of these subjects, to be able to provide the level of preparation, chairside support and help required during any likely complication that may arise.

Summary of tooth and root morphology, eruption dates, skull anatomy, nerve supply

Full details of the morphology of teeth and roots, and the eruption dates of the primary and secondary dentition are covered in Unit 6 (Chapter 7), but they are summarily covered in the following tables.

Tooth and root morphology of deciduous teeth

Tooth	Letter	Number of roots	Number of cusps (where applicable)
Central incisor – upper	A	One	N/A
Lateral incisor – upper	B	One	N/A
Canine – upper	C	One	N/A
First molar – upper	D	Three	Four
Second molar – upper	E	Three	Five
Central incisor – lower	A	One	N/A
Lateral incisor – lower	B	One	N/A
Canine – lower	C	One	N/A
First molar – lower	D	Two	Four
Second molar – lower	E	Two	Five

The three roots of the upper molar teeth are arranged like a tripod, with the largest root lying **palatally**, and the other two roots lying buccally, one in front of the other – so they are called the **mesiobuccal** and **distobuccal** roots. The two roots of the lower molars are arranged one in front of the other, so they called the **mesial** and **distal** roots.

As explained in Unit 6 (Chapter 7), the roots of all of the deciduous teeth undergo a process called **resorption**. In this process, the growth and movement of the underlying permanent teeth as they begin their eruption causes the 'eating away' of the roots of the deciduous teeth. This results in exfoliated deciduous teeth appearing to have no root structure at all. The length of remaining root of an extracted deciduous tooth will vary depending on how close to exfoliation it is at the time of extraction.

Eruption dates of deciduous teeth

Tooth	Letter	Eruption date (months)	
		Upper	Lower
Central incisor	A	10	8
Lateral incisor	B	11	13
Canine	C	19	20
First molar	D	16	16
Second molar	E	29	27

Tooth and root morphology of permanent teeth

Tooth	Number	Number of roots	Number of cusps (where applicable)
Central incisor – upper	1	One	N/A
Lateral incisor – upper	2	One	N/A
Canine – upper	3	One	N/A
First premolar – upper	4	Two	Two
Second premolar – upper	5	One	Two
First molar – upper	6	Three	Five
Second molar – upper	7	Three	Four
Third molar – upper	8	Three	Four
Central incisor – lower	1	One	N/A
Lateral incisor – lower	2	One	N/A
Canine – lower	3	One	N/A
First premolar – lower	4	One	Two
Second premolar – lower	5	One	Two
First molar – lower	6	Two	Five
Second molar – lower	7	Two	Four
Third molar – lower	8	Two	Four

The length of the roots of each tooth can vary from patient to patient, but the longest root in any person is usually the upper canine followed closely by the upper first molar.

Unlike the deciduous dentition, a full permanent dentition will contain eight premolar teeth, the upper first premolar having two roots while all the others have just one. These two roots are arranged across the arch so they are referred to as palatal and buccal. As with the deciduous dentition, the upper molars have three roots arranged in the tripod of palatal – mesiobuccal – distobuccal, and the lowers have two roots arranged mesially and distally.

It is often the case that the roots of permanent teeth are curved, and in multi-rooted teeth this can make their extraction extremely difficult. It is imperative that a radiograph is taken of any tooth that to be extracted, so that difficulties such as this can be detected and planned for before the extraction procedure.

Eruption dates of permanent teeth

Tooth	Number	Eruption date (years)	
		Upper	Lower
Central incisor	1	7–8	6–7
Lateral incisor	2	8–9	7–8
Canine	3	10–12	9–10
First premolar	4	9–11	9–11
Second premolar	5	10–11	9–11
First molar	6	6–7	6–7
Second molar	7	12–13	11–12
Third molar	8	18–25	18–25

Structures of the skull and oral cavity

The dental nurse requires a factual knowledge of the structures supporting and surrounding the teeth in the oral cavity. This is to enable the dentist to be fully anti-cipated and supported during an extraction or minor oral surgery (MOS) procedure.

Skull anatomy is covered in Unit 6 (Chapter 7), but an overview is given here. The skull is the bony structure that is referred to as the head, and can be separated into three distinct regions:

- **Cranium** – which holds the brain
- **Face** – which supports the eyes and the nose
- **Jaws** – which support the teeth and the tongue, and provide the openings for the respiratory and digestive systems

The areas of the skull that are of particular importance to the dental nurse are the jaws:

- **Maxilla** – the upper jaw, which is a fixed structure beneath the nose
- **Mandible** – the lower jaw, which is a moveable structure attached to the base of the skull at the temporomandibular joint (TMJ)

The maxilla:

- Is made up of two bones that form the roof of the mouth – **hard palate**
- Also forms the base of the nose
- Hollow space in between these two structures is filled with air, and called the **maxillary sinus** or **antrum**
- Nerves and blood vessels supplying the upper teeth and surrounding soft tissues run through the maxilla
- A horseshoe-shaped ridge of bone runs around the maxilla, called the **alveolar process** which ends at the back of the mouth as **tuberosities**
- The alveolar process holds the upper teeth in the dental arch

The mandible:

- Is made up of two bones joined in the middle to create a horseshoe shape
- Connected to the skull at the **TMJ** as a hinge joint, so that the mouth can be opened and closed
- Also has an **alveolar process** to hold the lower teeth in the dental arch
- Nerves and blood vessels supplying the lower teeth and surrounding soft tissues run through the mandible
- Supports a sheet of muscle running across the horseshoe to form the **floor of the mouth**
- The **tongue** lies above this muscle, within the oral cavity and enclosed by the mandible

The remaining soft tissue structures that complete the oral cavity are the surrounding muscles of the face (**muscles of facial expression**) and the muscles involved in closing the mouth and carrying out jaw movements, including chewing (**muscles of mastication**).

The blood and nerve supply to the teeth and supporting structures are very important when extraction or MOS procedures are being carried out. Poor technique by the dental team may cause damage to either the blood or the nerve supply with worrying consequences for the patient.

The blood supply to the teeth and gingiva comes from branches of the **external carotid arteries**, which travel into the area of the oral cavity within the neurovascular bundles. The blood vessels and nerves run together through the soft tissues, and in and out of the surrounding bony structures via natural openings (**foramina**) through the skull and jaw bones themselves.

The oxygen carried in the arterial blood passes into the surrounding cells to be used for energy, and the veins drain the deoxygenated blood from the area, ultimately joining the **superior vena cava**. It is then carried to the right side of the heart to be pumped back to the lungs for reoxygenation during the process of respiration.

The nerve supply to the teeth and gingivae is provided by the fifth cranial nerve (**trigeminal nerve**), which is one of the major nerves coming directly from the brain to supply the head and neck region. As stated previously, the blood vessels and nerves tend to run together as neurovascular bundles. Knowledge of their correct location is important during MOS procedures for the following reasons:

- To gain full local and regional anaesthesia for the procedure
- To avoid administering local anaesthetic into blood vessels
- To avoid cutting blood vessels during MOS procedures
- To avoid damaging nerves during extraction and MOS

Trigeminal nerve

This is so called because it splits into three divisions:

- **Opthalmic division** – supplies the upper face and soft tissues around the eyes
- **Maxillary division** – supplies the upper teeth and gingivae
- **Mandibular division** – supplies the lower teeth and gingivae

The maxillary division splits into five branches:

- **Anterior superior dental nerve** – supplies the upper incisors and canine, and their labial gingivae
- **Middle superior dental nerve** – supplies the upper premolars and the mesial half of the first molar, and their buccal gingivae
- **Posterior superior dental nerve** – supplies the distal half of the upper first molar and the other two molars, and their buccal gingivae
- **Greater palatine nerve** – supplies the palatal gingivae of the upper molars, premolars and distal half of the canine
- **Nasopalatine nerve** – supplies the palatal gingivae of the mesial half of the upper canine and the incisors

The mandibular division splits into four branches:

- **Inferior dental nerve** – supplies all the lower teeth and the buccal/labial gingivae of the premolars, canines and incisors
- **Long buccal nerve** – supplies the buccal gingivae of the lower molars
- **Lingual nerve** – supplies the lingual gingivae of the all the lower teeth
- **Motor branch** – to the muscles of mastication

Treatment option considerations

There are many reasons why a tooth may be electively extracted, as discussed previously. However, when the dentist decides that a tooth must be extracted it is for the following reasons:

- A carious or periodontally involved tooth is a continual source of infection in the patient's oral cavity, unless successful treatment to save it can be carried out
- Any infection may be intermittent, but often there are acute and very painful episodes that may require analgesic and antibiotic treatment
- Infection can spread into the blood stream (**bacteraemia**) and the patient can become generally unwell – this can be serious in older and medically compromised patients
- Repeat prescriptions of antibiotics to treat infection without tooth removal is considered poor practice
- No replacement of the tooth can be carried out to restore oral health until the tooth has been extracted

Once it has been determined that a tooth or root require extraction, the complexity of the procedure depends mainly on which tooth is involved, how much tooth or root is present, and its position in the jaw bone. The options available are:

- simple extraction
- surgical extraction involving soft tissue removal to expose an unerupted tooth or buried root
- surgical extraction involving dissection of the tooth in its socket and removal in sections
- surgical extraction involving the raising of a mucoperiosteal flap and bone removal to gain full access to a tooth or root

If it is a deciduous tooth, the following points need to be considered:

- **Resorption** – has root resorption occurred so that effectively just the crown of the tooth remains, attached merely to the gingivae
- **Permanent successor** – is the underlying permanent tooth present, and likely to be damaged during the extraction procedure
- **Infection** – is any dental infection present, that may make the procedure unnecessarily painful
- **Age and co-operation** – younger patients are usually less willing to undergo extraction procedures than older patients, and along with some of those with special needs, are less able to understand the need for the procedure or the consequences if it is not carried out
- **Medical history of the patient** – some medical conditions contraindicate extraction

- **Tooth status** – a grossly carious deciduous tooth may be difficult to extract simply and quickly, but a surgical procedure is not usually feasible in conscious younger patients; so some form of anxiety control will have to be considered

If it is a permanent tooth, the following points need to be considered:

- **Infection** – is any dental infection present, that may make the procedure unnecessarily painful
- **Medical history of the patient** – some medical conditions contraindicate extraction
- **Medications** – some adult medications will mean hospitalisation for extractions or MOS, because of possible serious side effects
- **Cooperation** – some adults and some patients with special needs will require some form of anxiety control to undergo these types of procedure
- **Age** – older patients have more friable soft tissues which are more easily traumatised during surgical procedures, and their jaw bones will be more brittle and more easily fractured
- **Tooth status** – a grossly carious tooth is more likely to require a full surgical procedure to complete its removal
- **Post-extraction** – will the missing tooth require replacement, and if so what are the options and cost implications

Simple extractions

Simple extractions are so called because the tooth or root is removed whole from the dental arch without involving tooth sectioning, flap raising or bone removal. Whether the tooth is still vital or has died from any associated infection, local analgesia will always be required to numb the surrounding gingivae at least. As in other units, the equipment required is as follows:

Item	Function
Topical analgesic gel	To numb the oral soft tissues at the site of injection, for patient comfort
Syringe – single-use or autoclavable	To hold the needle and cartridge together for use – may be aspirating type to avoid injecting into surrounding blood vessels
Needle – single-use	Long: 27 gauge for nerve block injections Short: 30 gauge for infiltration injections
Cartridge – single-use	Glass or plastic tube containing local anaesthetic; buffering agents; vasoconstrictor to prolong anaesthesia in some makes; sterile water

As discussed previously, the dental nurse needs a factual knowledge of the nerve and blood supply to the teeth and gingivae to be able to set up the correct equipment for administering the local anaesthetic (LA). The recorded medical history of the patient will highlight any precautions to consider for the specific

LA to be used, and this should be checked with the dentist. Any prescribed pre-treatment instructions should also be checked to ensure compliance, such as older patients taking prophylactic aspirin having stopped this medication beforehand to prevent excessive bleeding.

The specific instruments, equipment and medicaments that may be required for a simple extraction are:

Item	Function
Forceps	Range of sterile hand instruments used to grip a tooth or root at its neck before applying appropriate wrist actions to loosen the tooth/root in its socket during the extraction procedure. Various designs are available for use on upper or lower teeth, and for each individual tooth
Luxators	Sterile hand instruments used to widen the socket and sever the periodontal ligament attachment
Elevators	Sterile hand instruments used to prise the tooth/root out of the socket. Various patterns available – Cryer's, Warwick James', Winter's
Fine bore aspirator	Disposable item used to suck away all blood and maintain good moisture control during the procedure
Haemostats	Gelatine sponges or oxidised cellulose, inserted into the socket after extraction to aid blood clotting and achieve haemostasis

Forceps are used by being pushed along the sides of the root to sever the periodontal membrane. Once a reasonable position has been achieved, the root is gripped and gentle wrist movements are used to gradually loosen the tooth in the socket. The forceps are gradually worked further towards the apex of the tooth until it is loose enough in the socket to be removed. Unnecessary force during extractions often results in tooth or root fracture, although this can also occur anyway with grossly carious teeth.

Forceps are designed in various patterns, to be used individually for each type of tooth. Upper tooth forceps tend to have their handles and blades roughly in line with each other, whereas lower tooth forceps tend to be at right angles to each other for ease of access (Figure 12.1). Multi-rooted molar tooth forceps have blades, which are shaped as beaks so that they can grip the **furcation** area between the roots, but single-rooted tooth forceps are smooth (Figure 12.2). The commonest patterns of forceps used are shown in Figure 12.3. They are:

- **Upper incisor and canine forceps** are straight with single rounded blades and have both wide and narrow patterns
- **Upper root forceps** are similar in appearance, with narrow, straight blades
- **Upper premolar forceps** have slightly curved handles and single rounded blades
- **Upper left molar forceps** have curved handles and a beaked blade to the right, a rounded blade to the left to grip the buccal roots and the palatal root, respectively
- **Upper right molar forceps** have curved handles and the beaked blade is to the left

- **Upper bayonet forceps** have extended handles to gain access to third molars
- **Lower anterior forceps** have single, rounded blades at right angles to the handle
- **Lower root forceps** are similar, with narrow and straight blades
- **Lower molar forceps** have beaked blades at right angles to the handles, to grip the furcation of the two roots
- **Lower 'cowhorn' forceps** have curved and pointed blades at right angles to the handles, to grip the furcation of lower molar teeth
- **Smaller versions** of most patterns exist, for deciduous tooth extractions

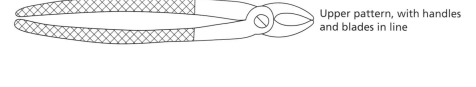

Upper pattern, with handles and blades in line

Cross-hatching on handles allows a firm grip

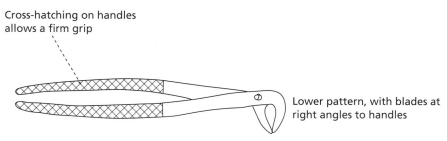

Lower pattern, with blades at right angles to handles

Figure 12.1 Upper and lower pattern of forceps.

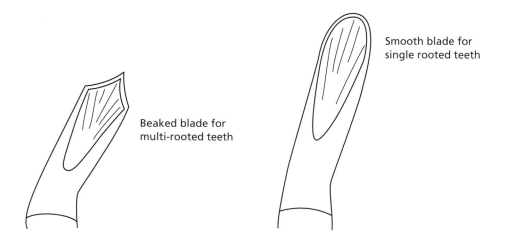

Smooth blade for single rooted teeth

Beaked blade for multi-rooted teeth

Figure 12.2 Blade patterns of forceps. Source: *Levison's Textbook for Dental Nurses*, 10th edn, C. Hollins, 2008, Wiley-Blackwell.

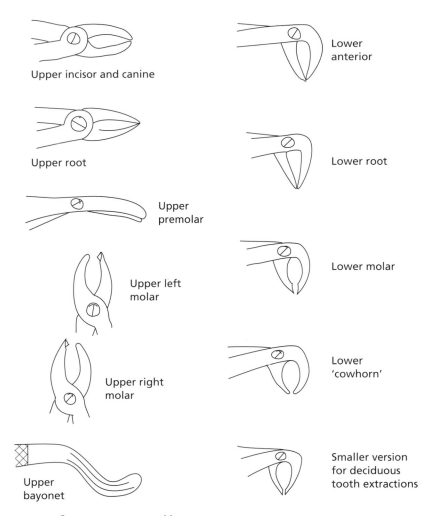

Upper incisor and canine

Lower anterior

Upper root

Lower root

Upper premolar

Upper left molar

Lower molar

Upper right molar

Lower 'cowhorn'

Upper bayonet

Smaller version for deciduous tooth extractions

Figure 12.3 Common patterns of forceps.

Similarly, elevators are available in a variety of patterns and are used to gradually sever the periodontal membrane and loosen the tooth in the socket. The more common types are shown in Figure 12.4.

(1) **Cryer's elevators** are available as left and right patterns, but can be used on either side of the mouth, depending whether they are engaged mesially or distally

(2) **Winter's elevators** have a similar blade design as Cryer's, but have a corkscrew style handle to give more leverage

(3) **Warwick James' elevators** are available as left, right and straight patterns

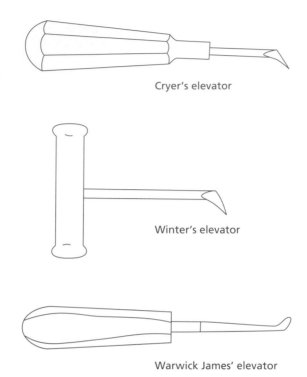

Cryer's elevator

Winter's elevator

Warwick James' elevator

Figure 12.4 Elevators.

Alternatively, the dentist may choose to use one of a variety of **luxators** that are available (Figure 12.5). These are used in a similar fashion to an elevator. A single-bladed chisel is also available in three sizes for splitting multi-rooted teeth. It is called **Coupland's chisel** (Figure 12.6).

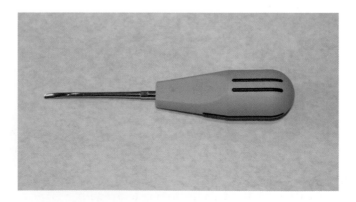

Figure 12.5 Luxator.

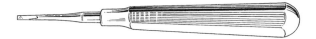

Figure 12.6 Coupland chisel. Source: *Levison's Textbook for Dental Nurses,* 10th edn, C. Hollins, 2008, Wiley-Blackwell.

Difficult extractions can be quite exhausting for the dentist and the patient, and it often helps both if the dental nurse supports the patient's head or mandible during the extraction. In this way, the dentist is not wasting energy by rocking the patient's head rather than loosening the tooth. It also allows the patient to relax more, rather than trying to hold their head still for the dentist.

Role of the dental nurse during extractions and MOS

There are some duties that are specific to extraction and MOS procedures, and others that are very similar in other areas of dentistry, but the good dental nurse must be competent and proficient in all. The role of the dental nurse can be summarised as follows:

- Have a good understanding of the procedure to be carried out
- Be aware of their position in the dental team for the procedure – this may be as the chairside nurse, or as a secondary nurse available for patient support and to fetch any extra instrument requirements, so that the surgical field is not breached
- Have all the patient records, charts, radiographs, consent forms completed and available for the appointment
- Have all the usual required instruments, equipment, materials and medicaments in good order, sterile, and available for the procedure
- Ensure the patient has followed all the prescribed pre-treatment instructions, and report any non-compliance to the dentist immediately
- Communicate effectively with the patient throughout the procedure, inspiring confidence and trust
- Assist during the administration of any anxiety control techniques, such as sedation or hypnosis
- Assist during the administration of local analgesia
- Provide support to the patient as instructed by the dentist during the procedure
- Monitor the patient throughout the procedure, and report any complications immediately
- Provide careful but efficient moisture control and soft tissue retraction throughout the procedure
- Anticipate and pass instruments, etc. to the dentist in the correct order during the procedure

- Correctly mix and pass any materials and medicaments as they are required
- Assist during the placement of any sutures
- Give accurate verbal and written post-operative instructions to the patient after the procedure
- Follow the infection control policy to fully decontaminate the surgical field after use – see Unit 4 (Chapter 5)
- Follow the health and safety policy with regard to disposal of hazardous waste – see Unit 1 (Chapter 2)
- Ensure that all records, charts, radiographs, etc. are correctly and securely stored for future use after being fully completed, maintaining patient confidentiality at all times – see Unit 6 (Chapter 7)

The dental nurse should have a full working knowledge of each item, including the full range of forceps available. This is to ensure the ability to provide close support and assistance to the dental team during the procedure.

Each instrument will be sterile and bagged, and should be carefully opened without touching it and then handed to the dentist with handles first, while holding the tips still within the sterile pouch – this is called the 'no-touch' technique (Figure 12.7). In this way, infection control is maintained.

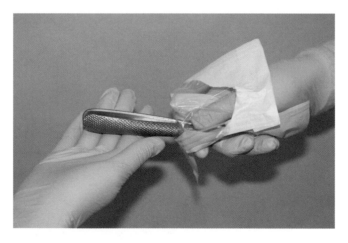

Figure 12.7 No touch technique of passing forceps.

As with any dental procedure, all the required instruments and equipment will have been made ready before the procedure begins, and laid out close to the dental chair for easy access but not in full view of the patient – this is likely to increase their anxiety. The dental nurse will anticipate the dentist and safely pass the instruments as required, using the technique described above.

Throughout the procedure, the dental nurse will monitor the patient for signs of distress (such as feeling pain) and notify the dentist accordingly. A calm, reassuring manner is required to put the patient at their ease and this must be adapted for the various types of patient that may be treated – whether a child, an adult or older adult, or a patient with special needs. When treating patients from different ethnic backgrounds, it is very useful to have a friend or family member present to interpret as necessary.

As the forceps, luxators and elevators used have to be pushed into the tooth socket, the dental nurse may also be required to stabilise the patients head or mandible so that the dentist's efforts are not wasted. The purpose of the support should be briefly explained to the patient beforehand.

Surgical field considerations

Whichever technique is used to extract a tooth or root the procedure is considered a surgical one, as bleeding will definitely occur and the tissues of the patient's oral cavity will be breached by instruments. If the working area is not treated as a sterile field during the procedure, there is a potential risk of cross-infection. This is more so with these types of procedure than with any other in dentistry. Consequently, the following special precautions are taken:

- **Sterile bagged instruments** – all instruments to be used must have been individually bagged and sterilised before the procedure
- **Protective personal equipment (PPE) for the dental team** – over and above the usual PPE requirements for dental procedures (see Units 4, 6, and 10 (Chapters 5, 7 and 11, respectively)) sterile surgical gloves must be worn by the team, as well as surgical gowns or single-use plastic aprons to prevent blood contamination
- **Disposable items** – wherever possible, disposable items should be used to prevent cross-infection, including aspirators, scalpel blades, needles, suture needles, etc.
- **Contamination policy** – any single-use items and materials that are opened but not used during the procedure should be disposed of anyway, to avoid contamination
- **Suction equipment** – must be run through with the required disinfectant solution after the procedure to remove all traces of blood from its inner workings
- **Operative field** – should be assumed to be blood contaminated and wiped down thoroughly with sodium hypochlorite (bleach) or another accepted decontaminant
- **Equipment coverage** – items such as the dental chair will obviously be re-used and are not sterilisable, so they must be covered before the procedure with a single-use impervious membrane, to prevent blood contamination
- **Sterile field** – the oral cavity and its immediate vicinity will be a sterile field during the procedure, and no team member who is not suitably gowned should enter it nor pass instruments into it without using a 'no-touch' technique

The aspects of infection control and health and safety that are relevant to these procedures, especially cleaning methods, infection control and sterilisation are fully covered in Units 1 and 4 (Chapters 2 and 5, respectively). In summary, these are:

■ All sharps are carefully disposed of in the sharps box – this includes LA needles
■ All autoclavable items are placed in a washer – disinfector unit, or an ultra-sonic bath, and treated before being placed in the autoclave for sterilisation
■ All contaminated waste is placed in hazardous waste sacks – this includes all impervious covers covering equipment items
■ All surfaces are disinfected using the correct solution

The patient records are completed and checked by the dentist before being filed away, and any radiographs used are similarly filed. As always, the records system must ensure the full confidentiality of the patient's details and notes, by being stored securely.

Pre- and post-operative instructions

Often, the patient will request information regarding the procedure itself in advance, and the dental nurse is ideally suited to allay their fears by giving advice beforehand as follows:

■ Local anaesthesia will always be necessary
■ The procedure will not be painful, as adequate LA will be given
■ If a surgical procedures is being undertaken, sutures will be necessary
■ Patient must take all medication as normal before the procedure unless the dentist informs them otherwise, except for aspirin which prevents blood clot-ting and could cause post-operative bleeding
■ Patient must have a light snack two hours before procedure, to avoid fainting
■ Full post-operative instructions will be given in writing, so the patient does not have to remember them
■ If the patient is a nervous adult or child, they should be escorted by a reassur-ing and competent adult

Similarly, after the procedure a full list of post-operative instructions (see below) should be given in writing. It is important that the patient understands that most post-operative complications occur because of disturbance to the blood clot which forms in the area, and that they should avoid this happening wherever possible. Post-operative instructions include:

■ Pain, swelling or bruising may occur after the procedure
■ Analgesics (**except aspirin**) may be taken as required
■ Alcohol, hot drinks, and exercise should be avoided for 24 hours

- No mouth rinsing should be carried out on the day of the procedure
- Hot salt water mouthwashes should be carried out after each meal, from the day after the procedure for up to one week
- If bleeding does occur, bite onto a cotton pack for up to 30 minutes
- Call the emergency telephone number given for care and advice if problems occur
- Details of further appointments if necessary, including suture removal

Surgical extractions

Under certain circumstances, a simple extraction cannot be carried out and either soft tissue alone, or soft tissue and alveolar bone have to be removed so that the dentist can gain access to a tooth or root. These circumstances include:

- When previous attempts at tooth extraction have left a retained root in the alveolar bone
- When a tooth is so grossly carious that attempts at simple extraction are impossible
- When the morphology of the roots makes it unlikely that the whole tooth can be removed simply, especially when the roots are curved
- When the tooth is only partially erupted and impacted, so that full eruption cannot occur
- When the tooth is unerupted and has associated pathology, such as a cyst
- When the tooth is unerupted and likely to cause future problems with either prostheses or orthodontic treatment
- When a deciduous tooth has failed to exfoliate because the root has become cemented to the alveolar bone (ankylosis) and natural loss cannot occur

Consequently, surgical extractions will fall into one of the following categories:

- Extraction involving tooth sectioning
- Extraction involving mucoperiosteal flap

The pre-operative and post-operative instructions given to the patient are detailed previously, as is the dental nurse's role during these procedures. What is different here from simple extraction procedures is the list of instruments that may be necessary to allow the dentist to gain access to the tooth or root.

Extraction involving tooth sectioning

This technique is a variation on the simple extraction technique for multi-rooted teeth that cannot be extracted whole. This is often indicated due to unfavourable root curvature or gross root caries that prevents simple forceps removal of the roots. The dentist can cut the tooth into a number of sections equal to the number of roots present, and then effectively extract each root separately in the usual way.

Sometimes, it may be necessary to remove some of the septal bone that lies between the roots and forms the individual socket walls. The only difference in the tooth sectioning technique from that of simple extractions is as follows:

- Use of high speed turbine and a suitable bur to cut the tooth into sections
- Use of Coupland's chisel to achieve the final separation of the roots
- Use of surgical handpiece and burs to remove septal bone
- Use of high speed suction to remove the water coolant of the drills
- Careful retraction of the patient's soft tissues during the cutting and sectioning procedures

All other points are as for the simple extraction technique, including instrument preparation and usage, dental nurse's role, and decontamination of the surgery afterwards.

Extractions involving mucoperiosteal flaps

Certain cases in which successful extraction cannot be carried out without gaining full access to a tooth or root by raising a mucoperiosteal flap are:

- **Unerupted tooth**
- **Buried retained root**
- **Root curvature** is excessive, and requires extensive bone removal
- **Gross root caries** prevents adequate instrumentation to extract the tooth in any other way

Teeth lie in sockets of alveolar bone, with a covering of mucoperiosteum over the bone which runs into the gingivae around each tooth. The mucoperiosteum is tightly held onto the bone, and has to be cut and separated to its full thickness before bone removal can be carried out. This is the **mucoperiosteal flap** (Figure 12.8). The flap thus raised has to have a wide base to ensure a good blood supply, so that full healing occurs once the procedure has been completed. It then has to be sutured accurately back into place for long enough so that reattachment can occur. This is a full surgical technique so all of the surgery and instrument preparation applies as described for simple extractions, but far more specific surgical instruments are required. These are detailed below.

The principle of the sterile field and the maintenance of thorough infection control are of great importance in preventing any contamination complications during the procedure. Depending on the patient, those with a compromised medical history may require the MOS procedure to be carried out in a hospital or dental clinic environment.

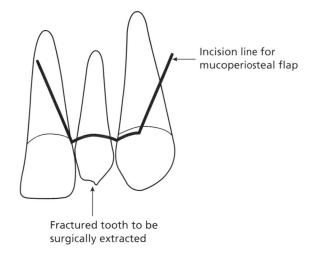

Incision line for
mucoperiosteal flap

Fractured tooth to be
surgically extracted

Figure 12.8 Surgical flap design.

Surgical instruments for flap procedures

Item	Function
Scalpel blade and handle (Figure 12.9)	To make initial cuts through the mucoperiosteum and around the necks of the teeth to create the flap
Osteotrimmer (Figure 12.10)	To raise the corners of the flap off the underlying alveolar bone
Periosteal elevator (Figure 12.11)	To complete the elevation of the flap off the bone
Handpiece and surgical burs	To remove alveolar bone and gain access to the tooth or root
Irrigation syringe	To irrigate the surgical field with sterile saline or sterile water
Austin and Kilner retractors	To protect and retract cheeks, lips and tongue from the surgical field, providing clear access for the dentist
Rake retractor	To retract the mucoperiosteal flap itself
Bone rongeurs	To nibble away bony spicules and produce a smooth bone surface for healing
Dissecting forceps (Figure 12.12)	To hold the loose flap edges taut during suturing
Needle holders (Figure 12.13)	To hold the pre-threaded needle firmly while suturing
Suture (Figure 12.14)	Half-moon needle, pre-threaded with either black braided silk or a resorbable suture material, to suture the flap back into position over the alveolar bone
Scissors (Figure 12.15)	To cut the suture ends after each stitch

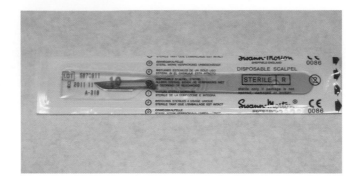

Figure 12.9 Scalpel blade and handle.

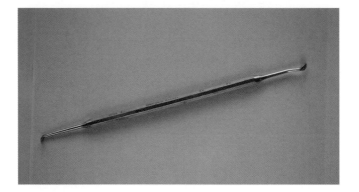

Figure 12.10 Mitchell's trimmer.

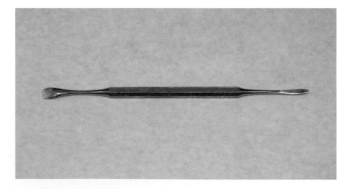

Figure 12.11 Periosteal elevator.

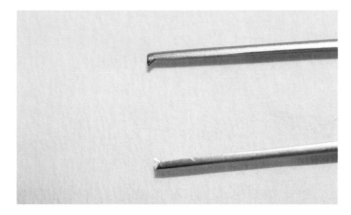

Figure 12.12 Tissue dissecting forceps – end detail.

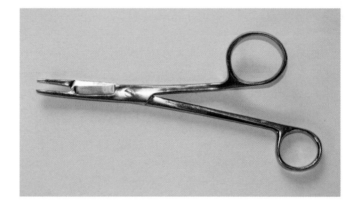

Figure 12.13 Needle holders.

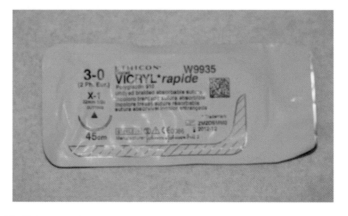

Figure 12.14 Suture pack.

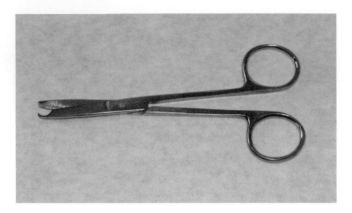

Figure 12.15 Suture scissors.

The dental nurse has specific roles to perform during the flap procedures, over and above all those previously identified. These are as follows:

- Correct and accurate use of suction equipment to remove water coolants and irrigation solutions
- Correct and accurate use of a fine-bore surgical aspirator to remove blood from the immediate surgical site
- Careful retraction of soft tissues for their protection and to provide a clear operative field, but without being so forceful that tissue damage occurs
- Assisting during the placement of sutures, which may include holding the flap taut and cutting the suture ends
- Preparation of bite packs to aid haemostasis
- Assisting in the placement of haemostats, such as oxidised cellulose or gelatine sponge

Again, full verbal and written post-operative instructions are given before the patient is discharged, and then the surgery is decontaminated as previously described. While the records are being written, the number of sutures used is specifically recorded so that all can be accounted for if they are of the non-resorbable type.

Tooth impaction

The most usual teeth to become impacted are the lower third molars, or 'wisdom' teeth. These are the last permanent teeth to erupt, and are often short of space to do so. The type of impaction that occurs will affect the difficulty of the removal of the tooth as follows:

- **Vertical impaction** – the tooth is upright but impacted into the ramus of the mandible

- **Horizontal impaction** – the tooth is lying on its side, facing forwards, backwards, or across the dental ridge
- **Mesioangular impaction** – the tooth is tilted forwards into the second molar tooth
- **Distoangular impaction** – the tooth is tilted backwards into the ramus of the mandible

Some dentists will refer patients with the more difficult types of impaction to a specialist oral surgeon for extraction, if the teeth are persistently infected or are causing food trapping and caries in adjacent teeth. However, if the impacted tooth is causing no problems (that is, it is **asymptomatic**) then it is usual for it to be left *in situ* rather than extracted, as there are risks involved in having the tooth surgically extracted. These are as follows:

- Extensive bone removal can weaken the mandible
- Post-operative pain and swelling are very likely to occur after a full surgical procedure
- The inferior dental nerve and lingual nerve lie close to the operation site, and temporary or even permanent damage can occur to them
- Limited mouth opening (**trismus**) can occur temporarily after surgery, and this will make eating and talking difficult

Patients must be warned of all these possible complications before undergoing the procedure.

Complications of extractions and MOS

Some complications can be highlighted as potential risks that may occur during an extraction or MOS procedure, the commonest one being the possibility of damage to one of the trigeminal nerve branches during the procedure. This risk can be identified by good pre-operative dental radiography and accurate planning of the procedure beforehand.

Where there is a potential for nerve damage to occur, the patient should be referred to a specialist for the procedure and warned of the possibility of it happening beforehand, so that informed consent may be given. Similarly, those medically compromised patients with conditions that may cause problems during extractions (such as haemophilia) should also be referred to specialist clinics or hospitals for treatment. Some other complications may occur during the procedure, despite all efforts to prevent them. These are as follows:

- **Unexpected tooth fracture** – especially if the tooth is heavily filled; this may result in a simple extraction becoming a more complicated one
- **Oral-antral fistula** – can occur while extracting upper premolar or molar teeth; the maxillary sinus lies over their roots and is often only separated by a membrane, so perforation of the sinus is not difficult

- **Loss of the tooth** – either into the respiratory or digestive tracts, or out of the mouth

Complications that can occur after the patient has left the surgery are:

- **Bleeding** – either within hours of the extraction (**reactionary haemorrhage**) or after 24 hours (**secondary haemorrhage**)
- **Infection** – following loss of the blood clot from the socket, the bony socket walls become infected (**localised osteitis**)

Tooth fracture

A grossly carious or heavily filled tooth is likely to fracture during extraction attempts. The dentist should be aware of the possibility and warn the patient regarding progression to a surgical procedure if necessary. This is likely to occur when the fracture extends subgingivally, as adequate access to the roots may be difficult. However, if small apical pieces of root fracture during extraction, they can be left *in situ* to either rise to the ridge surface themselves, over time, and be more easily removed, or to actually remain buried and cause no further problems. Whichever occurs, the patient must always be informed and a full explanation given.

Oro-antral fistula

An oro-antral fistula is an opening between the nasal antrum and the oral cavity. It occurs as a complication of the extraction of upper premolar and molar teeth, as the maxillary sinus lies over their roots. An inappropriate extraction technique can sometimes push the root into the sinus, where it will act as a foreign body and cause infection. The patient is best referred to a specialist oral surgeon for its removal. Long-rooted upper molar and premolar teeth sometimes impinge into the sinus naturally, and when they are extracted an oro-antral fistula is created, and if it is small in size it will close naturally.

Large openings require surgical repair by either direct suturing, or by raising a gingival flap off the palate and swinging it across to seal the fistula. The presence of a fistula can be confirmed by the appearance of air bubbles in the socket when the patient blows their nose. Again, the patient should be informed immediately, and told not to blow their nose until the fistula has healed.

Loss of the tooth

The tooth can be dropped during its removal from the mouth, or the force exerted during extraction can cause it to dislodge rapidly from the socket, before a firm grip has been achieved. If the tooth is swallowed, it poses no problem and should be allowed to pass naturally. However, if the tooth is likely to have been inhaled the patient should be sent to hospital immediately for chest and abdominal radiographs, to locate the tooth, as it could cause a serious respiratory infection. It may be removed using a bronchoscope if lodged in the main bronchi; if the tooth has descended further into the respiratory tract, thoracic surgery may be necessary to remove it.

Bleeding

Haemorrhage during extraction is a natural occurrence, as blood vessels in the periodontium are torn during the procedure. This usually stops within five minutes of completion of the extraction. It is called **primary haemorrhage**. The blood clots as follows:

(1)   Torn blood vessels constrict to slow the blood flow
(2)   **Platelets** circulating in the blood are exposed to air at the wound site. This causes them to become sticky, and clump together
(3)   Two complicated **clotting mechanisms** ensue, resulting in the protein fibrinogen being converted to fibrin
(4)   **Fibrin** chemically seals the cut vessels, and the haemorrhage ends

Bleeding that occurs several hours after the extraction is called **reactionary haemorrhage**. This is usually caused by the patient not following the post-operative instructions accurately and disturbing the blood clot. In healthy patients, it is easily controlled by re-application of pressure to the socket, reiteration of the post-operative instructions, or by suturing of the socket to compress the wound edges and promote clotting again.

In patients taking anti-clotting medication such as **aspirin**, **warfarin** or **heparin**, clotting will not occur so readily and the patient may need hospital treatment. Patients diagnosed as having haemophilia lack one of the vital components of the clotting mechanism. They could therefore bleed to death after even a simple procedure as tooth extraction, and must therefore only ever be treated in hospital. These patients should have been identified by a thorough medical history assessment, so that the complication does not arise.

The third type of bleeding complication is **secondary haemorrhage**, where the blood clot is lost early and the socket subsequently becomes infected, with break down of the healing mechanism. This occurs after 24 hours of the extraction being carried out.

Infection

Once the blood clot has been lost from the socket, the bone walls are bare and can become inflamed and subsequently infected from any of the bacteria normally present in the mouth. This is called **localised osteitis** ('dry socket') and occurs two to three days after the extraction. Patients with poor oral hygiene and smokers are particularly affected, although it can also occur after a difficult extraction, or where the patient has touched the socket with dirty fingers. To treat the condition, any food debris or necrotic clot tissue is removed then a sedative dressing is carefully placed (such as Alvogyl). The pain experienced by the patient can be relieved with the usual anti-inflammatory analgesics, and it is best if the post-operative instructions are reiterated.

Use of antibiotics with MOS procedures

As previously stated, many extractions are carried out because the patient presents with the pain of an acute infection. Previously, antibiotics were often prescribed for these patients as the first line of treatment (especially if the patient attended without an appointment), and the dental problem would be dealt with at a later date. Current thinking is that antibiotics:

- Are an adjunct to treatment only
- Should only be given if:
    - there is evidence that the infection is spreading locally
    - there is evidence that there is systemic involvement (raised body temperature is a good indicator)
    - the patient has a predisposing medical condition which necessitates antibiotics during treatment

Routine use of antibiotics is contraindicated for the following reasons:

- The source of the infection is better removed by extracting the tooth, or by lancing any abscess present
- Resistant strains of bacteria are more likely to develop if antibiotics are over prescribed
- The long-term consequences to the normal bacterial flora in the body, of a single course of antibiotics can last for months
- The dangerous potentiating action that antibiotics have on several drugs, especially oral anticoagulants
- The possibility of other drug interactions, especially with oral contraceptives and alcohol
- The development of hypersensitivity to the antibiotics by the patient, preventing their use in future
- All drugs should be avoided wherever possible during pregnancy

If antibiotics do need to be prescribed, the following are the current recommended choices:

- First choice – amoxicillin 250 mg, three times daily for five days
- Second choice – metronidazole 200 mg, three times daily for three days
- Third choice – erythromycin 250 mg, three times daily for five days

In severe infections, the first and second choices can be given together.

Patient monitoring

Any type of extraction procedure can be a worrying prospect for the patient. This is especially so for younger patients and some of those with special needs – when it may be difficult for them to appreciate why the procedure must be carried out – as well as those patients with an abnormal fear of the procedure (a **phobia**). A friendly, supportive and calming attitude throughout by the dental nurse will help to pacify the patient to some extent, as will talking to them and encouraging them when appropriate.

The patient should also be monitored for signs of any complication as follows:

- **Pain** – signs of pain include grimacing, wincing or crying, and should be pointed out to the dentist as the LA administered may not be sufficient
- **Colour** – the patient may feel faint and become pale and clammy, the procedure must be stopped while action is taken to restore their cranial blood flow (usually by dropping the dental chair so their head is below their feet)
- **Choking** – debris or the tooth may be lost to the back of the mouth, causing choking; immediate action is required by the team to prevent a serious medical emergency (see Unit 3 (Chapter 4))
- **Medical emergency** – anxiety can precipitate angina or a cardiac arrest in vulnerable patients, so patient response levels and vital signs should always be monitored by the whole team (see Units 3 and 6 (Chapters 4 and 7, respectively))
- **Tooth complications** – unexpected complications can occur, and the dental nurse should maintain a calm manner while assisting during the complication, especially by using suction and aspiration to retrieve debris, or applying pressure during primary haemorrhage
- **Bleeding** – immediately after the extraction, primary haemorrhage is quite normal but should stop after up to five minutes of pressure with a suitable dressing, so any recurrent bleeding must be reported to the dentist immediately, and the patient must not leave the surgery until all bleeding has stopped (this may involve assisting in placing haemostats or sutures)

Pain and anxiety control

Pain control during any dental procedure is provided by the administration of a suitable local anaesthetic, placed in the correct anatomical area to produce complete analgesia of the teeth and gingivae to be treated. However, some patients may require methods of anxiety control as well as local anaesthesia, before they are willing or able to undergo treatment; this is especially so with extraction procedures.

Only dental teams suitably trained in these anxiety control methods should use them, to ensure the safety of the patient. This is because part of the necessary training will involve the actions to take in the event of an emergency. This is particularly relevant when drugs have been administered to control anxiety and then an equipment failure occurs. In the hospital or dental clinic situation, back-up equipment and electrical supplies are available for these situations. This is not the usual case in general dental surgeries, so thorough training for all staff, and the exclusion of general anaesthesia techniques on these premises is the norm.

The anxiety control techniques available in general dental surgeries all rely on the patient remaining **conscious** throughout the procedure, and are summarised below.

- **Inhalation sedation** – patient breathes in a controlled mixture of oxygen and nitrous oxide ('laughing gas') through a nose piece, especially useful for younger patients
- **Intravenous sedation** – a sedative drug is injected into the patient's vein in a controlled manner, and their response and reducing level of anxiety is monitored until they are able to undergo dental treatment
- **Oral sedation** – a similar drug is given in tablet form one hour before the procedure, this produces less sedation and is especially useful in older patients
- **Hypnosis** – an altered state of awareness is produced by the verbal actions of the hypnotist, so that the patient is neither fully awake nor asleep and is more amenable to the power of suggestion
- **Acupuncture** – a branch of Chinese medicine that uses special needles placed in exact anatomical points on the body, to produce a local analgesic effect and to induce a form of hypnotic suggestion in the patient

Although the patient remains conscious throughout any of these anxiety control techniques, their mind is in an altered state until the effects wear off (whether due to drugs or hypnotic suggestion), and they must not be allowed to leave the dental surgery until it is safe for them to do so. This will be confirmed by the dentist alone, after assessing their level of responsiveness in one of various ways. Those patients who have had drugs administered must be escorted home by a responsible adult, and younger patients and those with special needs must be escorted by a parent or guardian. Failure to appreciate the level of fitness and awareness in the patient could leave them vulnerable and open to serious problems, such as assault, theft, personal danger or a medical emergency.

13 The VRQ and Question Examples

The formal part of the N/SVQ qualification is a 90-minute written paper covering four key areas of the syllabus:

- Principles of infection control in the dental environment
- Assessment of oral health and treatment planning
- Dental radiography
- Scientific principles in the management of plaque-related diseases

The question papers are set, marked and moderated by the National Examining Board for Dental Nurses. Each of the key syllabus areas has a stated aim and set learning outcomes, as shown below.

The VRQ questions are based on the underpinning knowledge required for each of these learning outcomes. They are set as a variety of multiple choice questions, lined or boxed short answer questions, and tick box questions. The marks awarded for each question are shown on the paper and will total 100, and candidates are required to achieve 65 marks (65%) to pass the paper.

Principles of infection control in the dental environment

The aim of this unit is to be able to describe infectious diseases, their routes of transmission and the methods of preventing cross-infection. There are five learning outcomes:

- Describe the process of infection control
- Explain the significance of micro-organisms
- Describe the management of infectious conditions affecting dental patients
- Describe the various methods of decontamination
- Describe the relevant health and safety legislation

The underpinning knowledge required for each of the five outcomes is as follows:

■ Outcome 1:

– Describe the causes of cross-infection
– Describe the methods for preventing cross-infection
– Explain the principles of standard (universal) infection control precautions

■ Outcome 2:

– Describe the main micro-organisms in potentially infectious conditions
– Explain the routes of transmission of micro-organisms
– Explain the significance of the terms 'pathogens' and 'non-pathogens'

■ Outcome 3:

– Describe infectious conditions which affect individuals within the dental environment
– Describe the actions to take to prevent the spread of infectious diseases in the dental environment
– Explain the importance of immunisation of dental personnel

■ Outcome 4:

– Describe the principles and methods of clinical and industrial sterilisation
– Describe the principles and methods of disinfection
– Explain the preparation of a clinical area to control cross-infection
– Explain the procedures used to decontaminate a clinical environment after use

■ Outcome 5:

– Identify health and safety policies and guidelines in relation to infection control
– Describe how to deal with a sharps injury
– Explain the use of personal protective equipment in the dental environment
– Describe ways of dealing with hazardous and non-hazardous waste

A sample of questions covering some of the underpinning knowledge for this area follows.

(1) Sterilisation is the killing of all:

(a) Fungi and bacteria
(b) Viruses, fungi and bacteria
(c) Bacteria and viruses
(d) Viruses, spores, bacteria and fungi

(2)   State three methods used in the dental environment to prevent cross-infection:

■   ....

■   ....

■   ....

(3)   Explain how a scalpel blade should be disposed off after use.

(4)   A micro-organism capable of producing a disease is known as:

(a)   Bacteriostatic
(b)   Pathogenic
(c)   Autoimmune
(d)   Bactericidal

(5)   List five diseases that dental personnel must be vaccinated against:

(i)   ....
(ii)   ....
(iii)   ....
(iv)   ....
(v)   ....

(6)   In the table below, put a tick to indicate the correct method of disposing of the following items:

Item	Non-hazardous waste	Hazardous waste	Special waste
Lead foil			
Empty local anaesthetic cartridge			
Patient bib			
Stock packaging			
Waste amalgam			
Endodontic file			

(7)   Define the term 'disinfection'.

(8)   Ultrasonic baths are used to:

(a)   Disinfect laboratory items
(b)   Sterilise hand instruments
(c)   Disinfect handpieces
(d)   Remove debris

(9)   State the first three actions to take in the event of a dirty sharps injury:

(i)   ....
(ii)   ....
(iii)   ....

(10)   Some dental products are sterilised industrially by exposure to:

    (a)   X-rays
    (b)   Steam at 160°C for one hour
    (c)   Ultraviolet light
    (d)   Gamma rays

Assessment of oral health and treatment planning

The aim of this unit is to understand the reasons and effective methods that can be used in oral health treatment planning. There are five learning outcomes:

- Describe the various methods of dental assessment
- Define the clinical assessments associated with orthodontics
- Explain the changes that may occur in the oral tissues
- Recognise medical emergencies that may occur in the dental environment
- Outline the basic structure and function of oral and dental anatomy

The underpinning knowledge required for each of the five outcomes is as follows:

- Outcome 1:

    - Identify the different types of dental records and charts
    - Describe methods of recording soft tissue conditions
    - Explain methods of recording periodontal conditions using periodontal charts

- Outcome 2:

    - Describe the classifications of malocclusion
    - Describe the types of orthodontic appliances in relation to treatment required
    - Explain pre- and post-operative instructions for orthodontic procedures

- Outcome 3:

    - Explain diseases of the oral mucosa
    - Describe the effects of ageing on the soft tissues
    - Outline the medical conditions that may affect the oral tissues

- Outcome 4:

    - Identify medical emergencies that may occur in the dental environment and how to deal with them
    - Describe the principles of first aid

■ Outcome 5:

  − Describe the structure, morphology and eruption dates of the primary and secondary dentition
  − Describe the structure and function of teeth, gingivae and supporting tissues
  − Describe the position and function of salivary glands and muscles of mastication

A sample of questions covering some of the underpinning knowledge for this area follows.

(1) The outer layer of compact alveolar bone is called:

  (a) Apical foramen
  (b) Lamina dura
  (c) Cancellous bone
  (d) Periodontal ligament

(2) State the first three actions to take if a patient faints:

  (i) ....
  (ii) ....
  (iii) ....

(3) List four functions of saliva:

  (i) ....
  (ii) ....
  (iii) ....
  (iv) ....

(4) Complete the table below to indicate the medical emergency when each drug would be used:

Drug	Emergency
Glyceryl trinitrate (GTN) spray	
Adrenaline 1:1000	
Salbutamol inhaler	
Aspirin 300 mg	

(5) State three factors that may aggravate a patient's periodontal condition:

  (i) ....
  (ii) ....
  (iii) ....

(6)   Enamel is formed by:

   (a)   Odontoblasts
   (b)   Lymphocytes
   (c)   Ameloblasts
   (d)   Erythrocytes

(7)   Dental caries can be detected by:

   (a)   Occlusal radiograph
   (b)   Transillumination
   (c)   Disclosing tablets
   (d)   Basic Periodontal Examination (BPE) probe

(8)   Functional orthodontic appliances work by using:

   (a)   Archwires to move the teeth
   (b)   Muscular forces to move the jaws
   (c)   Springs to move the teeth
   (d)   Muscular forces to move the teeth

(9)   Complete the following box to indicate the eruption date and correct charting notation for each of the following teeth:

Tooth	Eruption date (indicate months or years)	Palmer charting notation	FDI charting notation
Upper right first premolar			
Lower left permanent second molar			
Lower right deciduous canine			
Upper left deciduous lateral incisor			
Upper right permanent central incisor			

(10)   In Basic Life Support, 'DRSABC' stands for:

   ■   D   ....
   ■   R   ....
   ■   S   ....
   ■   A   ....
   ■   B   ....
   ■   C   ....

Dental radiography

The aim of this unit is to understand current radiography legislation, including the principles and techniques of taking and processing radiographs. There are four learning outcomes:

- Explain the regulations and hazards associated with ionising radiation
- Distinguish between the different radiographic films and their uses
- Describe the imaging process and the different chemicals used
- Explain the need for stock control of radiographic films

The underpinning knowledge required for each of the four outcomes is as follows:

- Outcome 1:

  - Outline the principles of the IRMER regulations
  - Explain the safe use of x-ray equipment
  - Explain the role of dental personnel when using ionising radiation in the dental environment
  - Identify the hazards associated with ionising radiation

- Outcome 2:

  - Identify different intra-oral radiographs and explain their uses
  - Identify different extra-oral radiographs and explain their uses
  - Outline the reasons for using digital radiography

- Outcome 3:

  - Explain the manual and automatic processing of radiographs
  - Describe the faults that may occur during the taking and processing of radiographs
  - Explain the chemicals used in radiography
  - Explain the safe handling and storage of chemicals

- Outcome 4:

  - Explain the importance of rotating film stock
  - Explain the methods of mounting radiographs correctly
  - Describe the storage of radiographs
  - Describe suitable quality control recording systems

A sample of questions covering some of the underpinning knowledge for this area follows.

(1) State three methods of achieving 'ALARA' with reference to dental radiography:

(i)   ....

(ii) ....

(iii) ....

(2) Briefly describe the image seen on the following radiographs:

Horizontal bitewing
Anterior occlusal
Periapical
Lateral oblique

(3) A lead foil is placed inside intra-oral film packets to:

(a) Allow easy bending of the packet
(b) Absorb unused x-rays
(c) Reflect x-rays back into the packet
(d) Produce an x-ray beam

(4) State four points that must be included in the 'local rules':

(i)   ....

(ii) ....

(iii) ....

(iv) ....

(5) The chemical deposits found in the bottom of the developing tank are:

(a) Bromine
(b) Silver
(c) Silver bromide
(d) Lead

(6) A substance that does not absorb x-rays when exposed to them is described as:

(a) Phosphorescent
(b) Radiolucent
(c) Translucent
(d) Radiopaque

(7)   State the expected appearance of a radiograph when the following processing faults have occurred:

Fault	Appearance
Over-developing	
Film opened in daylight	
Under-fixing	
Under-developing	

(8)   List three stages of an effective quality control system in relation to dental radiographs:

(i)   ....

(ii) ....

(iii) ....

(9)   Explain how intensifying screens reduce a patient's exposure to x-rays.

(10) A lid should cover the developing tank when not in use to prevent:

(a)   Evaporation of the developer
(b)   Developer spillages
(c)   Oxidisation of the developer
(d)   Films being dropped in

Scientific principles in the management of plaque-related diseases

The aim of this unit is to understand the aetiology and progression of oral diseases, methods of their prevention and restoration of the dentition. There are three learning outcomes:

■   Describe common oral diseases
■   Outline methods for the prevention and management of oral diseases
■   Describe how to manage and handle materials during restorative procedures in plaque-related diseases

The underpinning knowledge required for each of the three outcomes is as follows:

■   Outcome 1:

–   Describe the aetiology and progression of dental caries
–   Describe the aetiology and progression of periodontal disease
–   Outline the development of plaque
–   Describe the inflammatory process and effects of the disease process

- Outcome 2:
    - Identify effective oral hygiene techniques to prevent oral diseases
    - Describe how diet can affect oral health
    - Explain the advantages and disadvantages of the different applications of fluoride

- Outcome 3:
    - Identify the equipment, instruments and materials used during and finishing restorations
    - Describe the different matrix systems used during restorative procedures
    - Identify the hazards associated with restorative materials and equipment

A sample of questions covering some of the underpinning knowledge for this area follows.

(1) In the table below, put a tick to indicate the correct uses of the following periodontal instruments:

Instrument	Remove supragingival calculus	Remove subgingival calculus
Push scaler		
Ultrasonic scaler		
Periodontal hoe		
Sickle scaler		
Jaquette scaler		
Gracey curette		

(2) Explain the term 'non-milk extrinsic sugars' in relation to dental caries.

(3) Acid etchant used during the placement of composite restorations contains the following:

    (a) 25% lactic acid
    (b) 33% phosphoric acid
    (c) 35% hydrochloric acid
    (d) 50% polyacrylic acid

(4) List four methods available to the dentist to diagnose dental caries:

    (i) ....
    (ii) ....
    (iii) ....
    (iv) ....

(5) A Siqveland matrix system is required during the placement of a:

(a) Class I amalgam restoration
(b) Class III composite restoration
(c) Class II amalgam restoration
(d) Class V glass ionomer restoration

(6) Complete the table below to indicate the following:

Signs of generalised gingivitis
Symptoms of reversible pulpitis
Signs of acute lateral periodontal abscess
Symptoms of irreversible pulpitis
Signs of acute necrotising ulcerative gingivitis

---

(7) List and explain the use of four types of oral health aid available to patients:

(i) ....
(ii) ....
(iii) ....
(iv) ....

(8) Tooth surface loss associated with bruxing is called:

(a) Attrition
(b) Erosion
(c) Caries
(d) Abrasion

(9) Explain the term 'fluorosis'.

(10) Give a brief explanation of each of the following terms:

False periodontal pocket
Hidden sugars
Dental plaque
True periodontal pocket
Topical fluoride
Denture stomatitis

Glossary of Terms

Many words and phrases have been used throughout the text, whose meanings may not be clear to all, or which have pertinent meanings in the manner in which they have been used. To clarify each, and hopefully give a clearer understanding to readers, this glossary of terms has been compiled in alphabetical order for easy reference. The descriptions given are correct for the context in which they have been used here.

A

Abscess – a collection of pus and dead micro-organisms which forms in tissues, following infection of the tissues with the micro-organism

Aesthetics – relating to a pleasing appearance, as in the aesthetics of a crown or other prosthesis

AIDS – acquired immune deficiency syndrome, the disease process produced following infection with the human immunodeficiency virus or HIV

Alastik – a loop of elastic material used in fixed orthodontic appliances, to tie the archwire into the bracket

Allergen – a substance which produces an allergic reaction in the patient, such as pollen in hayfever sufferers, or penicillin in medicine

Analgesic – a drug which has the action of relieving pain

Antibody – a naturally occurring, or artificially introduced, substance in the blood which acts to destroy infectious micro-organisms in the body. They are artificially introduced by the process of immunisation

Anti-inflammatory – a drug which acts to reduce the effects of inflammation in the tissues

Apex locator – an electronic device used in endodontics, which is used to determine the position of the root apex of a tooth, so that a diagnostic working length can be determined during root canal therapy

Apical foramen – the hole at the end of the tooth root through which the blood vessels and nerve tissue enter and leave

Asepsis – the absence of all living pathogenic micro-organisms

Aspiration (injection) – the technique used to 'draw back' during the administration of a local anaesthetic, to ensure that a blood vessel has not been penetrated. It is a safety technique carried out to prevent intra-vascular injection of local anaesthetic solution

Aspiration (suction) – the use of high and low speed suction equipment during dental procedures, to remove fluid and small solid debris from the oral cavity

Asymptomatic – without symptoms, so used in dentistry as a description of a tooth with which the patient is experiencing no pain nor sensitivity problems

Autoclave – an electrical device used to sterilise dental instruments, by the application of heat under pressure to produce steam, which kills all micro-organisms and spores

Autoimmune disease – one which acts to destroy body tissue, by the action of antibodies produced by the patient's body itself

B

Bacteraemia – the condition of having bacteria in the blood stream, as often occurs after dental treatment, such as scaling, extractions, and endodontic procedures

Bone resorption – the natural action of osteoclast cells to eat away and reduce the alveolar bone, especially after extractions, to produce shape changes and reduction to the alveolar ridge

Bronchoscope – a medical device used to enter and view the bronchi of the respiratory system, often to take tissue for biopsies or to remove inhaled foreign bodies

Buccal – the surface of a posterior tooth (premolar or molar) which is against the cheek, or buccinator muscle

C

Cancellous bone – that which forms the open, sponge-like interior of bone, such as in the alveolar bone of the jaws, and through which blood vessels and nerves run

Cariogenic – a food or drink substance which is capable of producing caries in a tooth, and therefore is either acidic or containing a non-milk extrinsic sugar

Cermet – a dental material used for restorations, which contains glass ionomer cement with metal particles incorporated into it, for added strength. They are especially used in the build up of cores before a tooth is restored with a crown

Chromosome – a microscopic constituent of the nucleus of a cell, which contains the genetic material of the organism

Clinical audit – the systematic critical analysis of the quality of care in the clinical environment, such that techniques and procedures are constantly scrutinised, evaluated and improved on where necessary, for the benefit of the patients

Contemporaneous notes – clinical notes which have been written on the date specified, and which are unalterable so that they represent a true account of events. All clinical records should therefore be contemporaneous, to avoid medico-legal challenges as to their accuracy and truthful content

Cross-bite – a description especially used in orthodontic diagnosis, whereby the upper posterior teeth occlude (bite together) inside the lower teeth, rather than outside them, as they do in normal Class I occlusion

Cyst – an unnatural, fluid-filled sac within the tissues of the body. Cysts sometimes develop on the apex of a tooth due to a chronic infection of that tooth

D

Debility – to be in a state of poor or weakened health

Demineralisation – the action of weak organic acids on the enamel of the tooth, to produce areas where the mineral content is reduced and therefore more prone to attack by caries

Dentate – the condition of having some natural teeth present in the mouth

Diagnostic radiograph – the radiograph taken during root canal therapy whereby the length of the root is accurately determined so that canal preparation can be carried out to this established working length. In this way, under-instrumentation or apical perforation are avoided

Diastema – a natural space present between erupted teeth. When occurring between the upper central incisors it is called a median diastema

Direct restoration – a restoration made at the chairside by the dentist, rather than one which is produced in a laboratory by a technician, using models of the patient's teeth

Disclosing tablet – a chewable tablet of vegetable dye, which stains plaque to make it easily visible to the naked eye. They are used as an important oral health motivator, especially with children and young people

Disinfection – the destruction of bacteria and fungi, but not spores nor some viruses

Distal – the surface of a tooth which is furthest away from the midline of the dental arch, in other words, the 'back' of the tooth

Dysfunction – implying poor or unnatural function of a body part, as in the impaired function of the temporomandibular joint in patients who clench and grind their teeth

E

Edentulous – the condition of having no natural teeth

Eruption – the movement of the teeth through the alveolar bone and mucosa into the oral cavity

Exfoliation – the natural shedding of the deciduous teeth during childhood

F

Fluorapatite – a crystal structure of the enamel of teeth, whereby fluoride has been incorporated into normal enamel to produce this hardened structure, which is more resistant to attack by acid and therefore less likely to allow cavities to develop

Foramen/foramina – a natural anatomical opening, especially in bone, through which blood vessels and nerves can pass

Furcation – the natural point at which the roots of a multi-rooted tooth separate. It is therefore the point at which the tooth is usually held during extraction

G

General Dental Council – the governing body of the dental profession, with the power to ensure that professional standards are maintained, and to suspend or remove a dentist from the register of dental practitioners if they are found guilty of misconduct. It is currently in the process of introducing compulsory registration for dental care professionals

Gingival crevice – a 2-mm deep crevice around the necks of all healthy teeth, where plaque can accumulate when oral hygiene standards are poor

Grand mal – a serious type of epileptic fit, where the patient undergoes the convulsions of 'tonic-clonic' seizures

H

Haemostasis – the arrest of a flow of blood, especially after tooth extraction

Health and Safety Executive – a government body concerned with ensuring that all employers comply with the Health and Safety Act to maintain the health, safety and welfare of employees and members of the public. It must be notified when serious accidents and dangerous occurrences risk the safety of others, and it will carry out an investigation to determine the cause of the accident or occurrence

Hydroxyapatite – the usual crystal structure of enamel, and which can have fluoride incorporated to produce fluorapatite

Hypoxia – the condition of a lack of oxygen to the body tissues, and when occurring to the brain it usually results in a faint

I

Impaction – the condition of an unerupted, or partially erupted, tooth whereby its full eruption is prevented by being lodged against an adjacent tooth or a section of alveolar bone

Indirect restoration – a restoration produced by a technician in a laboratory, from models provided by the dentist of a patient's tooth (especially inlays)

Inoculation – the introduction of a micro-organism into the body tissues to cause a mild form of the disease, with the aim of producing immunity to that disease

Inorganic – not having the structure of a living organism, as in the mineral crystals which make up the non-living structure of enamel

Interproximal – the area between the mesial surface of one tooth and the distal surface of the tooth directly in front of it, as in interproximal caries

Irreversible pulpitis – inflammation of the pulp of a tooth which has progressed too close to the pulp tissue to be reversed by simple restorative treatment alone

L

Lancing – of an abscess, whereby the point of the infection is surgically pierced to allow the enclosed pus to be released, so that the infection can be dissipated and healing can begin

Lateral canal – a minor canal in the root of a tooth, running off the main pulp chamber usually to the root surface, the presence of which often causes failure of root canal therapy due to its inaccessibility to endodontic treatment

Lingual – the surface of all lower teeth closest to the tongue

Lymph node – a mass of tissue lying along the lymphatic vessels of the body, which are concerned with defence against infection and which are often felt as swellings (in the neck) when infection is present. Their enlargement can also indicate tumours associated with the lymph system, so they are checked for normality during routine dental examinations

M

Malaise – a general feeling of being unwell, or ill

Marginal leakage – an unwanted phenomenon which can occur microscopically down the sides of restorations, such that oral fluids penetrate beneath restorations, and either cause caries or dissolve any cements present so that the restoration is lost

Mastication – the correct term for the act of chewing

Maxillary antrum – the natural air filled space within the maxillary bones, where various branches of the trigeminal nerves run

Meniscus – the pad of cartilage which lies between the head of the condyle of the mandible, and the glenoid fossa of the skull in the temporomandibular joint. It acts as a protective cushion between the two bones

Mental symphysis – the joint between the two halves of the mandible, lying in the midline of the most anterior part of the lower jaw

Mesial – the surface of all teeth closest to the midline, in other words, the 'front' of the tooth

Mixed dentition – the stage in childhood where both deciduous teeth and permanent teeth are present in the mouth at the same time. It usually starts around 6 years of age and ends at around 12 years of age

Mucoperiosteum – the layer of tissue covering the alveolar bone, which consists of the alveolar mucosa, tightly attached to the underlying periosteum, which covers the bone surface

Mucous membrane – the covering epithelial surface of the soft tissues of the oral cavity

N

Necrosis – a section or area of dead tissue, as in necrosis of the pulp when a tooth has died

O

Occlusal – the surface of all posterior teeth (premolars and molars) which bite together in occlusion

Open drainage – the procedure whereby access has been gained to a necrotic pulp during endodontic treatment, and then the access hole has been left open to allow the necrotic contents (especially pus) to drain out of the tooth

Operculum – the flap of mucosa, which lies over partially erupted teeth, and which can become inflamed when third molars erupt. This is called pericoronitis

Opposing arch – during fixed restorative procedures, this is the arch which is not to receive the fixed prosthesis. An impression of the opposing arch will be taken so that the technician can determine the correct occlusion of the patient, so that the fixed prosthesis does not alter it in any way

Organic – a substance derived from living cells

Orthograde root filling – a root filling placed conventionally, through the crown of the tooth

P

Palatal – the surface of upper teeth closest to the hard palate, or roof of the mouth

Paraesthesia – the 'pins and needles' sensation experienced as local anaesthetics wear off, and sensation is returning to the affected area

Parallax – a radiographic technique whereby the same object is exposed to x-rays from different angles, so that the buccal or palatal position of unerupted teeth can be identified

Parkinson's disease – a progressive disorder of the brain, characterised by uncontrollable tremors

Peg lateral – an abnormally small upper later incisor tooth, said to be shaped like a 'peg'

Petit mal – a mild form of epilepsy where the sufferer often just appears to be daydreaming

pH – a measure of acidity, expressed as a value from 1 to 14, where 1 is strongly acidic, 7 is neutral (neither acidic nor alkaline), and 14 is strongly alkaline

Polyp – an overgrowth of mucous membrane tissue, which is attached by a stalk to the mass of tissue from which it originates

Post-dam – the most posterior border of a denture, which is raised into a ridge to aid the formation of the suction film of saliva necessary for good retention

Potentiation – the action of one drug increasing the effects of another drug, when both are given to a patient together. The increased action of anti-coagulation drugs caused by antibiotics, for instance, can have serious consequences for the patient

Proclined – in orthodontics, the angulation of the upper central incisor teeth in Class II division 1 whereby they protrude forwards from the mouth. The overjet will be increased

Prophylactic paste – a paste of pumice slurry used by dentists and hygienists to remove surface stains from the teeth, following scaling

Prophylaxis – the giving of antibiotics to susceptible patients to prevent disease, as in patients with a history of heart valve disease who are susceptible to bacterial endocarditis following dental treatment

Q

Quality assurance – a system to ensure that a consistently high standard of treatment or practice management is achieved

R

Radicular pulp – that part of the pulp tissue which lies within the root of the tooth, as opposed to that which lies in the crown of the tooth, in the pulp chamber

Radiolucent – a substance which does not absorb x-rays when exposed to them, so that it's image appears dark on the developed radiograph

Radiopaque – a substance which absorbs x-rays when exposed to them, so that its image appears light on the developed radiograph

Remineralisation – the action where fluoride is taken into areas of enamel which have been attacked and demineralised by acid, so that the crystal structure of the enamel is reformed and repaired

Resorbable suture – sutures (stitches) which are made from a material that gradually dissolves in the body tissues, so that they do not have to be removed at a later date

Retraction – the action of holding back soft tissues from a surgical site with special instruments called retractors, so that good vision and access are possible

Retroclined – in orthodontics, the angulation of the upper central incisor teeth in Class II division 2 cases, where they slope backwards into the mouth and the overjet is reduced

Retrograde root filling – a root filling which is placed from the root end of the tooth, during an apicectomy, rather than more conventionally from the crown end

Reversible pulpitis – inflammation of the pulp which can be resolved by the removal of caries and the restoration of the tooth, without the need for endodontic treatment

Risk assessment – a method of measuring the risks of injury during a procedure, or when using chemicals, so that a safe method can be developed to minimise the risks of injury to all

S

Serial extraction – in orthodontics, the technique of extracting certain deciduous teeth in a set order, to allow the eruption of the permanent successor into an acceptable position in the dental arch, to relieve crowding. Sometimes, the permanent teeth are extracted too, to allow eruption of other permanent teeth

Shellac – in removable prosthetics, a resinous material used warm and moulded into special trays over a patient's initial models

Silane agent – in fixed prosthetics, a coupling agent which allows resins to chemically attach to ceramics and metals, so that better adhesion is gained during the cementation of the prosthesis

Sinus tract – a suppurating connection from an infected area to the oral cavity, especially from a chronic periapical abscess

Sjögren's syndrome – an autoimmune disorder where the patient experiences reduced salivary flow, reduced tear flow, and rheumatoid arthritis

Social cleanliness – clean to a socially acceptable standard, but not disinfected nor sterilised

Stagnation area – any area of the mouth or of a prosthesis which prevents self cleansing to occur, so that plaque accumulates here

Standard precautions – those precautions taken when treating all patients in the dental workplace, as an infection control measure by assuming that any patient is a potential source of infection to others

Stensen's duct – the salivary gland channel connecting the parotid gland to the oral cavity. It opens against the buccal surfaces of the upper first and second molar teeth

Sterilisation – the process of killing all micro-organisms and spores to produce asepsis

Subgingival – beneath the gingival margin of the teeth, as in subgingival calculus

Supernumerary tooth – an additional tooth-like structure, often found on radiograph, lying between the roots of the upper central incisors. It can sometimes prevent their eruption

Supragingival – above the gingival margin of the teeth, as in supragingival calculus

Suture – a surgical stitch, used to close the edges of wounds following surgery or trauma, and can be made of various materials including silk

T

Tetracycline – an antibiotic which used to be given to alleviate the symptoms of acne, but which was found to be taken into the tooth structure of permanent teeth, to produce unsightly staining

Transillumination – the technique of shining the blue curing lamp through anterior teeth, to detect interproximal cavities

Trismus – the inability to fully open the mouth, due to swelling or inflammation of the surrounding muscles and soft tissues. This is often seen in patients with pericoronitis

Tumour – an unnatural swelling of a body tissue which is not due to inflammation, and which serves no purpose to the body. They can be benign (harmless) or malignant (cancerous)

U

Undercut cavity – one produced by the dentist during restorative procedures, whereby the inner surface is wider than that at the opening of the cavity. It is deliberately produced to aid the retention of non-adhesive filling materials, such as amalgam

V

Vaccine – a preparation of dead or harmless micro-organisms injected into the body to produce an immune response, and thus protect the patient from suffering from the disease at a later date

Vasoconstrictor – a substance added to local anaesthetic cartridges, which act to close the localised blood vessels to prolong the anaesthetic, and also to reduce bleeding in the immediate area

W

Wharton's duct – the channel connecting the submandibular salivary gland to the oral cavity. It opens beneath the tongue, at the front of the mouth

Z

Zoning – the technique of separating clinical areas in the dental surgery into 'dirty' and 'clean' zones, so that dirty instruments are not inadvertently placed where clean ones are, to prevent cross-infection and contamination

Index